A Dictionary of
Speech Therapy

Dedication

To my parents in recognition of their help, support and advice throughout the last 27 years.

A Dictionary of
Speech Therapy

David W. H. Morris

Dundee Royal Infirmary, Tayside Health Board,
Dundee, Scotland
formerly Senior Speech Therapist, Dalintart Hospital,
Argyll & Clyde Health Board, Oban, Scotland

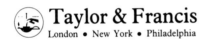

Taylor & Francis

London • New York • Philadelphia

UK   Taylor & Francis Ltd, 4 John St, London, WC1N 2ET

USA   Taylor & Francis Inc., 242 Cherry St, Philadelphia,
PA 19106–1906

British Library Cataloguing in Publication Data

Morris, David W. H.
   Speech therapy dictionary.
   1. Man. Speech disorders. Therapy.
   Terminology
   I. Title
   616.85′506′014

   ISBN 0-85066-444-6

Library of Congress Cataloging-in-Publication Data

Morris, David W. H.
   A Dictionary of Speech therapy/David W. H. Morris.
     p. cm.
   Bibliography: p.
   ISBN 0-85066-444-6 (pbk.)
   1. Speech therapy—Terminology—Dictionaries, etc.
   I. Title.
   RC423.M597   1988
   616.85′506′0321—dc19   87-35992
                                     CIP

Typeset by
Mathematical Composition Setters Ltd, Salisbury

*Printed in Great Britain by Taylor & Francis (Printers) Ltd,
Basingstoke*

Contents

Preface

An evil spirit seems to preside over all branches of clinical language studies. No one can escape his influence. He sets profession against profession, clinician against clinician, researcher against researcher. He tempts all to follow him, in the name of clarity and precision, but all who do, find only obscurity and quicksand. His name is Terminology.... (Crystal, D. 1984: 1)

This description of terminology by the Emeritus Professor of Linguistic Science at Reading University shows how mystifying it can be. And if this can be the case for someone experienced in this field, how much more so for someone new to the subject. Even speech therapists who completed their training before linguistic, phonetic and phonological terminology came into being can find it mystifying.

The aim of this book is to act as a guide to the essential terms used in speech therapy and its allied subjects. Suggested references are given at the end of each explanation, to direct the reader to further study of the terms as required.

It is hoped that this book will prove useful to students in helping to increase clarity and in providing some assistance to avoid 'obscurity and quicksand'.

David W. H. Morris
June 1987

Acknowledgments

I have greatly enjoyed writing this book. However, to produce a book of this magnitude, it requires work and encouragement from other people.

I should like to thank my parents, Rev. Dr and Mrs W. J. Morris, who, after I had put forward the idea of the book, having collected a few terms, persuaded me and encouraged me to develop the idea and try to find a publisher for it. Various parts of the initial manuscript were read by them and revisions made. In particular, I thank my mother, who, as a clinical psychologist, gave some very helpful suggestions in section 4. At another stage, part of their holiday was sacrificed for checking the cross-references both within and between the eight sections of the book.

Finally, my thanks go to Taylor and Francis for deciding to publish this work and for their help and advice in its publication.

How to use this book

1   The book is divided into eight sections, in which the terms appear in alphabetical order.

2   The explanation of each term appears under its main heading, eg., different forms of **aphasia** such as **acquired aphasia**, **developmental aphasia**, etc. appear under **aphasia**. The reader who turns first to **acquired aphasia** will find the appropriate reference, i.e., see **aphasia**.

3   Some terms appear in more than one section, e.g., **Alzheimer's Disease** appears in section 1 (Speech Pathology); section 4 (Psychology/Psychiatry); and section 5 (Medicine). In section 1 the speech and language disorders produced by Alzheimer's Disease are detailed; in section 4, the psychological effects of the condition; and in section 5, its medical aetiology. Where such a term appears in more than one section, the cross-references to the other sections are given at the end of each explanation.

4   In the explanation of any term, any other term which is explained elsewhere in the book appears in bold. If such explanation is to be found in the same section, there will be no section reference following it. If such explanation is to be found in another section, the section reference or references will be given in brackets.

5   The suggestions for further reading at the end of any explanation refer only to the term being explained.

Section 1

Speech Pathology

A

Acceptable stammer. The criterion of success used by speech therapists treating stammering patients using the **stammer more fluently** approach.

Acoustic agnosia.   See **agnosia**.

Acquired aphasia.   See **aphasia**.

Acquired apraxia.   See **apraxia**.

Acquired disorders. Any disorder not caused at birth, i.e., **congenital disorders**, or during childhood, i.e., **developmental disorders**. Acquired disorders usually have an **organic cause**, e.g., **CVA**, **head injury**, **meningitis**, etc. (all 5). The commonest acquired disorders are **aphasia**, **dysarthria**, **dyspraxia** and **dyslexia**. They can occur at any time in the person's life but it is the cause which differentiates them from other types of disorder. *See Crystal (1980): 50.*

Acquired dyslexia. Occurs following a **CVA** or **head injury** (both 5). There are four types:

1. **Phonological dyslexia**. The inability to read **nonwords** (2) aloud, e.g., 'dup', 'getuld' etc., while the ability to read everyday words aloud remains intact. The patient may produce other symptoms such as 'visual errors' in reading aloud nonwords, e.g. [dek] for /desk/. Derivational errors are also present when reading words aloud, especially when they contain **bound morphemes** (2).

2. **Deep dyslexia**. Semantic errors are present in the patient's reading. Other symptoms can also be present e.g., visual impairment, **function word** substitutions (2) and derivational errors. Low-imageability words are harder to read aloud than high-imageability words, verbs being harder to read than adjectives, which are harder to read than nouns when reading aloud. However, someone can only be diagnosed as suffering from this form of acquired dyslexia if there is the semantic error in reading aloud, even if he has none of the other symptoms.

3. **Letter-by-letter reader** (**word-form dyslexia**). Patients can only understand what they read aloud by reading one letter at a time. This is the only acquired dyslexia which can be explained neurologically. It can also be called **Dejerine Syndrome** (5). In general, writing is unaffected.

4. **Surface dyslexia**. A disturbance between the person's visual word recognition system and the semantic system. However, the patient can still say the word since the visual recognition system and phonemic system which produces voice are still intact. *See Ellis (1984): 38, 41–44, 83–84.*

Acquired dysphasia.   See **aphasia**.

Acquisition. Any learning process as opposed to certain types of **innateness** (4). The phrase **language acquisition** is used to describe the stages of language development in children between the ages of 9 months and 5 years. It can also be used to describe how children with specific learning difficulties, or adults with speech and language disorders, develop communication skills which they have hitherto lacked. *See Clark and Clark (1977): ch. 4.*

Action picture test. Devised by Renfrew in 1966 (rev. 1971), it is a quick means of finding out if a child suffers from **language delay**. The aim is to have the child produce examples of **expressive language** to be analyzed in two ways—information provided and grammatical forms produced. Five areas of the child's grammar are assessed, viz., use of nouns, verbs and prepositions; present, past and future tenses; irregular forms of plurals and past tenses; singular/plural forms of nouns and simple/complex sentences. It can be used with children of 3 years upwards although not.**standardized** (4) for children older than 7 years. An information score and a grammatical score can be obtained. *See test manual.*

Acute laryngitis. An inflammatory disease often occurring after a common cold when viruses or bacteria lodge in the upper respiratory tract. The symptoms are hoarseness leading to **dysphonia**, malaise, pain when speaking, redness and swelling of the **larynx** (5). Vocal rest is usually recommended and possibly a period of speech therapy. *See Pracy et al. (1974): 110.*

Adiodochokinesis. Inability to produce rapid sequences of movement by using the **articulators** (2). It exists with patients who suffer from **dysarthria**. It is opposed to **diodochokinesis**. *See Darley et al. (1975): 79*

Afferent (Motor) Aphasia. An aphasia described by Alexsander Luria in the 1960s. Similar to **dyspraxia**, the patient is unable to predict where or how to position the articulators for sound production. A severe afferent aphasia results in a global problem; in a mild form, only similar sounds may be confused, e.g., bilabials /p, b, m/, alveolars /t, d, n/ etc. There may be also a disorder in the patient's writing ability by confusing what Luria calls articulemes, i.e., sounds. The lesion causing such a disorder occurs in the secondary zones of the postcentral kinaesthetic cortex. *See Eisenson (1984): 107.*

Agrammatism. A disorder associated with **aphasia** affecting the use of **syntax** (2) rather than vocabulary. **Function words** (section 2) are either wrongly used or missed out completely. It is found in both the patient's **comprehension** and **expressive language** and diagnosed in the former using **formal assessments** such as the **Test for the Reception of Grammar (TROG)** or the **Token Test**. Most aphasic patients have some degree of agrammatism but it is particularly characteristic of **Broca's aphasia**. Such patients are therefore often described as **nonfluent** aphasic patients. Their speech sounds **telegraphic** or **telegrammatic**, i.e., without **function words**. *See Eisenson (1984): 23–24.*

Agnosia. The patient can still hear speech, see and touch objects but does not know what the speech means or what the objects are. Such a disorder could affect language rehabilitation of a person. There are four agnosias:

1. Acoustic—difficulty in sound discrimination.

2. Pure word deafness—a specific difficulty in recognizing speech sounds. The patient is unable to repeat what has been said but, with difficulty, can use some spontaneous speech, read or write. At times, by watching the therapist's face intently **lip-reading** (6) is possible for **auditory comprehension**.

3. Visual—inability to understand various situations by failing to recognize visual stimuli.

4. Tactile—inability to recognize objects by feel or touch.

Agnosia must be diagnosed early on, so that it can be taken into consideration when both assessing the patient and making a **treatment programme**. *See Eisenson (1984): 10–12.*

Alexia. See **acquired dyslexia** and **developmental dyslexia**.

Alexia with Agraphia. A disorder of both reading and writing, although they can occur separately, i.e., alexia without agraphia. *See Ellis (1984).*

Alternative Communication Systems. Sometimes referred to as argumentative communication aids (generally used in the United States) or supplementary communication systems. The latter term is usually preferred as the aids are to help a patient to produce speech to communicate when he has difficulty producing **expressive language**, and are not meant to be a substitute for speech. However, they may have to be used as an alternative device for communication with patients who cannot produce any speech at all. Such communication systems include the various **sign languages**, **gesture**, **electronic devices** (7) and **microcomputers** (8). *See Kiernan et al. (1982): passim.*

Alzheimer's Disease. According to Dr Ian Thompson's recent research (unpublished) patients suffering from this form of **dementia** (4 and 5) have the following speech and language problems. They have a mild disorder in copying; a moderate disorder in sentence construction and reading comprehension; a severe disorder in **comprehension** when they are given the **Token Test**; severe difficulties in using serial speech and word memory. Fluency, automatic writing, spelling and gesture are also severely affected. However, the worst affected modality is **comprehension**. Although these disorders may seem the same as those affecting **aphasic** patients, there is a difference produced by the aetiology. In **aphasia**, the onset is sudden as its aetiology is **emboli** or **Berry anneurysms** (both 5) producing specific damage to a particular part of the **brain** (5). However, the onset of dementia is gradual involving gradual changes to areas of the **brain**. A **factor analysis** (4) carried out to find the ranking of disorders in both the aphasic and demented populations found six factors in aphasic patients: **naming**, **fluency**, visuo-spatial, **comprehension**, recognition and reading; while seven were found in patients with dementia of the **Alzheimer's** type: visuo-constructional, writing, **agnosia**, **naming**, **comprehension**, reading, motor-gestural. These differences in the ranking prove there must be a difference between the disorders of **aphasia** found in **stroke** (5) patients and **aphasia** found in patients suffering from **dementia** of the **Alzheimer's** type. See also sections 4 and 5. *See Obler and Albert (1981).*

American Speech-Language Hearing Association. The governing body for those who work with speech/language and hearing disorders in America. Its equivalent in the United Kingdom is the **College of Speech Therapists**.

Amerind. This particular **sign language** is used, mainly, with patients having suffered a **stroke** or **head injury** (both 5) producing **aphasia**. Many suffer from a right **hemiplegia** (5), resulting in weakness down the right side of the body and thus difficulty in moving the right hand whilst control of the left hand may be retained. Amerind, developed by Skelly from the American Indians, has gestures which can be produced by using only one hand and so is ideal for this type of patient. *See Kiernan et al. (1982): 9–10.*

Anarthria. A severe form of **dysarthria**. The patient loses the ability to speak due to severe loss of the motor movements necessary for producing speech. *See Darley et al. (1975): 2.*

Anomia. Word-finding difficulties which may affect an aphasic patient. The patient cannot find the words required to finish a sentence. The lost word can be of any part of speech. Sometimes a patient will use circumlocution or find a synonym to express himself. In the sentence, 'Last night, I was watching television', the patient could not think of the word 'television'; he might say, 'Last night, I was watching the thing which shows moving pictures'. Anomia can occur in semantic fields (e.g., the patient says 'orange' for 'apple', or 'cat' for 'dog', etc.). Assessment of this condition is done by picture naming, sentence completion, a story to be summarized in the patient's own words or by asking the patient to supply a synonym for a word or phrase. *See Eisenson (1984): 21.*

Aphasia. Also known as dysphasia. Dysphasic patients have usually suffered a **stroke** or **head injury** (both 5) which has affected part of the **brain** (5), usually the left **cerebral hemisphere**, (5) which controls the use of **language** (2), both **comprehension** and **expressive language**. Both will be disordered to a greater or lesser degree. A more precise term for this disorder is acquired dysphasia. Children can also suffer from acquired dysphasia. The child suffers cerebral dysfunction which has been preceded by normal language development. The commonest cause is **open** and

closed **head injury** while **neurological tumours** (all 5) are also very common. The other main cause is convulsive illnesses which include **idiopathic (temporal lobe)**, **Sturge-Weber Syndrome** and **Landau-Kleffner Syndrome** (all 5). In the former cause, the child has a period of mutism, **word-finding difficulty**, an **auditory comprehension** problem and persistent **dyslexia** and **dysgraphia**. It is a **nonfluent** type of dysphasia. In convulsive aphasia, there is a fundamental auditory deficiency, auditory sequencing disorder, an auditory-verbal comprehension disorder, verbal-auditory agnosia and an **expressive language** disorder. The best assessments techniques are the **Test for Reception of Grammar (TROG)**, the **Bus Story** and the **Word-Finding Vocabulary scale**. The therapist may need to introduce some **alternative communication systems** and investigative therapy techniques.

In developmental dysphasia, the child has never been able to communicate well. It is also known as **specific developmental language disorder**. It has been defined as the '... slow, limited or otherwise faulty development of language in children who do not otherwise give evidence of gross neurological or psychiatric disability' (Zangwill 1978). Such a definition excludes children who suffer from **mental handicap, autism**, (4) minor brain damage. They suffer from **language disorder**. *See Eisenson (1984): passim (adult dysphasia); Satz and Bullard-Bates (1981) (acquired childhood dysphasia); Wyke (1978) passim (developmental dysphasia).*

Aphasiology. The study of aphasia in all its forms. Also the name of a new journal giving an interdisciplinary approach to **aphasia** research.

Aphemia. The old-fashioned term for **aphasia** used in the time of Paul Broca who discovered **Broca's Area** (5). *See Eisenson (1984): 106.*

Aphonia. See **dysphonia**.

Apraxia. An acquired disorder caused by a **CVA** (5) and characterized by the patient groping for the correct order of sounds, which produces trial and error realizations. The programming of the movements required to make sounds in a particular order becomes disordered, particularly, though not exclusively, with polysyllabic words. The patient also exhibits disruption in **prosody** (3), articulatory inconsistency and difficulties in initiating utterances. Developmental apraxia is found in children and may take the form of oral apraxia (see developmental articulatory apraxia), **articulatory apraxia** or **constructional apraxia**. *See Eisenson (1984): 12–13.*

Apraxia Battery for Adults. Devised by Dabul in 1979, it is an assessment to discover the severity of **acquired apraxia**. There are six subtests comprising **diadochokinesis**, increasing word length, limb and oral apraxia, latency and utterance time for polysyllabic words, repeated trials test and inventory of articulation characteristics of apraxia. It takes about 20 minutes to administer, longer if the patient's responses are slow. *See test manual.*

Articulation   Attainment   Test. Designed by Catherine Renfrew, it is not meant to be used as a diagnostic test of the child's articulation problems but rather is intended to find out how many consonants a child can produce. The test uses 38 words made up of 100 consonants. The child has to name the 38 objects spontaneously as well as produce some serial counting and phrases for repetition. If a child of **mental age** (4) 6.00 or older, scores under 70 per cent (less than the average child of 3.09), he will probably need speech therapy. *See test manual.*

Articulation delay. Many children suffer from an articulation difficulty, failing to produce a sound correctly because they cannot place their **articulators** (3) in the correct position. An articulation delay occurs when a child's **articulation** (3) development is below the child's **chronological age** (CA) (4). However, the child will catch up to his CA with regular therapy. To assess a child's articulatory difficulties, **articulation tests** are used. *See Grunwell (1982).*

Articulation disorder. A child who suffers from this condition requires a very systematic programme to improve his **articulation** (3). In other words, unlike an **articulation delay**, it will not improve with ordinary therapy. *See Grunwell (1982): 50–51, 199–205.*

Articulation tests. Assessments used by speech therapists to find out the severity of the **articulation disorder** or **delay** from which the child suffers. Two of the commonest tests used in the UK are the **Edinburgh Articulation Test** and the **Goldman-Fristoe Articulation Test**.

Articulatory   apraxia. See **developmental articulatory apraxia**.

Artificial larynx. There are several artificial laryngae available to patients who have undergone **total laryngectomy** (5). With the **larynx** (5) removed, to produce

voice the patient requires artificial techniques such as the Barts vibrator, the Medici speech vibrator, the Siemens Servox, the Rexton laryngopophone, the Weston electronic No. 5A (male) and No. 5B (female). Each works by being next to the neck; a button on the side is pressed, which starts a diaphragm vibrating on top of the device; this produces a voiced sound as the patient mouths the sounds. There are facilities to control volume, pitch and tone of the voice produced. Most have rechargeable batteries. There are also two pneumatic devices available—the Tokyo and Osaka. These consist of a tube which leads from the **tracheastoma** (5) passing through a cylindrical unit which contains a rubber membrane. The membrane is vibrated by air from the **lungs** (5) as a sound source and directs the sound into the mouth by the mouth tube. *See Edels (1984): 146–152.*

Asemantic jargon. See **jargon**.

ASHA. **The   American   Speech-language Hearing Association**.

Assessment of phonological processes. Tests which show the number of **phonological processes** (3) which a child possesses at a particular age. Weiner has produced such an assessment in his **Phonological Process Analysis** (3).

Assessments. These are tests used by speech therapists to find out what **communication disorders** the patient may have and their severity. There are assessments for almost all problems but since some patients may have a mixture of problems, e.g., **dysphasia** with some **dysarthria**, two or more tests may be required. Most assessments are made up of smaller tests called subtests. The two main types of assessment are the **formal** and **informal assessments**. The former type is a published assessment like those described in this book while the latter are assessments made up by the therapist to assess certain parts of the therapy programme devised for each patient.

Aston Index. This test was developed in Birmingham by Newton and Thomson. It is a 'classroom screening test' for 5–14 year olds. Level 1 is suitable for the screening of 5–6 year olds while level 2 is for use with the older children. It contains six tests to measure general ability, the results providing **age equivalent scores** (4) and ten performance tests which measure the **ability** (4) necessary for learning to read and write; these include two visual sequential memory tasks, an auditory sequential task, sound-blending and sound discrimination sub-tests, a motor dominance subtest and two subtests concerning the child's writing ability. The results of the first six tests of general ability (picture recognition, vocabulary, Goodenough draw-a-man test, copying geometric designs, Schonell reading test and Schonell spelling test) are plotted onto the graph provided, as are the results of the ten performance sub-tests. Thus, the therapist can discover any delay in development or the most signifi-cant difficulties a child may possess. *See test manual.*

Ataxic dysarthria. The speech disorders resulting from this type of **dysarthria** are caused by a lesion in the **cerebellum** (5). The symptoms are **consonants** (3) which become imprecise, problems with stress patterns, irregular articulatory breakdown, distorted vowels, harsh voice, prolonged sounds, prolonged intervals, monopitch, monoloudness and slow rate. *See Darley et al. (1975): ch. 7.*

Auditory aphasia. *See Wernicke's Aphasia.*

Auditory comprehension. An activity used in therapeutic programmes to either test or train the patients' ability to under-stand what is heard. Tests designed to assess this type of disorder are the **Token Test**, **TROG**, some subtests in the **Boston Diagnostic Aphasia Examina-tion**, and some subtests found in **MTDDA**. In very severe cases, it may appear that the patient is deaf rather than simply not understanding what is being asked of him. Various therapeutic tech-niques can be used to help such patients, including **sign systems**, **sign languages**, and some **PACE** activities. *See Riedel (1981): ch. 8.*

Auditory Discrimination Screening Test. Designed by Catherine Renfrew, it assesses the phonological feature con-trasts and semantic confusions often found in children with speech and lan-guage problems. It can be used with children of 5 years and upwards but as long as the therapist covers up the bottom row of three pictures on each page, the test can be used with children between the ages of 3 and 4 years. In scoring, errors in auditory discrimination must be distinguished from vocabulary errors. If a child of 5 years or older makes two or more discrimination errors on any page, the child will require a period of auditory training. *See test manual.*

Augmentative communication aids. See **alternative communication systems**.

B

Babbling. An early stage in **language acquisition**. The child will babble when he is comfortable and this is reflected in the type of sounds the child produces, e.g., **velars** (3), sounds made by the tongue against the top of the mouth, and open vowel sounds. By nine months, babbling has become more human. Strings of sounds follow put together in a CVCVCV structure. The pitch pattern is similar to the one used in normal English, i.e. ⋏ Cooing and vocal play where the child experiments considerably with voice quality and **airstreams** (3) are also produced. *See Cruttenden (1970).*

Baby talk. A phenomenon which occurs in **language acquisition** which refers to the special use of a simplified language used by a mother to communicate with her child. At first, she may use simple words to refer to objects, animals or people, e.g., [brm, brm] = 'car'; [hor-sie] = 'horse'; [doggie] = 'dog'; [mama, dada] = 'mummy, daddy', etc. As the child's language develops, he begins to use two-word phrases, e.g., [cake allgone] = 'there is no more cake'; [dada shoe] = 'there are daddy's shoes'. The mother seems to know intuitively at what level to pitch her language, so that she is always one step ahead, thus encouraging the child to reach another stage in his language development. It is also described as parental speech. *See Cruttenden (1979): 75–79.*

Bangor Dyslexia Test. Designed by Professor T. R. Miles as a **screening test** to find out if the difficulties from which a child suffers are those typically found in **dyslexia** or not. It is not to be used with children under 7 years of age and even when used with 7–8 year olds, the results should be treated with caution. The test results are unhelpful if the test has been used with a child of limited ability, as such subjects tend to have a general and not a specific learning difficulty. There are ten subtests: knowledge of left/right body parts, repetition of polysyllabic words, subtraction, multiplication tables, months forwards, months reversed, digits forward, digits reversed, b–d confusion and familial incidence. *See test manual.*

Base 10. A therapeutic technique for showing the success of a treatment programme, usually in **aphasia** therapy. It was devised by Lapointe in the mid-1970s. It comprises a printed form on which the aims of the therapy are entered and baseline scores are recorded. Progress is shown graphically, thus giving positive feedback to the patient and providing the therapist with a record of success. The activities can be modified if improvement occurs. It is very useful for intensive therapy. *See Code and Muller (1983): 10, 11, 47–50.*

BDAE. **Boston Diagnostic Aphasia Examination**.

Biber's Test. Used for assessing the comprehension of aphasic patients. In the single form of the test, the patient has to select a picture showing single word comprehension. The stimuli can be presented auditorily or visually and the patient has to indicate by whatever means whether the heard/seen word corresponds to the picture. In the 'three-somes' version, selection is made from three pictures, two semantically related and an unrelated distractor. The rest of the procedure is the same as for the 'single' form of the test. *See test manual.*

Bilateral abductor paralysis. See **laryngeal nerve palsies**.

Bilateral adductor paralysis. See **laryngeal nerve palsies**.

Blissymbolics. This **sign system** was developed by Charles Bliss in Canada in 1971 and was first introduced into the United Kingdom in 1974. It helps those patients who either have no or limited **expressive language** to communicate their needs. It comprises symbols, which when used in a particular order and combination represent words, phrases and sentences. The symbols are set out on a chart. If the patient is too handicapped to draw the symbols, then the patient can either point or eye-point to the desired square on the chart. *See Kiernan et al. (1982): 10–11, 42–44, 47–52.*

Blocking behaviour. See **block modification**.

Block modification. A patient who stammers is often described as exhibiting blocking behaviour. This is the actual act of stammering, i.e., the repetition of sounds. Van Riper proposed block modification as a therapeutic technique to reduce the amount of blocking behaviour produced by the patient. It is part of the **stammer more fluently** theory, so the criterion for success is not necessarily total fluent speech but an **acceptable stammer** where the speaker is happy to speak despite his **dysfluency** and where the listener is aware of some **dysfluency** but is not annoyed by it. The first stage of this technique is to identify the stammer, i.e., what it sounds like, then desensitize the patient's fear and panic when he anticipates a stammer. Block modification has three stages:
1. cancellation—the patient corrects his speech after the block has occurred;
2. pull outs—the patient recognizes he is in the middle of a block, stops and repeats the word or phrase in which his blocking took place;
3. preparatory blocks—the patient anticipates a block and prepares himself to speak as fluently as possible. *See Dalton (1983): 144–145.*

Blom-Singer oesophageal prosthesis. A device in the **fistula** (5) following a **laryngectomy** operation. If successful, the patient can regain voice and communicate almost normally. The voice is usually fluent and sounds more normal than **oesophageal voice** . It is powered by pneumatic air pressure; the duration in speech is better; the voice is louder and greater change in pitch is possible than with a normal oesophageal voice, in allowing greater scope and variability. If, however, the patient does not like the resulting voice, the prosthesis can be removed and the tracheo-oesophageal fistula will close completely. *See Édels (1984): 272–282.*

Boston Diagnostic Aphasia Examination. Devised by Goodglass and Kaplan in 1972, it is an **assessment** for testing an aphasic patient. A formal assessment which has undergone **standardization** (4), which incorporates what the authors describe as the 'three general aims' of any **aphasia** test:
1. diagnosis of presence and type of aphasic syndrome, leading to inferences concerning cerebral localization;
2. measurement of the level of performance over a wide range of both initial determination and detection of change over time;
3. comprehensive assessment of the assets and liabilities of the patient in all language areas as a guide to therapy.

From a practical point of view, the test does not give hard and fast guidelines for therapy. It highlights all the possible areas where the patient may find varying difficulties such as **articulation** (3), loss of verbal fluency, word-finding difficulty (see **anomia**), repetition, **serial speech**, loss of **syntax** (2), **paraphasia**, **auditory comprehension**, reading and writing. The authors do not accept that there is a disorder called **dyspraxia** and so the term is not used in this **assessment**. *See Eisenson (1984): 137–139*.

Boston School. A group of people, of whom the authors of the **BDAE** are part, who believe that aphasic patients can be categorized according to which part of the left **cerebral hemisphere** (5) is damaged. Often known as the **locationist theory**, since its proponents attempt to locate the damaged part of the brain. The Boston School propose seven major types of **aphasia** and four pure aphasias: major aphasias: **Broca's aphasia, Wernicke's aphasia, conduction aphasia, anomia, transcortical sensory** and **motor aphasias, alexia with agraphia**; pure aphasias: **aphemia, pure word deafness, pure alexia, pure agraphia**. *See Goodglass and Kaplan (1972): ch. 1*.

British Picture Vocabulary Scales. A **formal, standardized assessment** (4) to test the auditory vocabulary of a patient. It is suitable for children with learning difficulties, patients who cannot produce an oral or written response, or as a screening test for new school entrants. The patient is given a page of four pictures, only one of which corresponds correctly to the auditory stimulus. The patient need only finger point or eye point. **A ceiling score** and a **basal score** (both 4) must be found. It is quick to administer and can be given either as a detailed test using the 'Long Form' or as a quick **screening test** using the 'Short Form'. *See test manual*.

British Sign Language. Used by the deaf in the UK. It is a natural language, which has been developed by deaf people, having a grammar of its own, unlike any other **sign language** such as **Makaton**, which is not grammatical in its structure. However, the grammar of BSL does not match that of spoken English. *See Kiernan et al. (1982): 6–7*.

Broca's aphasia. Discovered by a French doctor Paul Broca in the nineteenth century. A major **aphasia** proposed by the **Boston School** for a language defect caused by a **CVA** or **head injury** (5) to **Broca's area** (5). This is part of the left **cerebral hemisphere** (5) or, more precisely, the third frontal convolution in the pre-central **gyrus** (5). A sufferer of Broca's aphasia has **nonfluent** conversational speech, varying degrees of **comprehension** difficulty, inability to repeat what is said, difficulty in confrontation naming, problems with reading out loud, varying degrees of difficulty in reading comprehension and a disorder in writing. Although the authors of the **Boston Diagnostic Aphasia Examination** show in the test manual a typical picture of this type of **aphasia**, not all aphasic patients will fit into such a neat picture. *See Goodglass and Kaplan (1972): ch. 4*.

BT. Baby Talk.

Bus Story. Devised by Catherine Renfrew in 1969 to test a child's use of continuous speech. Other tests such as **RDLS** test only the **comprehension** and use of words, phrases and sentences. The bus story may be used with 3–8 year old children. The child is presented with a picture book containing four pages with three pictures on each, telling the story of a 'naughty bus'. The picture book is in the form of a strip cartoon. Two scores can be obtained—one for sentence length and one for information. *See test manual*.

C

CADL. Communicative Abilities in Daily Living.

Cancellation. See **block modification**.

Carryover. When a speech therapist has given the patient certain techniques to overcome a **communication disorder** and knows it can be used well in the speech therapy situation, the patient must go out and continue to use these techniques in his everyday **communication**. This process can also be called **maintenance**.

Case history. A summary of the patient's **communication disorder** from its onset to the condition as presented to the therapist. This will include details of the relevant parts of the patient's medical history, his leisure activities and feelings about his present condition. The amount of information required for a case history is determined by the severity of the disorder from which the patient is suffering. *See Brown (1981): 12, passim.*

Cerebral palsy. A medical condition producing physical handicaps, such as weakness in the limbs as well as in the muscles of the face which are used for **articulation** (3) and **chewing** (5). In severe cases, the patients can neither produce **expressive language** nor feed themselves. The speech therapist can help with both these disorders. In the former, either the muscles have to be strengthened to improve articulation or an **alternative communication system** has to be found. A programme for helping the patient to feed correctly can also be devised by the therapist. (See also section 5). *See Darley, Aranson, Brown (1975): 135, 137.*

Chronic non-specific laryngitis. A condition caused by nasal discharge into the **nasopharynx** (5) and thence to the **larynx** (5) which becomes irritated. In many cases, the only symptom is persistent **hoarse voice**. The primary problem, i.e., nasal disorder, should be put right first before the secondary problem, i.e., the laryngitis. *See Pracy et al. (1974): 113.*

Cleft palate. As surgical procedures have improved in closing a cleft in the child's palate and/or lip, the need for speech therapy to improve the child's **articulation** (3) is not as great as in the past. However, the therapist's main purpose is to counsel the parents about the child's future speech, efficacy of future surgery and to give advice on the best types of feeding techniques available at the time. There may be problems with articulation, for which speech therapy may be required. (See also section 5). *See Edwards and Watson (1980): chs 8 and 14.*

Cluttering. A particular type of **dysfluency** in which the patient is unaware of any problems which may include a short attention span, problems with **articulation** (3), incoherent speech impeded by an amazing speed of delivery. Many authors have given their view as to what cluttering is, but the diagnosis can only be made by close examination of the symptoms, *viz.* repetitions, excessive speed, drawling and interjections, vowel stop, articulation and motor disabilities, poor breathing, monotonous voice, poor concentration, inner language, reading disorders, writing problems, grammatical difficulties, unawareness of symptoms, restlessness and hyperactivity and delayed speech development. Therapy for this disorder is aimed at relaxing the patient and slowing down the speech **rate** (3) to a more acceptable level. *See Dalton and Hardcastle (1977): ch. 7.*

College of Speech Therapists. The professional body organizing the **speech therapy** service throughout the United Kingdom. The College sets out a code of ethics which every therapist has to follow. Until recently, it organized the 'diploma' examinations before speech therapy became a 'graduate' profession. It organizes 'working parties' to study all the **communication disorders** for which therapists provide treatment. These working parties can be approached at any time for advice on treatment programmes for a specific disorder. Membership of the College is open to all qualified therapists as well as to speech therapy students. College is financed by a yearly membership subscription and in return therapists receive the *British Journal of Disorders of Communication*, the *Bulletin* (a monthly magazine for therapists by therapists), a Directory (a list of names and addresses of members of College) and a twice-monthly list of vacancies in Health Boards in the UK. Information pamphlets are also available. College is not a salary-negotiating body. Such matters are taken up by the Association of Scientific and Technical Managerial Staff (ASTMS). *See Jennings (1984).*

Communication. The ability to spread information from one person to either another person or to a group of people. There has been much discussion as to the form the communication process takes. Thus, the **speech chain** (3) came into being. When a link breaks in this chain, the result is a **communication disorder** and the therapist has to find ways to mend the links so the chain will function normally. A breakdown in the way people communicate is probably one of the biggest handicaps anyone can suffer. *See Denes and Pinson (1973):1, passim.*

Communication disorder. See **communication**.

Communication profiles. Different types of **assessment** for **stroke** (5) or **head injury** (5) patients. These are not formal **assessments** which have undergone **standardization** (4) nor do they test the actual breakdown in **communication** but rather the potential use of language in various situations such as 'greeting' 'understanding', 'social conventions' and so on. *See Eisenson (1984).*

Communicative Abilities in Daily Living (CADL). A test of **functional communication** which takes the form of a **communication profile**. There are ten functional categories:

1. reading, writing and use of numbers;
2. **speech acts** (3);
3. verbal and non-verbal contexts;
4. **role playing** (4);
5. divergencies;
6. relationship dependent communicative behaviour;
7. non-verbal symbolic communication;
8. **deixis** (2);
9. humour, absurdity;
10. use of metaphor.

There is an attempt to relate CADL to type, cause and severity of **aphasia**. The rating is on a three-point scale. Administration takes the form of a structured interview utilizing props and situational contexts. It is designed for all age groups. CADL has two objectives:
1. to gain a valid reflection of **communication** skills;
2. to obtain a reliable assessment of these skills. It is a test of talking behaviour and communication, assessing more than just propositional and linguistic content. It does not discriminate against patients who may use an **alternative communication system**. *See Eisenson (1984): 142–144.*

Comprehension. The process used by children and adults to understand both spoken and written language. Speech therapists have to understand this process as **communication disorders** such as **aphasia** will probably involve a disorder of comprehension. With children, comprehension is often better than their **expressive language**. Many people think, often erroneously, if the child can understand what is said to him, he will be able to produce a similar **utterance** (3).

Conduction aphasia. A major type of **aphasia** described by the **Boston School**. It is caused by damage to the **arcuate fasciculus** in the **left hemisphere** (both 5). The patient produces **fluent** conversational speech, has normal **comprehension** except for complex grammatical structures, abnormal repetitions with many **literal paraphasias**, abnormal confrontation naming, abnormal reading out loud although reading comprehension is normal and there is a difficulty in writing. *See Goodglass and Kaplan (1972).*

Congenital disorder. A disorder which appears at birth, perhaps as a result of a problem during the **prenatal period**, **perinatal period** or **postnatal period** (all 5). It is opposed to a **developmental disorder** which occurs during childhood and an **acquired disorder** which has an organic cause.

Constructional apraxia. A disorder of movement which affects the person's ability to dress, build, feed and so on.

Constructs. See **personal construct therapy**.

Contact ulcers. Growths which appear on the **vocal cords** (3) producing **hoarse voice**. The symptoms of contact ulcers are extreme localized and generalized tension on the cords, explosive speech patterns, sudden glottal stops, restricted pitch and habitual clearing of the throat. They are produced by the hard cartilagenous surfaces of the vocal processes hitting the opposite vocal cord. Therapy takes the form of reducing the effort in **phonation** (3), reducing the pitch level of the voice, getting the patient to speak with a relaxed mouth and jaw and at a lower volume and stopping the patient from using hard glottal attack. *See Fawcus (1986).*

Cued speech. Devised by Cornett in 1966 as an **alternative communication system** for those who either cannot or have difficulty in expressing their needs. It is not a **sign language** as such, but rather an oral approach supported by hand signs. The instructor can show the patient the sound orally while the shape made by the hand clearly 'shows' which sound has been made. *See Kiernan et al. (1982): 5, 165.*

Cues. Techniques used by the therapist to help the patient succeed during therapy. These cues may be signing, i.e., giving a clue to the correct response; semantic, i.e., giving the meaning of the word; phonemic, i.e., giving the first sound of the correct response; repetition, i.e., the therapist says the response for the patient to repeat; and visual, i.e., the therapist produces a picture of the correct response, perhaps with some distractors for the patient to choose the correct response.

D

DAF. Delayed auditory feedback.

Delayed auditory feedback. See section 7.

Delayed echolalia. See **echolalia.**

Deep dyslexia. See **acquired dyslexia.**

Derbyshire Language Scheme. Devised by Masidlover and Knowles in 1977 for use with children who suffer from **language delay/disorder.** It has non-**standardized** assessment (4) procedures to test the severity of the delay and teaching procedures based on the preceding **assessment.** It is based on the natural communication of the child by playing with toys and looking at pictures. **Language** (2) is taught through the medium of play. The criterion for success is the child using what he has learnt during the therapy sessions at home and in the community. The **assessment** is divided into two parts—the **rapid screening test (RST)** and the **detailed test of communication (DTC).** The results of these assessments can be plotted onto an assessment summary. There is a progress record to show graphically the child's performance, and to reveal areas of language development which still require therapy. Before using the scheme, therapists are required to go on a three-day training course to become registered users. Any therapist can use the scheme under the guidance of a registered user.

Detailed Test of Comprehension. This is an **assessment** procedure used in the **Derbyshire Language Scheme.** It is used after the **rapid screening test** has been administered so that the therapist can assess more accurately the problems which the child has in both **comprehension** and **expressive language.** These two aspects of communication are tested in natural contexts with everyday toys and pictures. The authors introduce the concept of information-carrying words, i.e., how many words the child requires to understand a command. In the

example below, the sentences are from different levels of the DTC.

In other words, the child has to show his comprehension at different levels by ignoring similar distractors. When testing the child's **expressive language,** the therapist writes down everything that the child says during the test even if it is unconnected with the toys or pictures used in the test. *See test manual.*

Developmental disorder. Any disorder which occurs after birth, during childhood, unlike a **congenital disorder** which occurs during pregnancy or at birth.

Developmental aphasia. See **aphasia.**

Developmental articulatory apraxia. A cause of **articulation disorder** which occurs during childhood. The difficulty is in placing the tongue in the correct position to produce certain sounds. This may be due to some muscle weakness in the tongue or to some other disorder of the **articulators** (3). Therapy consists of training the patient to place the articulators in the correct position to produce the sounds with which there is difficulty. The **Nuffield Dyspraxia Programme** is one possible treatment technique. *See Grunwell (1982): 201–205.*

Developmental dyslexia. A reading and writing disorder which occurs during childhood. In general, the child has difficulty in learning to read and write. There is a particular difficulty in learning to spell despite the child having an above-average IQ. The term 'dyslexia' is used to describe only a child whose reading and spelling are unexpectedly poor. The **Bangor Dyslexia Test** is a **screening test** to find out the severity of the disorder. *See Hornsby (1984).*

Diadochokinesis. The average rate used by patients to move their **articulators** in producing certain sequences of sounds. The sequences are produced in all positions in the mouth, e.g., /p, p, p/, /t, t, t/,

INSTRUCTION	NO. OF ITEM	COMP. LEVEL
Wash the teddy	TEDDY	0
WASH the TEDDY	CLOTH, BRUSH,	
	TEDDY, DOLL	2
WASH the TEDDY'S FOOT	SAME AS ABOVE	3
WASH the LITTLE	LITTLE TEDDY, BIG	
TEDDY'S FOOT	TEDDY, LITTLE DOLL	
	CLOTH, BRUSH	4

/k, k,, k,/, /p, t, k, p, t, k,/, /oo ... ee ... oo ... ee/, etc. This test can be used with both adults and children. It is opposed to **adiadochokinesis**. *See Robertson (1982): (adults); Canning and Rose (1974): (children)*.

Diagnosis. The decision made by the therapist of the patient's condition, after thorough examination, investigation and **assessment**. It is important to make sure the decision is correct and no other diagnosis is likely. This is known as a **differential diagnosis**. It is possible, for instance, for some aphasic patients to suffer also from **dysarthria**, so it is necessary to test each patient to find out if **aphasia** or **dysarthria** alone is present or a mixture of the two conditions. Assessment will show also the differing severities of the two disorders where both are present in the one patient. Before treatment begins a sound diagnosis must be made. *See Brown (1981): 5, 34, 36, 116, 118*.

Differential diagnosis. See **diagnosis**.

DLS. **Derbyshire Language Scheme**.

DTC. **Detailed Test of Comprehension**.

Dysarthria. A disorder which interferes with the muscles controlling the mechanism used for producing speech. Such an impairment may also involve poor breathing patterns, poor vocalization, and, with some patients, there are feeding problems. The sounds may also be distorted, so the patient's speech can sound slurred. There are three types of dysarthria—**flaccid**, **spastic** and **ataxic**. There are two **assessments** commonly used in the United Kingdom to establish a **diagnosis—Robertson Dysarthria Profile** and the **Frenchay Dysarthria Assessment**. *See Darley et al. (1975): passim*.

Dysfluency. The general term for describing **stammering/stuttering** behaviour as well as **cluttering**. It can also describe other forms of speech which includes a lot of repetitions, hesitations and so on. It is also called **nonfluency**. When a speaker hesitates during a conversation for effect or while thinking of something else to say, this is described as normal dysfluency or normal **nonfluency**. *See Dalton (1983): passim*.

Dysgraphia. A disorder of writing caused by **CVA** or **head injury** (5) and associated with **aphasia**. Such disorders in writing may mirror other disorders caused by **aphasia**, e.g., **anomia**, **agrammatism**. However, the condition may involve only minor spelling mistakes or difficulty in copying and writing to dictation. Writing disorders are not always associated with **aphasia**. Sometimes, they are caused by a loss of power in the dominant hand, requiring the patient to be retrained to write with the non-dominant hand—a slow process requiring much counselling and encouragement. *See Eisenson (1984): 22–23*.

Dyslalia. An old name for **articulation disorder**, no longer used. It was used as a blanket term to cover all such disorders. Since it failed to be as precise in definition as **articulation disorder** and **phonological disorder**, these terms have now replaced it.

Dyslexia. A general description for a disorder affecting a person's ability to read, write and spell. For a child, it is the unexpected failure to learn to read and write as he reaches the appropriate age (see **developmental dyslexia**) while for an adult, it refers usually to the difficulty found in reading after a **CVA** or **head injury** (5) (see **acquired dyslexia**).

Dysphagia. A disorder in swallowing caused by a **CVA**, **tumour of central nervous system**, **head injury** (all 5), degenerative disease or lesions to the **upper** and **lower motor neurones** (5). These causes produce difficulty in swallowing liquids. Dysphagia can also be caused by **organic** and **anatomical** disorders such as structural abnormalities, e.g., **cleft palate**, disease, radiography, surgery, e.g., partial/total **glossectomy**, **laryngectomy**, etc. (5), neck or facial trauma and burns. When these occur the patient has difficulty swallowing solids. Therapy depends on what the patient cannot swallow and which part of the **swallowing system** (5) does not function. *See Silverman and Elfant (1979)*.

Dysphasia. See **aphasia**.

Dysphonia. Those who have **voice disorders** suffer from dysphonia. It has many causes which can be classed under five headings:

1. localized lesions of the **larynx** (5) e.g., **vocal nodules**, **contact ulcers**;

2. neuropathologies, e.g., paralysis of one/two **vocal cords** (3);

3. **endocrine disorders** e.g., hypothyroidism, etc.

4. drugs, mechanical and chemical irritants and alcohol;

5. indirectly through **hearing loss** (6).

Assessment and therapy will be described under the heading of each cause. *See Fawcus (1986)*.

E

EAT. **Edinburgh Articulation Test**.

Echolalia. A phenomenon found in many **communication disorders** where patients repeat almost word for word what the therapist says to them. **Delayed echolalia** occurs when the repetition of the word, phrase or sentence is made after an interval of time has passed or after another of the patients' utterances.

Edinburgh Articulation Test. Devised by Antony in 1971, it is a formal test which has undergone **standardization** (4) aimed at finding out which sounds a child finds difficult to produce. It consists of 41 common pictures which are easy for a child to name. If the child has difficulty with the pictures, the therapist can use the objects of the pictures. The child is only asked to name the pictures without reference being made to the fact that it is a test for assessing his **articulation**. There are two ways of scoring, the first is mandatory while the second is optional. The quantitative assessment is where the therapist marks the sounds the child makes as either correct or wrong. For those which have · been produced wrongly, the therapist writes down the child's **realization** (3) next to the **target sound** (3). If the child's **standard score** (4) is 85 or below, then the child's articulation should be further examined and therapy given. An **age equivalent score** (4) can also be found for the child. The qualitative assessment, which is optional, is divided into six columns—adult form, i.e., correct form, minor variations, almost mature, immature, very immature and atypical substitutions. This assessment is important for checking the child's progress each time the child is retested. For example, when the form is scored, there may be a lot of marks in the right-hand column, i.e., atypical substitutions; the more these marks move to the left the better the child's **articulation** (3) is becoming. Retesting may take place six months after the initial test, so test learning does not take place. *See test manual.*

Edinburgh Functional Communication Profile. A test for assessing the patient's **functional communication**. There are twelve interaction situations, grouped into six 'communicative contexts':

1. greeting
2. acknowledging
3. responding
4. requesting
5. propositions
6. verbal problem-solving.

It is designed to be used with elderly patients as well as **aphasic** patients who have difficulty in coping with aspects of daily **communication**. Rating is on a seven-point scale of carefully defined responses. Administration takes the form of **observations** (4) either by the therapist, spouse or medical staff. The profile looks at the **total communication** (6) of the patient including the use of signing, computers, etc., to help him communicate, for which he still receives credit. It can also discriminate between the non-language modes used by the patient. *See profile manual.*

EFCP. **Edinburgh Functional Communication Profile**.

Elective mutism. An **emotional disorder** (4). However, it is a problem for which speech therapists can provide therapy. The child should be desensitized to the situation in which he does not speak. This may take some time but following this, the child should be put in as many speaking situations as possible to gain confidence. Whispering should be allowed although the child should be encouraged to use his normal voice as soon as possible. (See also section 4). *See Rutter (1978): 224–227.*

Endocrine disorder. Some **communication disorders** are caused by a disorder of the way the **endocrine system** (5) functions in the body. **Dysphonia** is such a disorder and is caused by:

1. Castrati voice;
2. Eunochoid voice—could respond to hormone treatment;
3. Incomplete vocal mutation—failure of voice to break at the normal time; it either breaks earlier or later than average. The voice may be hoarse or weak. The vocal range is very low and chest resonance is limited. The patient will probably complain of vocal fatigue because he is trying to lower his voice. The vocal cords show a varying degree of hyperaemia, congestion and irritation. The cords also show a 'mutational triangle' where they fail to adduct. Treatment takes the form of **voice therapy**, hormone treatment and **psychotherapy** (4);

4. Delayed maturation of pituitary gland or it is of thyrogenic origin;
5. **Puberphonia**;
6. Precocious vocal mutation—when patient shows true sexual precocity before 8 years of age;
7. Perverse mutation—this occurs in females when there is a change from the infantile female voice to the abnormal male voice by the excessive secretion of androgenic **hormones** (5);
8. Perello—after six months of pregnancy, there are physiological changes in breathing and a slight thickening of vocal folds which become oedematous. This can also happen when menstruation occurs;
9. Menopausal voice changes—these are caused by adreno-cortical activity after the ovarian oestrogens have been reduced. This can produce a decrease in the **fundamental frequency** (Fo) (3), the glottal membrane becomes thicker, the mass of the vocal cords increases in size and there is a decrease in voice pitch;
10. Hemaphroditic voice—can occur in **schizophrenia** (4);
11. Voice disorders caused by **thyroid** disorder:
    a) cretinism—the patient has a **larynx** (5) similar to an infant. The voice is without **intonation** (3) and has a very limited range of less than one octave:
    b) myxoedema—hypothyroidism produces voice loss. It could be referred to as hyperfunctional but it is myxoedema. The patient puts on weight, there is a decrease in the activity of the basal mechanism, the face becomes dry and puffy and there is a loss of hair, and there is a bowing of the **vocal cords** (3);
    c) hyperthyroidism—slight weakness and huskiness in the voice but nothing really noteworthy.

All these causes can be treated by **voice therapy** and relaxation. *See Fawcus (1986)*.

English Picture Vocabulary Test. Devised by Brimer and Dunn, it is a **formal**, **standardized** test (4) to find out the extent of a child's 'listening vocabulary'. The child is asked to choose the correct picture from a selection of four and the resulting score measures what the child can understand semantically. *See test manual*.

Environmental deprivation. A possible cause of **language delay**. When taking a **case history**, the therapist should establish to what extent the mother plays with the child or takes time to talk with him about pictures and toys or how frequently she or the father tells the child stories. Unless the child has the experience of talking through play, then he may have difficulty in acquiring language. *See Garvey (1977)*.

EPVT. **English Picture Vocabulary Test**.

Establishment Programme. See **Monterey Fluency Programme**.

Expressive aphasia. A patient who suffers from **Broca's aphasia** is expressively aphasic as his speech will be **non-fluent**. The amount he says will be reduced by the lesion in the brain. There will also be an element of **agrammatism** for those who can produce more than a few words. As with other types of **aphasia**, each patient will be affected differently depending on the severity of the lesion. It is most apparent with those patients who have **word-finding difficulties**. Some patients will suffer from both **comprehension** and expressive aphasia. It is part of **expressive-receptive aphasia**. In this condition **comprehension** of language is also affected to some extent. *See Eisenson (1984): passim*.

Expressive language. Language which is used in everyday conversation. It is not exactly synonymous with speech, which refers to the way in which people produce sounds, i.e., **articulation** and other motor problems. Expressive language is opposed to **comprehension**. An aphasic patient may have a disorder of expressive language, i.e., **expressive aphasia** and children who suffer from **language delay** will exhibit immature expressive language, i.e., the language of a younger child.

Expressive-receptive aphasia. See **Expressive aphasia**.

Extraneous movement. Any movement used by patients which is inappropriate to the situation in which they find themselves. This often happens with patients who **stammer**. To try and hide their **blocking behaviour**, they will use distracting movements such as waving their arms, kicking their legs, eye twitches, odd facial expressions or writhing on the seat. These movements have to be checked usually before therapy can begin on the actual **blocking behaviour**. A behavioural programme such as a simple **token economy** (4) can be used effectively with such patients.

Eye contact. Some patients who have a **stammer** or a **voice disorder** are so embarrassed when they speak, they fail to look directly at the therapist or person to whom they are talking. It is an important part of the initial assessment of these **communication disorders**. *See Dalton (1983).*

F

Facilitation. A phenomenon which describes the way in which a therapist helps patients with **communication disorders**. It is the **therapy programme** which will facilitate or allow the patient to relearn skills which have been lost, for example, by a **CVA**, **head injury**, **degenerative disease** (5). Elements of such a programme may include **alternative communication systems**, **PACE**, **MIT** and so on. The type and quantity of therapy which is given is important as it is these two elements which will determine the patient's facilitation to cope in situations which he has found difficult since the onset of his illness. *See Eisenson (1984): 195–196 (facilitation in* **aphasia**).

FAST. **Frenchay Aphasia Screening Test**.

FCP. **Functional Communication Profile**.

Feeding Check List. Devised by Jennifer Warner (1981), it is aimed at improving the child's feeding behaviour. It comprises five sections:

1—General
2—Head and trunk control
3—Food and feeding utensils
4—Control of tongue and lips for feeding and drinking
5—General features.

Each of these sections has questions which are to be answered with a 'yes/no' response. It can be used by either a therapist or a parent.

First word stage. A stage in a child's development of language. It lasts from about 1 to almost 2 years of age. A child's one-word **utterances** (2) are sentences of one word which name objects, describe actions, make requests or, with proper **intonation** (3), express emotional states or surprise at seeing something unexpected. The sort of items used in this stage are:

1. Familiar things and objects
   (a) important people, e.g., dada, mama
   (b) animals
   (c) clothing
   (d) household items
   (e) body parts
2. Action/event
   (a) name of movers (agents)
   (b) movables (objects affected by action)
   (c) some children pay particular attention to names of objects while others to names of people
3. Intonation used meaningfully (occurs later during this stage)
   (a) recurrence
   (b) negation
   (c) location.

Although the child may not use these completely with meaning, the meaning can be taken from their use of gesture and the context of the utterance. *See Cruttenden (1979): 13–15.*

First Word Language Programme. A language programme developed by William Gillham in 1979. It can be used with children who suffer from **language delay** or **language disorder**, those with learning difficulties and those who cannot produce speech for physical reasons. The child is taught using short structured sessions either once a day or more often. There is also the possibility of using informal settings for therapy where they occur. The therapist should keep records of the progress made by the children. *See Gillham (1979).*

'Fis' phenomenon. A situation in which a child refuses to repeat an adult's **utterance** (2) although it is the same as the child's incorrect utterance. It was found by Berko and Brown in 1960. When they were speaking to a child who called his 'fish' a [fis], they repeated this wrong utterance to the child, e.g., 'that's your "fis"', and the child said it was not 'fis' but 'his fis'. Such dialogue went on until the adults produced the correct form 'fish' and the child agreed it was his 'fis'. Thus, it was assumed the child had a very keen auditory perception whereby the child could recognize the difference between the words auditorily but not produce it correctly. *See Clark and Clark (1977): 384–385.*

Flaccid dysarthria. A type of **dysarthria** caused by a disorder in the **lower motor neurones** (5). The principal speech characteristics comprise four noises:

1. **hypernasality** (5);
2. nasal emission of air;
3. continuous breathiness during **phonation** (3);
4. audible inspiration.

The **consonants** (3) are also distorted and the patient speaks in short phrases because of breathing problems. *See Darley, Aranson and Brown (1975): ch. 5.*

Flow. See **prolonged speech**.

Fluency. A description of normal speech which has little or no **nonfluency** or **dysfluency** in it. There may be hesitation while the speaker thinks of his next utterance, i.e., normal **nonfluency**. Fluency is the ultimate aim of all who **stammer**. *See Dalton (1983); 77–78.*

Fluent aphasia. See **Wernicke's aphasia**.

Formal assessments. See **assessments**.

Frenchay Aphasia Screening Test. Devised by Enderby (1977), it is a fast way of finding out the existence and type of **aphasia**. It examines the patient's **comprehension, expressive language**, reading and writing. FAST consists of a composite picture, pictures of shapes and five graded sentences from which a non-speech therapist, because of its simplicity and speed to administer, could diagnose aphasia. The test has been **standardized** (4). When the scores are obtained, they are compared to a cut-off score. If the patient's score is lower for his age level than the cut-off score, aphasia is diagnosed and the patient should be referred to a speech therapist.

Frenchay Dysarthria Assessment. Devised by Enderby (1977), it is a **formal, standardized assessment** (4) to examine the severity and indicate the type of the patient's **dysarthria**. The **assessment** includes eight sections:

1. Reflex
2. Respiration
3. Lips
4. Jaw
5. Palate
6. Laryngeal
7. Tongue
8. Intelligibility.

All eight sections are scored on a nine-point scale. The test takes about 30 minutes to administer. The author believes it has fulfilled six criteria:

1. it is applicable to therapy;
2. it can demonstrate changes in the patient's speech;
3. it is easy and short to administer;
4. it has been standardized;
5. no training is necessary for administering it;
6. the results are easy to read and other professionals can understand them easily. *See test manual.*

Functional communication. The type of communication used, especially, in the treatment of aphasic patients. **Communication profiles** are used to find the type of functional communication a patient lacks. In the past, aphasic patients have been treated with such activities as sentence completion and picture naming which, nowadays, are not thought to be as effective as allowing the patient to communicate naturally. 'As language is used to establish interpersonal relationships, regulate the behaviour of others, satisfy material needs or desires, explore and organise environments and exchange messages and information (Halliday in Cole, 1982), therapy for the language impaired also needs to focus upon such functions'. (Green) Thus, the therapist should devise context-orientated therapy for these patients. *See Green (1984).*

Functional Communication Profile. A test of **functional communication**, devised by Sarno in 1969 for all age groups. It tests five functions:

1. movement
2. speaking
3. understanding
4. reading
5. other.

The 45 items divided into these five functional categories have been selected according to what are considered functions of everyday urban life. The rating which is based on a nine-point scale is very subjective. Administration takes the form of an unstructured interview. It can be used for prognosis and is designed for all age groups. The profile describes residual skills rather than deficits and yields a quantifiable measure of **functional communication** regardless of severity of impairment. It is a test primarily of language in a natural setting rather than all modes of **communication**. *See Sarno (1969).*

Functional dysphonia. There are different types of functional dysphonia:

1. Misuse and abuse of the patient's voice which produces **vocal nodules, contact ulcers**, etc.;
2. Learned patterns of **maladaptive behaviour** (4);
3. **Psychogenic** (4):

(a) those with a psychiatric history, having **psychosomatic** (4) symptoms and who are very vulnerable to physical and mental stress;

(b) in those with no history of psychiatric problems but who suffer from prolonged life stress.
See Fawcus (1986): 2, 7, 8, 9, 11.

G

Generalization. Synonymous with **carryover**.

Gesture. Either a recognized **sign language**, **sign system** or a series of gestures made up by the therapist which may be easier for the patient to understand. It has been found that, with practice, aphasic patients can cope with gesture and use it effectively for communication, although some therapists dispute its efficacy. *See Stuart-Smith and Wilks (1979).*

GILCU. **Gradual Increase in Length and Complexity of Utterance**.

Global aphasia. A patient who has suffered a severe **CVA** (5) has both **comprehension** and **expressive language** severely affected. Global aphasia produces **nonfluent** speech, inability to repeat words, phrases or sentences, inability to understand what is being said to him or asked of him and a difficulty in naming objects, pictures or people. Sometimes, the **stroke** (5) patient fits this classification immediately following a **CVA** (5) but may begin to recover various communication skills through **spontaneous recovery**. The degree of recovery depends on the size of lesion and its locus in the brain. *See Eisenson (1984): 110, 112, 113.*

Glossectomy. The surgical removal of part of the tongue due to a disease of the tongue, an accident to the tongue or natural wasting. The therapist has to retrain the patient in tongue placement and timing. Similar exercises to those given to a **dysarthric** patient are used. Quite intelligible speech can result, although the patient has to speak more slowly and carefully than before surgery. Most patients regain reasonable tongue mobility—it can be protruded, kept in the midline, can be moved to touch the left corner of the mouth and towards the right corner but not touching it. Patients should be counselled before surgery, that it is possible to **facilitate** intelligible speech after partial or complete **glossectomy**. *See Travis (1971).*

Goldman-Fristoe Articulation Test. This test is designed to discover which sounds a child has difficulty in producing. However, this test is different from the **EAT** in that the authors have put the emphasis on finding out in which part of the word the child makes an error. The results are scored in one of three columns headed **word-initially, word-medially** and **word-finally** (3). Not only are 'sounds-in-words' tested but also 'sounds-in-sentences'. Then the child has to retell a story from pictures after hearing it from the therapist. The scoring is carried out as in the first part of the test. *See test manual.*

Gradual Increase in Length and Complexity of Utterance. A structured programme to establish fluency in the **Monterey Fluency Programme** (**MFP**) for patients who **stammer**. The therapist asks the patient to say one word fluently and then extends this through the highly structured programme until he can speak fluently in the three modes of MFP. Fluent speech is reinforced by saying the word 'good', for those under 12 years; coloured tokens and the word 'good' is used for reinforcement. If the client stutters, the therapist says 'stop' and gets up to say the word fluently. *See programme manual.*

Group therapy. Now used quite widely in place of individual therapy. It has many advantages:

1. Patients discover others with similar problems, thus, creating support for one another;

2. Conversational situations can be created for context-oriented therapy so that the group can have some **functional communication**;

3. More intensive therapy can be given;

4. **Carryover** or **maintenance** is more likely;

5. A more stimulating environment is created, yet the patient is less tired than when given individual therapy since the burden of responding is spread around the group;

6. The patient finds a social purpose;

7. The patient becomes more involved in therapy;

8. A potentially more effective learning situation is created. Group therapy is used mainly with those who **stammer**, and suffer from **aphasia** or **dysarthria**. *See Fawcus (1979): 113–119.*

H

Harsh voice. A cause of **dysphonia** with the essential feature being tension in the **vocal cords** (3). Therapy is aimed at decreasing tension in the patient generally as well as particularly in the vocal cords. General relaxation or relaxation by suggestion can be used effectively so that the patient can learn how to relax spontaneously when in stress-provoking situations. The **yawn/sigh technique** or chewing technique can be used to decrease tension in the vocal cords. *See Fawcus (1986).*

Hoarse voice. A cause of **dysphonia** produced by the patient straining to speak against the tension of the vocal cords. Wilson (1975) has described it as a 'combination of harshness and breathiness with harsh voice predominating in some cases and breathy elements in others'. *See Fawcus (1986).*

Hysterical dysphonia. See **functional dysphonia** (3a, b). *See Fawcus (1986).*

I

Illinois Test of Psycholinguistic Abilities. A **formal, standardized assessment** (4) devised by Kirk in 1969. It can be used with children aged 2–10 years old, although it is less useful for children below the normal 4-year-old level. The twelve subtests assess:

1. auditory reception
2. visual reception
3. visual sequential memory
4. auditory association
5. auditory sequential memory
6. visual association
7. visual closure
8. verbal expression
9. grammatical closure
10. manual expression
11. auditory closure
12. sound blending

The **raw scores** (4) from these subtests together produce a psycholinguistic age or separate scaled scores. These scores can be produced on a graph to show each child's psycholinguistic abilities. *See test manual.*

Informal assessments. These **assessments** do not have a fixed format. They are evolved by the therapist to assess a patient's difficulties, if the patient is unable to cope with a **formal assessment**, or used during therapy to assess the efficacy of a therapy programme. Such tests allow more latitude to the therapist who may, by giving **cues**, discover how much and what kind of help the patient requires to succeed. Material used in such tests must be different from the material used in **formal assessments** so as not to invalidate their results if used later in therapy.

Inhalation. See **oesophageal voice.**

Injection. See **oesophageal voice.**

Insufflation. See **oesophageal voice.**

ITPA. **Illinois Test of Psycholinguistic Abilities.**

J

Jargon. See **jargon aphasia**.

Jargon aphasia. Butterworth described
jargon as a 'rare and spectacular manifestation of an aphasic condition'. There
are four types of jargon aphasia:

1. Undifferentiated jargon: a disorder
of **language** (2) where the patient uses
phonemically (3) possible words, i.e., the
structure of the words follows the rules
for word-formation in English. However, they do not come out as real words.

2. Phonemic jargon: where the patient
does produce real words but sometimes
substitutes nonwords which are related
phonologically to the target word.

3. Asemantic jargon: where the patient
uses real words in possible syntactic contexts but the sequences produced do not
make sense.

4. Neologistic jargon: when the
patient uses nonwords (unrelated to the
target) placed in possible syntactic structures.

Patients who produce jargon are unaware
they are not communicating satisfac-
torily. Jargon does not contain the
hesitations, **word-finding difficulties**
and self-corrections, etc., found with
other aphasic patients. *See Butterworth
(1984): 61–93.*

L

LAD. **Language Acquisition Device**.

Laddering. See **personal construct
theory**.

Landau-Kleffner Syndrome. A possible
symptom of those children who suffer
from **specific developmental language
disorder**. Such children have severe
problems in **comprehension**, it is not
just delayed. The errors they make are
usually consistent and not found in
normal children of the same age. These
comprehension problems do not only
appear with auditory stimuli but also
with written or signed stimuli. Thus, the
way in which the sentence is presented is
of no matter to them. Their problem in
comprehension could be due to the fact
that they fail to understand the **hierarchy**
(2) of structures used to form the utterances. The **Test for the Reception of
Grammar** has been used with such
children as the hierarchy of structures are
presented in progressively more difficult
subtests. *See Bishop (1982).*

Language acquisition. See **acquisition**
and Appendix B.

Language acquisition device (LAD). A
psycholinguistic theory (2) proposed by
Noam Chomsky (see **Chomskyan
linguistics**: section 2) to explain how
children learn **language** (2). He believes
children's **language acquisition** is an
innate (4) process. Chomsky believes
humans to be born with several areas in
their brains which allow them to develop

various skills. **Language** is one such skill
and it is LAD which sparks off this
hypothetical language area in the child's
mind. *See Steinberg (1982): 94–100.*

Language imitation test. An **assessment** devised by Berry and Mittler in
1981. It assesses the **expressive language** of mentally handicapped children
of 2½–4 years, using six subtests:

1. sound imitation

2. word imitation

3–4. syntactic control (two subtests
are used)

5. word organization control

6. sentence completion.

The child has to repeat words and sentences after the therapist has said them.
The child's production is scored so that a
numerical score can be obtained or a
score which will reveal the child's
strengths and weaknesses in this area of
expressive language. *See test manual.*

**Language Assessment, Remediation and
Screening Procedures (LARSP)**. An
assessment devised by David Crystal in
1976 to discover the extent of the child's
expressive language. It shows how the
child organizes his **language**, the main
stages of **language acquisition** reached
by the child as well as the way the child
interacts with the therapist. There are no
rules for carrying out the **assessment**.
The procedure is to have a 30-minute
taped play session, discussion, picture
description, free conversation or a com-

bination of all these. The tape is analyzed and the grammatical structures summarized in a single profile chart. Any delay in grammatical development of the child can be discovered and the missing structures can be taught to the child. A computerized version of LARSP has been produced by Dorothy Bishop for both the **BBC** and **Apple microcomputers** (8). The **program** (8) has been written so that the child's **utterances** (3) can be analyzed into word, phrase and clause. Each part of the program runs automatically from the other and a summary sheet is given with all the calculations having been done by the computer. *See Crystal (1982): ch. 2; Bishop (1984).*

Language delay. One of the commonest problems among children as they acquire language. The child produces **language** (2) of a much younger child, i.e., below his **chronological age** (4). The therapist uses **assessments** such as **RDLS** or **DLS** to find out how significant is the delay. Language delay can have various causes:
1. **hearing loss** (6)
2. **mental handicap** (1, 4, 5)
3. visual impairment
4. severe **emotional disorders** (4)
5. gross neurological problems
6. **environmental deprivation**.

This differentiates children who suffer from **SDLD** who should not suffer from any of the six causes given above. *See Rutter (1978); 280–281.*

LARSP. Language Assessment, Remediation and Screening Procedure.

Laryngeal nerve palsies. Neuropathologies (5) can produce a paralysis of one or both **vocal cords** (3). Both the **abduction** and the **adduction** (5) of the cords can be affected and it can occur unilaterally or bilaterally. There are several types of laryngeal nerve palsies:
1. Unilateral adductor paralysis, caused by a disorder in the **arytenoids** (5) which bring the vocal cords together;
2. Bilateral adductor paralysis, where both the vocal cords take up a paramedial position, i.e., halfway between being fully closed and fully open in the **larynx** (5);
3. Unilateral abductor paralysis, which produces temporary hoarseness as the affected cord is held in the midline of the **larynx** (5). A **teflon injection** is given to the vocal cord;
4. Bilateral abductor paralysis, perhaps the most serious condition when both cords remain in the midline of the **larynx** (5). The patient must undergo a permanent **tracheostomy** (5) otherwise

the patient will be unable to breath. He may also have to undergo an arytenoidectomy in which the arytenoids are removed;
5. Right recurrent laryngeal palsy, which is caused by a **carcinoma** in the **oesophagus** (both 5), thickening of the pleurae at the apex of the right **lung** (5), anneurysm in the right subclavian artery or pneumonectomy, i.e., part of the lung removed. Symptoms are a very weak, breathy voice. Straining to produce voice will make the patient hoarse.
6. Left recurrent laryngeal palsy, which is commonly caused by an aortic anneurysm with similar symptoms.

Treatment for all these is aimed at **facilitation** of the spontaneous compensatory movement of the non-affected cord, helping to decrease the amount of air waste, improving breathing patterns and discouraging unnecessary effort in using the patient's voice. *See Fawcus (1986).*

Laryngectomy. An operation which may have to be carried out if the patient has a **malignant tumour** in the **larynx** (both 5). Such a tumour can sometimes be removed by **radiotherapy** (5) but, failing this, a laryngectomy may be carried out, resulting in the loss of the mechanism for producing voice. A **stoma** (5) is made in the neck so that the patient can breath. Patients and relatives should be counselled about the loss of voice and advice given as to the type of voice which the patient can be trained to develop post-surgery by using **artificial laryngae** or the three methods for producing **oesophageal voice**. *See Edels (1984).*

Laryngitis. A cause of **dysphonia**. (See **acute laryngitis** and **chronic non-specific laryngitis**).

Laryngofissure. The removal of one vocal cord which allows the other to compensate completely. *See Fawcus (1986): 61, 64.*

Letter-by-letter reader. See **acquired dyslexia**.

Lexical Understanding with Visual and Semantic distractors. Devised by Dorothy Bishop, it is a picture selection test to assess the patient's ability to understand single words presented auditorily or visually and to match them with a choice of pictures. The pictures have been selected so that a number of subtests are formed:
1. target + stimuli unrelated in any way;
2. target + one semantically related and the rest unrelated;

3. target + visually alike and the rest unrelated.

Each subtest is further divided so that the patient has to select one of four or eight pictures. *See test manual.*

Light contacts. See **prolonged speech**.

Linguistic profiles. **Assessment** procedures proposed by David Crystal in 1982. His first profile concerned the syntactic development of the child's language—**LARSP**. His later profiles concerned the child's development of sounds: **profile of phonology**, of prosody: **profile of prosody**, and of semantics: **profile in semantics**. All these profiles provide a means of analyzing the patient's language sample obtained from play sessions, free conversation, picture description or a mixture of these three speaking situations. The results are intended to provide the therapist with a comprehensive view of the child's language development and provide information for a remediation **treatment programme** for any delay in the child's language development. *See Crystal (1982).*

Literal paraphasia. Although the patient's **articulation** (3) is unaffected, syllables can be produced in the wrong order or wrong sounds are placed in a word producing confusion. *See Kahlan and Goodglass (1972);* 8.

Living Language. A remedial package, devised by Locke, for children who suffer from **language delay**, which can be used with children from pre-school age to 16 years of age. It is designed to help children to develop their use of **expressive language** normally. The package is divided into three parts:
1. Before words
2. First words
3. Putting words together.
These three subdivisions match the main stages of the child's normal **language acquisition**. *See handbook.*

Locationist theory. Proposed by the **Boston School** in their discussion of **aphasia**. The theory itself dates from the 1860s when Paul Broca, Karl Wernicke and their contemporaries proposed groups of **language disorder** produced by lesions in certain parts of the **brain** (5) producing specific **aphasic** characteristics. *See Eisenson (1984);* 57–68.

Logopaedics. Another name for **speech and language pathology**.

LUVS. **Lexical Understanding with Visual and Semantic distractors**.

M

Maintenance. See **carryover**.

Maintenance programme. See **Monterey Fluency Programme**.

Makaton. A **sign language** devised by Margaret Walker in 1977 for mentally handicapped adults. It contains about 350 words placed in nine developmental stages, and is the only **sign language** which follows closely the normal **acquisition** of vocabulary. Makaton symbols, pictorial representations of the signs, have been developed so that it will be easier for children to use and understand the original signs. Computer programs have also been written for use with Makaton. Learning Makaton increases the child's **eye contact**, attention, sociability, vocalization and **expressive language**. Far from interfering with the child's acquisition of speech and language, it can encourage it. *See Kiernan et al. (1982): 7–8 and passim.*

Management. Includes all the decisions which a therapist makes concerning the patient, from the taking of a **case history** through to decisions concerning the best method of **assessment**, the **diagnosis**, **treatment programme** and possible prognosis. However, there must be flexibility and willingness to change the treatment programme if the patient does not make a positive response. *See Brown (1981): 13, 14.*

Mean Length of Utterance. A theory used in **language acquisition**, proposed by Brown, which compares the child's age to the length of **utterances** (2) measured in **morphemes** (2). They give a more precise idea of the complexity of the utterance than counting words. He put forward five stages of development of MLU:

STAGE	MLU	AGE
I	1.75	1;6 –2;3
II	2.25	1;9 –2;6
III	2.75	1;11–3;1
IV	3.50	2;2 –3;8
V	4.00	2;3 –4;0

Age is not a good guide to development, as the rate of acquisition is so variable among children. However, MLU is a good guide to grammatical development especially until stage V. With children who have a **language disorder**, the MLU can show up mismatches between the child's order of acquisition and the normal order. Age plus MLU is important as they can give indicators to the size of the delay from which a child is suffering. *See Cruttenden (1979): 49.*

Melodic Intonation Therapy. Devised by Sparks, Helm and Albert (1974), Sparks and Holland (1976) and revised by Sparks (1981), it is a therapeutic technique used **asphasic** patients who have a lesion in the left **cerebral hemisphere** (5) of the **brain** (5). They make the hypothesis that **intonation** (3) and other musical phenomena remain intact in the right **cerebral hemisphere** (5), which can somehow transfer information provided by intonation from it to the left hemisphere. It has been used successfully with patients suffering from **oral apraxia** or with those who are severely **nonfluent** patients but with good **auditory comprehension**. The therapist provides a model of an **utterance** (3) intoned in the form of 3–4 notes emphasizing the **prosodic** (3) pattern. The aim is to allow the patient to produce the utterance with as normal a **prosody** (3) as possible. Common song tunes should not be used as this will encourage the patient to sing the utterance rather than say it with its correct **prosodic** (3) pattern. *See Eisenson (1984); 227–228.*

Mental handicap. 'A condition of arrested or incomplete development of mind which is especially characterised by subnormality of intelligence' (World Health Organisation 1967). The work of **speech therapists** has increased greatly with mentally handicapped patients, especially with those who have **communication disorders**. Children with little or no **expressive language** can be given **alternative communication systems**. The aim of therapy is to give the patients a better quality of life by enabling them better to communicate their everyday needs. *See Clarke and Clarke (1974): passim.*

MH. Mental handicap.

Minnesota Test for the Differential Diagnosis of Aphasia. Devised by Schuell in 1965 and revised in 1973, it is a **formal assessment** to test **aphasic** patients. The five modalities tested are:

1. auditory
2. visual–reading
3. speech/language
4. visuomotor/graphic
5. numeric/arithmetic functions.

The test is American but in some of the subtests British amendments have been made so it is possible to use the test **reliably** (4) in Britain. There are two rating scales to establish the functional ability of the patient and the severity of his condition. The severity scale is from 0 (no impairment) to 4 (severe impairment). The five types of communicative behaviour are rated on a severity scale of 0–6. It has a prognostic potential. *See Eisenson (1984): 130–134.*

MIT. Melodic Intonation Therapy.

Mixed transcortical aphasia. A particular **syndrome** (5) used in the classification of **aphasia**. The symptoms from which patients suffer include nonfluent language, impaired **comprehension** and **naming** while repetition is intact. *See Eisenson (1984): 112, 113.*

MLU. Mean Length of Utterance.

Modification. The therapy programme, devised by the therapist, is aimed at modifying the patient's impaired **communication** ability.

Monterey Fluency Programme. Devised by Ryan and Kirk in 1978 and based on the ideas of those who follow the **speak more fluently** approach to the treatment of **stammerers**, it is a highly structured **behaviour modification** (4) programme following the principles of **operant conditioning** (4). Its main aim is to establish complete **fluency**; an **acceptable stammer** is not regarded as success. It begins with a fluency interview lasting 30 minutes during which the patient is put into as many communication situations as possible. The next stage is a criterion test in which the patient is asked to perform for 5 minutes in three modes—reading, monologue and conversation. If the **stuttering** rate is <0.5 stuttered words per minute in any of the three modes, the patient is put through an establishment programme in a particular mode using two techniques **GILCU** and **DAF**. There is another criterion test, and if the patient stutters >0.5 stuttered words per minute, he progresses to the transfer programme, but if it is <0.5 the patient is recycled through the establishment programme. Following the transfer programme, there is another criterion test with similar requirements as in the last one. If the patient succeeds, he is placed on a maintenance programme which can last several months. If the patient maintains fluency over a period of 22 months, he can be discharged. *See Dalton (1983): 56–58, 91–92.*

Motivation. The therapist must motivate the patient, so that the patient will succeed during therapy. There must be something which sparks the patient into life so that he will respond to therapy.

Motor aphasia. See **Broca's aphasia** and **dyspraxia**.

Motor neuron disease. A progressive disease which produces **dysarthric** elements in the patient's speech. It affects the patient's breathing pattern and **articulation** (3). (See also section 5.) *See Darley et al. (1975): 230–235.*

MTDDA. Minnesota Test for the Differential Diagnosis of Aphasia.

Multiple sclerosis. A progressive disease which produces **dysarthric** elements in the patient's speech, among which are problems with volume, **harsh voice**, and poor **articulation** (3). Therapy follows a similar procedure to that used for other **dysarthric** patients. (See also section 5.) *See Darley et al. (1975): 235–243.*

Munchausen syndrome. A type of

dementia (4 and 5) which can be accompanied by **dysarthria**. In one recent case a patient presented with severely dysarthric speech. Most **consonants** (3) were substituted by **glottal stops** (3) and, although he claimed to suffer from **multiple sclerosis** (5) his speech had none of the characteristics associated with MS. It seemed his speech disorder was **functional** (4). He was put on a **treatment programme** of having his speech taped followed by his listening to it. Having listened to it, he began using normal speech quickly. His response to such therapy was very much like the response of those suffering from **functional dysphonia**. *See Kallen et al. (1986): 377–380.*

Myaesthenia Gravis. A disease which produces particular **dysarthric** elements in the patient's speech, which worsens as the amount of speaking increases. The muscles used for speech become tired, **hypernasality** (5) increases, **articulation** (3) becomes worse, **dysphonia** sets in and the voice becomes quieter. *See Darley et al. (1975): 125–126.*

N

Naming. An assessment procedure as well as part of a **treatment programme** used with aphasic patients. There are four stages used by the patient—picture recognition, retrieval of the **semantic** (2) relation corresponding to the picture, accessing a phonological form using the semantic relation and, finally, producing the spoken word to name the picture. If the patient suffers from an **aphasia** compounded either by **agnosia** or by a difficulty in retrieving **semantics** (2), naming will become difficult. *See Benson (1979): 293–327.*

Nasalization. A disorder found in both children and adults. With children, it is usually caused by inflamed **adenoids** or **tonsils** (both 5) while with adults, the usual cause is a **CVA** or **head injury** (both 5) or progressive disease which produce **dysarthric** elements in the patient's speech. Therapy is aimed at finding a way for the patient to use the **soft palate** (5) which has become immobile through any of these causes.

See Edwards and Watson (1980): ch. 8.

Natural Process Analysis. Devised by Shriberg and Kwiatowski in 1980 to obtain a **sample** of **spontaneous speech** for the therapist to discover which **phonological processes** (3) are used by the child when he produces sound changes. The **elicited** (3) words are transcribed and then coded into **stops, nasals/glides, fricatives/affricates** (3) and the information can be summarized. *See test manual.*

Neologism. See **jargon**.

Neologistic jargon. See **jargon**.

Nonfluent aphasia. A type of **aphasia** found in **Broca's aphasia, global aphasia, transcortical motor aphasia** and **mixed transcortical aphasia** where the patient's language is impeded by **word-finding difficulties** to varying degrees of severity. *See Eisenson (1984): 103–104, 111–113.*

Nonword. See **nonsense word**.

Nonsense word. A word which follows the **phonotactic** (3) structure of a true word in English but it does not have any meaning, e.g., dup, sep, mib, etc.

Northwestern Syntax Screening Test. Devised by Lee in 1969, it is a quick test to find out the **comprehension** and **expressive language** abilities, which can be tested independently, of children between the ages of 3 and 7 years. In the **comprehension** section, two sentences are read out to describe a picture and the child has to point to the correct picture. The picture with the asterisk is always read first to cue-in the child. If an error is made with the first sentence, then both sentences are scored wrong. In the **expressive language** section, there are only two pictures from which to choose. Two sentences are given, the therapist points to the two pictures and the child has to say what the pictures are. In essence, this is a language **imitation** (2 and 4) test based on the idea, children will

repeat only the syntactic utterances in their syntactic repertoire. The same syntactic structures are used in both subtests. *See test manual.*

Nuffield Dyspraxia Programme. A programme designed to help the child with **articulation delay/disorder**. Most of the **consonant** (3) sounds are depicted by pictures of objects which make the sound. For example:

snake	= /s/	lollipop	= /l/
tap	= /t/ (dripping)	pram	= /ʃ/
drum	= /d/	train	= /tʃ/

It is aimed at improving the accuracy and speed of the child's articulatory movements. The therapist works on two or three sounds at a time, includes exercises for oral muscles and varies the **place of articulation** (3). Therapy will be successful if the child can articulate with ease and fluency. There are ten steps to achieve this end. *See programme manual.*

O

Oesophageal voice. When a patient, having undergone a **laryngectomy**, is trained to produce a voice from the top of the **oesophagus** (5). There are two techniques for producing oesophageal voice:

1. Inhalation/insufflation requires patient relaxation so that the appropriate airways are open, i.e., **nose, mouth** (both 5) and pseudo-glottis. The patient has to be able to open the **oral, nasal** (both 5) and pharyngeal cavities adapt his breathing using the **stoma** (5) in his neck.

2. Injection is the commoner technique. Air is pushed down into the **oesophagus** (5), the tongue is positioned firmly against the **hard palate** (5) and the pressure released with the voiced sound /ae:/, sometimes described as 'squeezing a bubble of air gently backwards down into the throat followed by immediately attempting to voice /ae:/'. (Edels, 1983). Adaptations can be made to the stoma with the **Blom-Singer prosthesis** or the **Panje voice button**. *See Edels (1983): 116–119, 119–124.*

Open class word. See **pivot grammar**.

Oral apraxia. See **developmental articulatory apraxia**.

Overextension. At the two word stage of **language acquisition**, overextensions may occur. A child learns a new word, but may only recognize some particular aspect of it, e.g., shape, movement, size, sound, texture and, sometimes, taste, so that every time he sees a similar object, he uses the same name. For example, he may call all four-legged animals with a tail 'dog', as the first time he saw such an animal it was a 'dog'. *See Clark and Clark (1977): 492–494.*

Overgeneralization. Another stage in **language acquisition**; a child learns how to use syntactic functions, e.g., how to make the past tense, make singular nouns into plurals, etc. The regular way to form the past tense is to add [d] or [ed]. However, there are irregular ways of making the past tense, e.g., [went], [gone], [ran], etc. Once the child has learnt how to use the regular form of the past tense, he is likely to overgeneralize its use to irregular forms, e.g., [wented/goed], [ranned/runned], etc. *See Cruttenden (1979): 61–62.*

P

PACE. **Promoting Aphasic's Communicative Effectiveness**.

PACS. **Phonological Assessment of Child Speech**.

PACS Pictures: Language Elicitation. Designed by Grunwell to give a complete description of the child's **sound system** (3) with several examples of each sound. It can also be used as a **screening test** with a sample of 100 words including 41 words from the **EAT**, and can also be used with the actual PACS assessment. *See manual.*

Paget-Gorman Sign System. One of the earliest **sign systems** to have been developed. Designed by Paget in the early 1930s and developed into the 1950s, by which time he and his colleagues had made up a 3000-word sign vocabulary. When Paget died, his work was carried on by Dr Pierre Gorman and Paget's widow. The original signs were revised and the system was called 'A Systematic Sign Language'. In 1971, Lady Paget changed the name to 'The Paget-Gorman Sign System' in recognition of Gorman's help in its development. The **sign system** has one sign corresponding to one word and a sign for each **morphological** (2) ending in English, i.e., plurals, tense endings, etc. The system has 21 standard hand positions and 37 basic signs used in different combinations. The basic signs represent groups of words with a common concept, e.g., time, position, animal life, etc. One hand gives the concept, while the other hand is used to modify the concept to make the required communication clear. *See Kiernan et al (1982): 8–9, 135–136.*

Palilalia. The patient's continual repetition of the end of his own phrases and sentences. It is part of the **communication disorders** suffered by **psychiatric**, e.g., **schizophrenic** patients (4).

Panje Voice Button. It is made of silicone and has two flanges. It is placed in the tracheo-oesophageal wall. The operation is reversible but the patient for whom the voice button is suitable is limited by the diameter of the **stoma** (5), dexterity of the patient and thickness of the tracheo-oesophageal wall. Placement is completed by out-patient surgery and no special instruments are required. The button is self-contained in the tracheo-stoma. *See Edels (1983): 282–286.*

Papillomata. The commonest laryngeal tumours occurring before 6 years of age. They are non-malignant, and can be removed by surgery. Speech therapy may be necessary post-surgery. They can cause **hoarse voice** due to excessive air-waste. Therapy should be aimed at obtaining the best voice level possible. *See Fawcus (1986): 61, 79, 86, 87.*

Paraphasia. An error usually found in the **language** of **aphasic** patients, where they substitute a word, sound or **morpheme** (2) for another in the spoken or written form of **language** (2). This condition is produced in aphasic patients due to the **degeneration** (5) of the **brain** (5) while other people these errors may be caused by **stress** (4), fatigue or lack of attention. In the subtests of the **expressive language** section of the **BDAE**, it is possible to score paraphasic errors. *See Eisenson (1984): 14–16.*

Parental speech. See **baby talk**.

Parkinson's disease. Patients with this disease show three main symptoms—tremor, rigidity, bradykinesia. The final two symptoms affect the muscles which control the speech mechanism. This produces **dysarthric** speech characteristics since the **vocal cords** (3), respiration muscles, and pharyngeal muscles are all affected. There is also a slowing down of lip and tongue movement in speech and a loss of fine movements as in writing. (See also section 5.) *See Darley et al. (1975): 174–195.*

Pausing. See **prolonged speech**.

Peabody Picture Vocabulary Test. A **formal assessment** devised by Dunn for children over 2½ years of age. It has a booklet of 150 pages, each with four pictures. The child has to choose the correct picture from the four at the request of the therapist. *See test manual.*

Perceptions of Stuttering Inventory. A personality inventory used to discover situations in which patients expect to stammer, or produce struggling behaviour and which they try to avoid. It was devised by Wolff in 1967. There are five reasons for carrying out this inventory:

1. to describe what the stammerer does;

2. to give greater understanding of why he **stammers**;

3. to give insight into his emotional states;

4. to give a check on progress;

5. to provide a profile for working out goals and expectations.
See Dalton and Hardcastle (1977).

Perseveration. The persistence of an abnormal response made by a brain-damaged patient even when the stimulus which induced the initial response is removed. It may take the form of continuous repetition or blocking, where the patient makes repeated efforts to make a sound. *See Eisenson (1984): 186–187.*

Personal Construct Theory. A psychological theory proposed by Kelly in 1955. The Centre for Personal Construct Psychology in London organized by Dr Fransella practices PCT. The basis of the theory is put into the form of a fundamental postulate. According to Kelly, this refers to the way in which a person views the world and this depends on how much experience the person has of the world and what that experience has taught him. Human personality does not stand still but is an ongoing process which goes forward from construct to construct. Constructs are always being revised, validated, invalidated, thrown out, added to and so on. It is anticipated that constructs will allow a person to foresee his own behaviour and the reaction of others. 'Yet constructs themselves undergo change. And it is in the transitions from theme to theme that most of life's puzzling problems arise' (Kelly). In therapy, the therapist has to discover how the patient views the world from his experience, i.e., what constructs he uses. If the therapist deems these constructs require revision, then therapy will be given. **Assessment** techniques used in PCT are **repertory grids**, laddering and **self-characterization**. *See Dalton (1983): 112–114, passim.*

PGSS. **Paget-Gorman Sign System**.

Phases of stuttering. A possible course of stuttering (**stammering**) showing how a stutter can become severe. There are four phrases proposed by Bloodstein:
    1. shows mild repetitive stammering which becomes worse in communicative stress;
    2. occurs at school where the disorder becomes chronic and **blocking behaviour** becomes more common;
    3. shows the child is still **blocking** and has secondary symptoms;
    4. is the full-blown pattern of stammering found in adolescents and adults with the ensuing avoidance of speaking situations.
See Dalton and Hardcastle (1977).

Phonemic jargon. See **jargon**.

Phonological Assessment of Child Speech. Devised by Grunwell in 1985, it is an assessment of the child's **sound system** (3) and the means of comparing it to the adult system. There are two types of analysis possible of the data obtained—**contrastive analysis** and/or **phonological processes** (both 3). The aim is to give an exhaustive analysis of the child's speech and a basis on which the therapist can produce a **treatment programme**. *See test manual.*

Phonological delay. This should not be confused with an **articulation delay**. The child can produce the sound but not place it in the correct position in the word. It is a delay because a child may produce /g gi/ for [d gi] at the age of 3½–4 years when he should have stopped doing this between 2 and 3 years of age. *See Grunwell (1982).*

Phonological disorder. A very severe form of **phonological delay** in which the child may have a **sound system** (3) which is abnormal. For example, he may have no **fricatives** (3) in his system except those not used in normal English. Such a system for children of 4–5 years of age or older would be described as a phonological disorder. *See Grunwell (1982).*

Phonological dyslexia. See **acquired dyslexia**.

Phonological Process Analysis. Devised by Weiner in 1979 for use with children between 2 and 5 years to discover the **phonological processes** (3) used in their speech. The child responds to action pictures rather than picture naming, using single words and sentences. These are taped and transcribed so that the process accounting for any sound changes within the words can be identified. *See test manual.*

PICA Porch Index of Communicative Abilities.

PICAC. Porch Index of Communicative Abilities in Children.

Pivot Grammar. A grammatical system proposed in the 1960s by Braine. He found that when children were acquiring language, they produced **sentences** (2) containing repeated words in one position while other words were used less often. The former process was called a pivot word while the latter was an open class word. The system was used to explain the two-word stage in language acquisition. *See Cruttenden (1979): 40–42.*

Pivot word. See **pivot grammar**.

Polyps. Organic growths which can appear in the nasal cavities (see **nose**: 5) and the **vocal cords** (3). They occur on the latter unilaterally; they may be round, vascular, oedemitis and inflammatory. A polyp may produce **hoarse voice**, coughing and perhaps even choking, interfering with the patient's **phonation** (3). Therapy takes the form of **voice rest** and a complete ban on smoking. *See Fawcus (1986)*.

Porch Index of Communicative Abilities. Devised by Porch in 1967, it is a formal **assessment** which has undergone **standardization** (4), to test the language function of **aphasic** patients. Porch changed the aim of **aphasia** testing. He wanted to find out which of the patient's responses could be reliably and objectively quantified. The 16-point scoring system, unique to Porch, is based on four variables:

1. the responsiveness of the patient;
2. the accuracy of the patient;
3. the promptness of response;
4. the efficiency of response, i.e., evidence of motor delay.

Such a test provides the therapist with an extremely detailed performance record for each patient. There are at least 18 test tasks in the form of four verbal tasks, eight gestural tasks and six picture tests. Ten objects are also used and must be presented in a required order. The therapist must attend a 40-hour workshop to become a registered user. Porch does not follow any particular theory of **aphasia** and his approach cannot be placed under any particular classification of aphasia. *See Eisenson (1984): 134–137*.

Porch Index of Communicative Abilities in Children. Devised by Porch in 1971, it is designed for use with children having learning difficulties, requiring special education and suffering from **SDLD**. It has two scales, one for the age group 2–6 years and the other for those of 6–12 years of age. As with **PICA**, Porch was concerned only with the child's **communication**, not necessarily with **linguistic** (2) and **phonological** (3) aspects of the child's language. The basis of this test is the same as for **PICA**, as is the scoring system. *See test manual*.

Portage Checklist in Early Education. A means of finding out the different abilities of children with the **mental ages** (4) of 0–6 years. It is used mainly with those children who will require special education, severely physically handicapped children and those suffering from a severe delay in acquiring various skills. It is designed for use in the home by parents under the supervision of a **speech therapist**, **psychologist** (4) or

district nurse. After analyzing the results, the therapist can give the parents a programme to work on with the child. It assesses motor skills, cognitive skills, language skills, social skills, self-help skills and, for young children, infant stimulation. The language skills are not particularly appropriate for British children, so a new language section has been devised—the Wessex revised portage language checklist. *See Shearer and Shearer (1974)*.

PPVT. **Peabody Picture Vocabulary Scale**.

Preparatory blocks. See **block modification**.

PRISM.   **Profile In Semantics**.

Profile in Semantics. Devised by Crystal (1982) to analyze the child's use of **semantics** (2). It is the most experimental of the profiles as very little research has gone into the acquisition of semantics. The profile is based on the acquisition of **semantics/grammar** and **semantics/lexicon** (2). PRISM-G is a three-page chart which analyzes the relationship between meaning and grammatical elements of a sentence. PRISM-L has a 16-page analysis because of the amount of vocabulary it has to cover. It is possible for one chart to be used without the other but if the two are used together, an in-depth analysis of the child's semantic system can be discovered. *See Crystal (1982): ch. 5*.

Profile of Phonology. Devised by Crystal (1982), it is a means of analyzing the English **sound system** (3) of a child. There is a transcription page plus a separate three-page section on ways of summarizing the data. The therapist takes a language sample of about 100 words but need only transcribe as much of the sample as is necessary to work out the child's phonological problem. First, the sample must be transcribed onto the transcription page, using one line for each word-type. The next step is to fill up the two pages where the **segments** (3) used by the child can be shown within the **syllable** (3) and the phonetic type of segment. Following this, there is the interpretation sections of the profile where the therapist can work out the error realizations in single consonants, single vowels and consonant clusters. All three types of segments are divided into errors of **place** and **manner of articulation** (3). Altogether this profile gives an in-depth analysis of the child's sound system. *See Crystal (1982): ch. 3*.

Profile of Prosody. Devised by Crystal (1982) to analyze the **suprasegmental**

patterns (3) in the child's speech. It comprises a one-page chart on which is put the **pitch, loudness, rate,** and **rhythm** patterns (all 3) of the patient's speech. It is supposed to complement **PROPH.** A large part of the profile is devoted to the child's use of **intonation** (3) since most linguistic errors come from this variable. The **intonation** section is divided into **tone units** and **tones** (3). A summary section is also provided. *See Crystal (1982): ch. 4.*

Prolongation. See **prolonged speech.**

Prolonged Speech. A treatment technique for use with patients who **stammer.** It has five parts:

1. Prolongation which is intended to slow down the rate of articulation and allows the patient to become **fluent.** This process simplifies the movement from one sound to another which is usually difficult for a person who stammers.

2. Flow requires the patient to run the words together, thus reducing the stopping and starting in a stammerer's speech. Flow is normal in fluent speech but it is not so to the stammerer.

3. Light/soft contacts are encouraged between the **articulators** (3) to reduce the tension in the mouth when producing a particular sound.

4. Pausing is encouraged as stammerers hate pauses even when it is a normal characteristic of fluent speech. It is often suggested they purposely take a breath to produce a pause.

5. Slowing down is encouraged to help the stammerer produce what is required in 1–4 above. All these are intended to encourage the feeling of using **fluent** speech which some stammerers have never experienced. *See Dalton (1983): 80–82.*

Promoting Aphasic's Communicative Effectiveness. Devised by Davis in 1980, it is a treatment technique used with aphasic patients. It has been designed to produce more meaningful interaction between the therapist and patient. Speech therapy sessions should resemble everyday face-to-face conversations. PACE is based on four principles:

1. equal participation between therapist and patient;
2. new information is conveyed between therapist and patient;
3. there is a free choice of communicative modalities;
4. the feedback from the therapist sounds more natural.

When PACE is used effectively, the patient enjoys therapy because it is he who is communicating some new information to the therapist or another member of a group. *See Eisenson (1984): 228–229.*

PROP. **Profile on Prosody.**

PROPH. **Profile on Phonology.**

PSI. **Perceptions of Stuttering Inventory.**

Puberphonia. The persistent falsetto voice in a male who has developed a **larynx** (5) of normal adult proportions. It may be caused by psychological factors such as **neuroses** (4), a denial of adolescence, or a defect in the **vocal cords** (3) resulting from habitual misuse. A patient will possibly require both speech therapy for exercises to lower the voice and psychological intervention. *See Fawcus (1986).*

Pull-out. See **Block modification.**

Pure agraphia. A type of **pure aphasia** identified by the **Boston School.** Patients have problems with writing and spelling. *See Goodglass and Kaplan (1972).*

Pure alexia. A type of **pure aphasia** identified by the **Boston School.** Patients have problems with reading, although objects presented to the patient may still be recognized without difficulty. *See Goodglass and Kaplan (1972).*

Pure aphasia. A type of **aphasia** identified by the **Boston School.** Only one language modality is affected while all other allied modalities remain intact. *See Goodglass and Kaplan (1972).*

Pure word deafness. A type of **pure aphasia** identified by the **Boston School.** The patient's **auditory comprehension** fails although his **expressive language** remains unimpaired, as do his reading and writing. *See Goodglass and Kaplan (1972).*

R

Rapid Screening Test. This test forms part of the **assessment** techniques used in the **Derbyshire Language Scheme.** It is a quick way to find out the child's level of **comprehension**. After analyzing the scores, if it is found the child requires further assessment for **comprehension**, the therapist will administer the **detailed test of comprehension**. *See DLS manual.*

Raven's Progressive Matrices. Devised by Raven during 1938–1977 to assess the patient's non-verbal **comprehension**. The black and white version was published in 1938 for use with adults. The coloured version was published in 1949 for use with young children and adults suffering from **mental handicap** (also 4 and 5) or other impairment. The advanced version was published in 1962 for use with those patients of above-average ability between the ages of 11 years and adulthood. The patient is presented with a progression of abstract patterns and in each one a part is missing. The missing piece is reproduced at the bottom of the page with other distractor pieces. The patient has to choose the correct piece. Although designed for use by **psychologists** (4), it can be used successfully in **speech therapy**. Patients who suffer from a **CVA** or **head injury** in the right **cerebral hemisphere** (all 5) will probably have difficulty carrying out the matrices successfully, so it can provide limited evidence of where the lesion site is in the **brain** (5). It can be used as an alternative to the **Token Test**. *See test manual.*

RDLS. Reynell Developmental Language Scales.

Rebus. Devised by Woodcock in 1969 in the form of The Rebus Reading Series for use with mildly mentally handicapped children. A rebus is any pictorial representation which acts as a symbol to represent either individual words, phrases or sentences. It has been developed to help those children with **language delay** or **language disorder** and who may or may not be mentally handicapped. The **Makaton Symbols** are of a rebus type. A computer program of rebus symbols has been produced for **BBC microcomputers** (8). *See Kiernan et al. (1982): 12, 44–45.*

Receptive aphasia. A description of the condition suffered by a patient whose **comprehension** (how language is 'received') has been affected by a **CVA** or **head injury** (5). Its characteristics are similar to **Wernicke's aphasia**. It is the opposite of **Expressive aphasia**. The degree of severity of receptive aphasia can be determined by administering the **Token Test**, the **Reporter's Test** or the

Test for the Reception of Grammar as well as the comprehension subtests of the **Boston Diagnostic Examination of Aphasia**. *See Eisenson (1984): 19–20, 212–215.*

Repertory Grids. An **assessment** technique used in **personal construct theory**. If this theory is to be used effectively, the therapist has to find out how the patient views the world and so the patient's constructs have to be elicited. The patient is provided with role constructs, e.g., someone you look up to, someone you dislike, someone who is successful, someone who is not successful, etc., and gives the names or initials of the people he thinks about. The patient, however, should include himself in the role constructs, e.g., me as I am now, me as I would like to be. Once the people have been identified, three are chosen and the patient is asked the following question: 'Can you tell me in what important way two of these people are alike and thereby different from the third'. By doing this constructs are found. The constructs which the patient gives can be divided into subordinate constructs, e.g., helpful/unhelpful, and superordinate constructs which the therapist finds out using the technique of laddering. In laddering, the therapist takes one of the bipolar constructs, e.g., helpful/unhelpful, and asks the patient questions to obtain a more in-depth analysis of the patient's personality. The therapist would stop the interview when it was thought a superordinate level had been reached. Both types of constructs (both subordinate and superordinate) are placed on a grid by the patient using a rating system of 1–9. Correlations between the ratings of the constructs are worked out by a computer. *See Dalton (1983); 120–128.*

Reporter's Test. Devised by De Renzi and Ferrari in 1978, it is a **formal assessment** derived from the **Token Test**. Its full name is 'The Reporter's Test: A Sensitive Test to Detect Expressive Disturbances in Aphasics'. Although the **Token Test** is essentially a test for **auditory comprehension**, the same stimuli are used to test the patient's **expressive** abilities. So that the patient becomes accustomed to the material, the 36-item **Short Token Test** is given first. Following this, the 20 tokens are laid out in the prescribed manner. The patient is told to pretend there is someone else next to him, with board placed between the patient and this 'other person'. The therapist indicates by pointing to a token which the patient has to tell the 'other person' to point to. If the tokens are all the same size, only the colour need be distinguished but if they are of different size and different colour, then both size and colour have to be differentiated. The scoring is based on whether the report would or would not allow a correct reproduction by the 'other person'. One point is scored if the response is correct after the first presentation and half a point after the second presentation. The correct names and adjectives must be used. If the patient scores 18–35 or less, he may be diagnosed as suffering from **expressive aphasia**. The weighting score scale measures the patient's verbal output. If he scores 54 or less, he will be diagnosed as suffering from **aphasia**. *See Eisenson (1984): 146.*

Renfrew Test Battery. Devised by Catherine Renfrew in the late 1960s to assess various modalities of the child's communication. There are five tests:
1. **Bus Story**—a test of continuous speech;
2. **Action Picture Test**—a test of expressive language;
3. **Word-Finding Vocabulary Scale** —a test of the use of words;
4. **Auditory Discrimination Screening Test**—a test of **auditory comprehension**;
5. **Articulation Attainment Test**—a test for the use of English consonants.

Revised Token Test. See **Token Test**.

Reynell Developmental Language Scales. Devised by Reynell in 1966 (revised 1977), it is a **formal, standard-** ized assessment (4) to assess the child's development of **expressive language** and **comprehension**. Although it can be used with children between the ages of 1 and 7 years, it is most sensitive for assessing children between the ages of 1 and 5 years. It can also be used with physically and visually handicapped children as well as with those who have a **hearing loss** (6). The **raw score** (4) on the **comprehension** and **expressive language** tests can be converted to a **standard score** (4) from which an **age equivalent score** (4) can be derived. *See test manual.*

Right recurrent laryngeal nerve palsy. See **laryngeal nerve palsies**.

Robertson Dysarthria Profile. Devised by Robertson in 1982, it is a **formal assessment** to assess the severity of a patient's **dysarthria**. It concentrates on testing the patient's **articulation**, **rate**, **prosody** and other **suprasegmental** phenomena (all 3). There are seven sub-tests:
1. **voice** (3)
2. **respiration** (5)
3. **facial musculature** (5)
4. **diadochokinesis**
5. reflexes
6. **articulation** (3)
7. **rate, prosody, intelligibility** (3).

Unlike the **Frenchay Dysarthria Assessment**, the profile will not produce an aetiology but, instead, will give an in-depth analysis of the problems facing a sufferer from **dysarthria**. *See Robertson et al. (1986): passim.*

RST. **Rapid Screening Test**.

S

S–24. An **assessment** to find out the attitudes of a stammerer to his **communication**. The patient has to give a true/false answer to 24 statements, e.g., I often ask questions in groups. The higher the score, the more the patient's **communication** is disordered. It is a shortened form of Erikson's (1969) S-scale. *See Dalton (1983): 33–36, 37–38.*

Sample. A sample of **language** (2) is often taken by a therapist for analysis as the patient's language in a free situation is often more natural than in an **assessment** situation. It is an **informal assessment**. It can be analyzed by any of the **linguis-** tic profiles devised by Crystal or just by the therapist's **intuition** (2) and experience. *See Crystal (1980); 29.*

Schizophrenia. Some patients who suffer from schizophrenia (4) have associated problems in **communication**. These include:
1. **perseveration** in syntax
2. repetition of words and syllables
3. disruption of semantic memory
4. clang associations
5. **echolalia** and **palilalia**
6. echopraxia
7. mutism
8. poverty of thought and speech

9. concreteness
10. **phonation** (3)
11. **flattening of affect** (4).

A therapist will have to take a **sample of communication** for analysis and plan a **treatment programme** accordingly. *See Davison and Neale (1982).*

Schuell. In 1964, Schuell and her colleagues put forward a classification of **aphasia** comprising five major categories and two minor syndromes:

1. simple aphasia—a breakdown in the symbolic use of language, resulting in a reduction in language, **word-finding difficulties** with syntactic problems plus phonemic or **jargon** errors depending on the severity of the aphasia and **comprehension** errors depending on the length and complexity of what is said;

2. aphasia with visual involvement;

3. aphasia with persistent **dysfluency**;

4. aphasia with scattered findings—the patient has some functional language, not severely handicapped but may suffer from **dysarthria**;

5. aphasia with sensory motor involvement—mild aphasia with persisting dysarthria.

The two minor syndromes are:

a) aphasia with intermittent auditory imperception;

b) irreversible aphasia syndrome—there is a sudden loss in all modalities and loss of all functional language. Schuell believed aphasia was not modality-specific but affected all language modalities. Following this theory, she devised the **MTDDA**. *See Eisenson (1984); 111.*

Screening. The carrying out of quick tests to discover the disorders from which the patient is suffering. Screening tests are **formal assessments** used for such a purpose. *See Brown (1981); 154.*

Screening test. See **screening**.

SDLD. **Specific Developmental Language Disorder**.

Self-characterization. An **assessment** technique used in **personal contact therapy**. It is part of the 'credulous' approach. The patient is asked to describe himself in a non-threatening way as if his best friend were making the description. The request is presented to the patient thus: 'I want you to write a character sketch of (patient's name), just as if he were the principal character in a play. Write it as it might be written by a friend who knew him very intimately and very sympathetically, perhaps better than anyone ever really could know him. Be sure to write it in the third person. For example, start out by writing, "(patient's name)"'. *See Dalton (1983): 120–128.*

Sensory aphasia. An **aphasic** disorder identified by Luria in 1966, producing problems of **auditory comprehension** which affects **comprehension** of what is said to the patient and disorders in **expressive language** with similar problems in writing. *See Eisenson (1984): 107, 108.*

Sentence Comprehension Test. Devised by Wheldall, Hobsbaum and Mittler in 1977, it is a **formal assessment** to test the child's understanding of grammatical constructions. Having discovered the type of sentence which the child finds difficult to understand, systematic remediation can begin. It can only be used with a limited group of children, of 3–5½ years for normal children and for children with comparable **age equivalent scores** (4) in their language development. It comprises 15 subtests, each of which tests a different grammatical structure. Each subtest has four items from which the child has to choose the correct one. A subtest is passed if he scores three or more in each subtest which produces a profile score out of 60 items from which the therapist decides whether or not therapy is required. A new edition of the test was published in 1986. Five subtests have been left out as well as several items (there are only ten subtests now) and the pictures have been redrawn. *See Wheldall (1987): 72–86.*

Serial speech. The type of **language** (2) which is automatic to most people, e.g., ability to produce the days of the week, months of the year, counting and the alphabet. With some **aphasic** patients, it may be the only language which remains intact. Thus, in many **assessments** for testing **aphasia**, subtests for serial speech are included. *See Eisenson (1984): 9, 195.*

Short Token Test. See **Token Test**

Sigh/yawn technique. See **yawn/sigh technique**.

Sign languages. A type of **alternative communication system** taught to patients who have difficulty in using **expressive language**. A sign language has its own grammar and has similar characteristics to any oral language, i.e., historical change, puns, humour, arbitrariness, etc. Such languages include **British Sign Language** and American Sign Language for use with patients suffering from a **hearing loss** (6). *See Kiernan et al. (1982): passim.*

Sign systems. A type of **alternative communication system** taught to patients who have difficulty in using **expressive language**. A sign system is not a language in itself although it has signs to represent words and **morphological** (2) endings in a spoken language. It does not have its own grammar, but follows the spoken language as there is one sign per word, e.g., **PGSS, Makaton**. *See Kiernan et al. (1982): passim.*

Signed English. This **sign system** is designed to represent oral English. The hand signs are used with speech which makes the message to be communicated very clear. It can be used with children suffering from a **hearing loss** (6). Each sign has a semantic relationship with each English word. There are about 2500 sign words and 14 sign markers for plurals, past tenses, etc. *See Bornstein and Hamilton (1982).*

Simple aphasia. A reduction in the ability to use all **language** (2) modalities without signs of **dyspraxia** or **dysarthria**. It is a term defined by Schuell in the 1960s. *See Eisenson (1984): 111.*

Singer's nodes/nodules. See **vocal nodules**.

Spastic dysarthria. A type of dysarthria caused by a disorder in the **upper motor neurones**(5). The muscles used for breathing and moving the **articulators** (3) become stiff, move very slowly and can become quite weak. The patient's speech is slow and requires much effort to produce. *See Darley et al. (1975): 134–148.*

Speak more fluently. A technique of remediation for patients who **stammer**. Little attention is paid to any underlying psychological causes. It concentrates on removing the **stammer** and making the patient totally **fluent**. Therapists using this theory aim for total **fluency**—an **acceptable stammer** is regarded as failure. The **Monterey Fluency Programme** is based on this theory as is **prolonged speech**. *See Dalton(1983): 76–77, 78–92.*

Speaker's nodes/nodules. See **vocal nodules**.

Specific Developmental Language Disorder. A disorder affecting children. The causes are dissimilar to those which produce **language delay**. The child will suffer from one of the following:

1. a **phonological delay** during the child's early years;
2. a grammatical problem in **expressive language**;
3. a high non-verbal IQ and a low verbal IQ;
4. disorder of **prosody** (3) and rhythm (see **prosody**, [3]);
5. limited symbolic play;
6. visual sequential memory is superior to auditory sequential memory;
7. degree of frustration from producing a language performance below his intellectual level.

If a child is to be diagnosed as suffering from SDLD, he may or may not present with some of these causes:

1. **developmental articulatory, verbal** or **constructional dyspraxia**;
2. minor neurological problems;
3. **comprehension** involvement;
4. **Landau-Kleffner Syndrome**;
5. **dyslexia or dysgraphia**.

This **differential diagnosis** can only be made by a speech therapist. SDLD must be differentiated from **language delay**. *See Wyke (1978).*

Speech pathology. Another name for **speech therapy**, commonly used in the US.

Speech pathologist. Another name for a **speech therapist**, commonly used in the US.

Speech therapist. The person who assesses, diagnosis and treats people who present speech and language disorders.

Speech therapy. The profession in the UK which is responsible for assessing, diagnosing and treating the speech and language disorders suffered by both children and adults. *See Crystal (1984): 24–28.*

Spontaneous recovery. Spontaneous recovery occurs without the intervention of professional skills such as **physiotherapy** (5) or **speech therapy**. It can occur during the first 2–6 months following the onset of a disorder such as **aphasia**, but some such patients do not have spontaneous recovery. *See Eisenson (1984): 162–164, 168–169.*

Spontaneous speech. A description of **language** (2) which a patient uses every day. It is opposed to language produced in picture description, object naming or when reading. A language **assessment** whether it is **formal** or **informal** should always include a subtest from which an analysis can be made of the patient's spontaneous speech.

Stammer. A disorder which is characterized by an impediment in a person's speech. Although efforts have been made in the past to distinguish stammering from **stuttering**, they are now regarded as being synonymous. The cause of stammering has not yet been fully established. There have been many hypotheses; however, there are just as many patients who force researchers to withdraw or modify these hypotheses. It is very dangerous to state that there is only one cause. Some have hypothesized that a stammer is caused by **organic** (5) factors such as minimal brain damage, a forced change in **cerebral dominance** (5), heredity or IQ level. Others have proposed a **neurotic** (4) cause in the form of an emotional predisposition, a **compulsion neurosis** (4) or a **conversion neurosis** (4) while others believe it to be part of some learnt behaviour. This last cause makes use of **classical** and **operant conditioning** (4). Avoidance reaction is another psychological cause which has been proposed. However, nowadays it is argued that stammering could be caused by a combination of some of these factors. Treatment techniques fall into two main theories—**speak more fluently** and **stammer more fluently**. *See Dalton (1983): passim.*

Stammer more fluently. A treatment theory used with those who suffer from a **stammer**. It takes into account the underlying psychological symptoms from which the stammerer may suffer. One of the major therapeutic techniques used is Van Riper's **block modification**. This can also be called stutter more fluently. *See Dalton (1983): 93–99.*

Stutter. See **stammer**.

Stuttering stages. A description, proposed by Van Riper, of the sequences found in stammerers as their **dysfluency** progresses:

1. primary stuttering stage—easy repetitions of words, syllables, of a sentence without emotion or stress;

2. secondary stuttering stage—the patient becomes more conscious of his **dysfluency** and begins to anticipate the situations in which he will **stammer**;

3. transitional stuttering stage—this occurs between the primary and secondary stages in which emotions accompany the easy repetitions of the primary stuttering stage. *See Dalton and Hardcastle (1976).*

Stuttering theories. See **Stammer**.

Supplementary Communication Systems. See **Alternative Communication Systems**.

Surface dyslexia. See **acquired dyslexia**.

Symbolic Play Test. Devised by Lowe and Costello in 1976, it is a formal, **standardized assessment** (4) to test a child's symbolic play. It can be used with very young children of 1–3 years of age. The development of concept formation and symbolization is a prerequisite for the successful development of language. This is a test of the child's non-verbal playing in a structured situation. It is a short test, taking 10–15 minutes, and does not rely on the child's ability to use **comprehension** or **expressive language**. The scoring system is based on the number of meaningful responses and connections the child makes among the objects presented to him. *See test manual.*

T

Teacher's nodes/nodules. See **vocal nodules**.

Teflon injection. An injection of teflon into the paralyzed vocal cord, to enlarge it so that the other will be able to cross over and compensate for the loss of the paralyzed cord. It is used in the treatment of **laryngeal nerve palsies** of the vocal cord. *See Fawcus (1986): 144.*

Temporary tracheostomy. See **tracheostomy**.

Test for Auditory Comprehension of Language. Devised by Carrow-Woolfolk in 1976 (revised 1985), it is an **assessment**, which has undergone **standardization** (4), to test the child's auditory understanding of semantic relations (see **semantics**, section 2) **syntax**, **morphology** (both 2) and complex sentence structures. The therapist presents the child with a series of pages, each with three line-drawings; the child has to point to the correct drawing when given the auditory stimulus. The original test (1976) was used with children of 3–6 years, but the revised edition can be used with children of 3–10 years. The therapist obtains a **raw score** (4) which can be converted into a **standard score** (4), **age equivalent scores** (4) or **percentile rankings** (4). *See test manual.*

Test for Reception of Grammar. Devised by Bishop in 1984, it is a formal, **standardized assessment** (4) to test children's **comprehension**. However, it can be used to gain a more in-depth analysis of an aphasic patient's **comprehension**, although it has not been standardized for this population. Eighty grammatical constructions are tested, each being represented by four colour pictures. The patient has to point to the correct picture after receiving the auditory stimulus. Each construction is tested in blocks of four stimuli. To be credited with a 'pass', all four stimuli must be answered correctly. *See test manual.*

Testing. See **assessments**.

Token Test. Devised by DeRenzi and Vignolo in 1962, it is a **formal assessment** to test the **auditory comprehension** of aphasic patients. The test material comprises 20 tokens which differ in size, shape and colour. The original Token Test was divided into five parts, the first four used auditory commands of increasing length while the fifth contained commands of increasing grammatical complexity. The Revised Token Test devised by McNeil and Prescott in 1978 looks at auditory comprehension from a linguistic viewpoint. The Short Token Test was devised by Spellacy and Spreen in 1969. *See Johns (1978): 115–116, 120, 121.*

Tracheostomy. An operation carried out on the **trachea** (5) to restore a good breathing pattern to those who have undergone breathing problems. An opening is made into the trachea. There are two types of tracheostomy:
1. temporary tracheostomy.
2. permanent tracheostomy.

In (1) an opening is made in the anterior wall and is kept open by a tracheostomy tube. This operation is required if there is an obstruction in the upper airway, long-term artificial ventilation or if the lower airway needs protection due to an incompetent **larynx** (5). The last two disorders require a tracheostomy tube with an inflatable cuff. When the disorder has improved, the tube can be removed and the hole produced by the operation will close. In (2) the trachea is stitched to the edge of the **stoma** (5) in the neck skin after a **laryngectomy** has taken place. When the **stoma** is established, there is no need to wear a tube. As this operation takes place after **laryngectomy**, a new way of producing voice has to be given to the patient. *See Fawcus (1986): 53, 59, 60, 66, 77.*

Transcortical motor aphasia. A major form of **aphasia** described by the **Boston School**. It produces **nonfluency**; repetition and **comprehension** remain relatively intact while **naming**, reading out loud and writing are impaired. It is the perisylvian areas of the **brain** (5) where the lesion occurs. *See Goodglass and Kaplan (1972).*

Transcortical sensory aphasia. A major form of **aphasia** described by the **Boston School**. It produces **fluent** language full of **neologisms** and **paraphasias**, impaired **comprehension**, **naming**, reading **comprehension** and writing while reading out loud is affected to varying degrees and repetition remains unaffected. *See Goodglass and Kaplan (1972).*

Transfer programme. See **Monterey Fluency Programme**.

Treatment programme. The plan of therapy produced by a therapist for each individual patient based on the **assessments** which have been carried out. This may include some published therapy techniques, e.g., **PACE**, **MIT** etc., **alternative communication systems**, or therapy devised by the therapist and based on experience of what has worked best with patients suffering from similar disorders, although the same therapeutic techniques cannot necessarily be used in exactly the same way even with patients suffering from the same disorder.

TROG. **Test for Reception of Grammar**.

U

Underextension. The opposite of **overextension**. During the stage of underextension, the child uses one word for a particular object. So, the child may use the word 'teddy' for his own teddy but not for the teddies belonging to his siblings or friends. However, at a later stage, he could call other teddies by their correct name and overextend its use to objects which may have similar characteristics to a teddy bear, but is another object. *See Clark and Clark (1977): 491.*

Understanding. See **comprehension**.
Undifferentiated jargon. See **jargon**.
Unilateral abductor paralysis. See **laryngeal nerve palsies**.
Unilateral adductor paralysis. See **laryngeal nerve palsies**.
Unintelligible speech. The speech of a child who suffers from a very severe form of **articulation/phonological delay** or **disorder** . With such children, the parents can usually make out what the child says but for the therapist and other people it is almost impossible.

V

Verbal dyspraxia. See **developmental articulatory apraxia**.
Verbal paraphasia. Occurs in **aphasia**. A word is mistakenly used as a substitute for another. See *Goodglass and Kaplan (1972): 8*.
Vocal abuse. See **vocal nodules**.
Vocal misuse. See **vocal nodules**.
Vocal nodules. Growths which appear on the posterior third of the **vocal cords** (3). They can occur in both children and adults through **vocal abuse** or **vocal misuse**. This takes the form of excessive shouting, abnormal **phonation** patterns (3) and excessive strain. on the vocal cords. The nodules increase in size because of the persistent rubbing together of the strained cords (cf. the appearance of corns on the feet after wearing ill-fitting shoes). The nodules prevent the cords from closing normally during phonation and **harsh voice** and **hoarse voice** characteristics appear. Treatment takes the form of relaxation exercises and voice exercises which prevent the cords from coming together harshly, e.g., **yawn/sigh technique**. **Vocal rest**, where the patient has to use the voice as little as possible may also be necessary. This could result in the patient having to take time off work. *See Fawcus (1986)*.
Voice disorders. See **dysphonia**.
Voice rest. See **vocal nodules**. *See Fawcus (1986): 167, 181, 205*.

W

Wernicke's aphasia. A type of **aphasia** described by Wernicke in 1874 and one of the major types of **aphasia** identified by the **Boston School**. It occurs in **Wernicke's area** (5) which allows people to process **comprehension**. Its other main characteristic is **fluent** language with an almost normal syntactic construction but completely meaningless. Repetition, **naming**, reading out aloud, reading comprehension and writing are all severely impaired. *See Goodglass and Kaplan (1972)*.
Whurr Screening Test. Devised by Whurr in 1974, it is a **screening test** to test the severity of the **aphasia** suffered by patients. It covers all modalities of **communication** in both **comprehension** and **expressive language**. Each subtest is scored out of five. The scores are plotted onto a profile chart to give an instant idea of the patient's difficulties and where treatment can begin. In some cases, it may be necessary to use a more formal, **standardized** (4) **assessment** such as the **BDAE** or **MTDDA**. *See test manual*.
Word-finding difficulty. See **anomia**.
Word-Finding Difficulty Scale. Devised by Renfrew in 1968 (revised 1977), it tests the child's correct usage of vocabulary. Children between the ages of 3 and 8 years can be tested. The therapist must treat all dialectal pronunciations as being correct and ignore articulation errors as long as the therapist is sure the child is aiming at the correct word. If the child fails the word or says 'don't know', but later says the correct word, the child should be passed for that word. The total of words correctly used by the child is made, as is the total of 'don't know'

responses. If the score is in the lower middle range of scores for his age, this may be due to **mental handicap** (also 4 and 5), **environmental deprivation** or specific **word-finding difficulty**. *See test manual*.

Word-form dyslexia. See **acquired dyslexia**.

Wug. An imaginary bird-like creature used in an experiment to find out the order of **acquisition** of grammatical **morphemes** (2). In 1958, Berko proposed that if a child had learnt the correct morphological affixes for **nouns** and **verbs** (2), then he could put the correct ending on imaginary words. She drew pictures of imaginary creatures, of which the 'wug' was one. The picture was presented to the child, who was told what it was, and then another picture of the same creature was presented. To the first one, the child was told 'This is a wug, here is another, we have two ...', and usually the child replied correctly: 'wugs'. *See Clark and Clark (1977): 344.*

Y

Yawn/sigh approach. A technique advocated by Boone in 1977 for treating **vocal nodules**. It is a means of producing voice without the hard **glottal attack** (3) which produces the nodules. The patient is advised to relax completely, take in a deep breath and let it out as a sigh or yawn and during this stage begin to **phonate** (3), thus preventing the **vocal cords** (3) from clashing together harshly. *See Fawcus (1986): 182.*

REFERENCES

Benson, D. F. (1979). 'Neurologic Correlates of Anomia'. In Whitaker, H. A. and Whitaker, H. (Eds) (1979), *Studies in Neurolinguistics*, vol. 4. Academic Press.

Bishop, D. V. M. (1979). 'Comprehension in Developmental Language Disorders'. In *Developmental Medical Child Neurology* (1979) 21; 25–238.

Bishop, D. V. M. (1982). 'Comprehension of Spoken, Written and Signed Sentences in Childhood Language Disorders'. In *Journal of Child Psychology & Psychiatry* (1982) 23;1 1–20.

Bishop, D. V. M. (1984). 'Automated LARSP: Computer-assisted Grammatical Analysis'. In *British Journal of Disorders of Communication* 19;1 (1984) 78–87.

Bornstein, H. and Hamilton, L. B. (1978). 'Signed English'. In *Ways and Means* (1978). Globe Education.

Brown, B. B. (1981). *Speech Therapy: Principles and Practice*. Churchill Livingstone.

Butterworth, B. (1984). 'Jargon Aphasia: Processes and Strategies'. In Newman, S. K. and Epstein, R. (Eds) (1985), *Current Perspectives in Dysphasia*. Churchill Livingstone.

Canning, B. A. and Rose, M. F. (1974). 'Clinical Measurements of the Speed of Tongue and Lip Movements in British Children with Normal Speech'. In *British Journal of Disorders of Communication*, 9;1 (1974) 45–50.

Clark, H. H. and Clark E. V. (1977). *Psychology and Language: An Introduction to Psycholinguistics*. Harcourt Brace Jovanovich.

Clarke, A. M. and Clarke, A. D. B. (1974). *Readings in Mental Deficiency: The Changing Outlook*. Methuen.

Code, C. and Muller, D. J. (1983). *Aphasia Therapy*. Edward Arnold.

Cruttenden, A. (1970). 'A Phonetic Study in Babbling'. In *British Journal of Disorders of Communication*, 5 (1970) 110–117.

Cruttenden, A. (1979). *Language in Infancy and Childhood*. Manchester University Press.

Crystal, D. (1976). *The Grammatical Analysis of Language Disability*. Edward Arnold.

Crystal, D. (1980). *Introduction to Language Pathology*. Edward Arnold.

Crystal, D. (1982). *Profiling Linguistic Disability*. Edward Arnold.

Crystal, D. (1984). *Linguistic Encounters with Language Handicap*. Blackwell.

Dalton, P. (1983). *Approaches to the Treatment of Stuttering*. Croom Helm.
Dalton, P. and Hardcastle, W. J. (1977). *Disorders of Fluency and their Effect on Communication*. Edward Arnold.
Darley, F. L., Aranson, A. E. and Brown, J. R. (1975). *Motor Speech Disorders*. W. B. Saunders.
Davison, G. C. and Neale, J. M. (1982) *Abnormal Psychology: An Experimental Clinical Approach*. John Wiley.
Denes, R. B. and Pinson, E. N. (1973) *The Speech Chain: The Physics and Biology of Spoken Language*. Anchor.
Edels, Y. (Ed.) (1984). *Laryngectomy: Diagnosis to Rehabilitation*. Croom Helm.
Edwards, M. and Watson, A. C. H. (Eds) (1980). *Advances in the Management of Cleft Palate*. Churchill Livingstone.
Eisenson, J. (1984). *Adult Aphasia*. Prentice Hall.
Ellis, A. W. (1984). *Reading, Writing and Dyslexia: A Cognitive Analysis*. Erlbaum IBD.
Fawcus, M. (1979). 'Group Therapy: A Learning Situation'. In Code, C. and Muller, D. J. (1983). *Adult Aphasia*. Edward Arnold.
Fawcus, M. (Ed.) (1986). *Voice Disorders and their Management*. Croom Helm.
Fransella, F. (1972). *Personal Change and Reconstruction*. Prentice Hall.
Garvey, C. (1977). *Play: The Developing Child*. Fontana/Open Books.
Gillham, W. (1979). *The First Words Language Programme*. George Allen and Unwin and Beaconsfield Publishers.
Goodglass, H. and Kaplan, E. (1972). *The Assessment of Aphasia and Related Disorders*. Lea and Febiger.
Green, G. (1984). 'Communication in Therapy: some of the procedures and issues involved'. In *British Journal of Disorders of Communication* 19, (1984) 35–46.
Grunwell, P. (1982). *Clinical Phonology*. Croom Helm.
Hornsby, B (1984). *Overcoming Dyslexia*. Dunitz.
Jennings, A. A. (1984). 'What Do I Get for My Money?' In *CST Bulletin*, February 1984 No. 382.
Johns, D. F. (1978). *Clinical Management of Neurogenic Communicative Disorders*. Little, Brown and Company.
Kallen, D., Marshall, R. C. and Casey, D. E. (1986). 'Atypical Dysarthria in Munchausen Syndrome'. In *British Journal of Disorders of Communication* (1986), 21; 3 377–380.
Kiernan, C., Reid, B. and Jones, L., (1982). *Signs and Symbols*. Heinemann Educational Books.
Obler, L. K. and Albert, M. L. (1981) 'Language in the Elderly Aphasic and in the Dementing Patient'. In Sarno, M. T. (ed.) (1981) *Acquired Aphasia*. Academic Press.
Pracy, R., Siegler, J. and Stell, P. M. (1974) *A Short Textbook of Ear, Nose and Throat*. Hodder and Stoughton.
Riedel, K. (1981) 'Auditory Comprehension in Aphasia'. In Sarno, M. T. (ed.) *Acquired Aphasia*. Academic Press.
Robertson, S. J. and Thomson, F. (1986). *Working with Dysarthrics*. Winslow Press.
Rutter, M. (1975). *Helping Troubled Children*. Penguin.
Sarno, M. T. (1969). *The Functional Communication Profile: Manual of Directions in Rehabilitation Monograph 42*. New York: Institute of Rehabilitation Medicine.
Satz, P. and Bullard-Bates, C. (1981). 'Acquired Aphasia in Children'. In Sarno. M. T. (ed.) (1981) *Acquired Aphasia*. Academic Press.
Shearer, D. E. and Shearer, M. S. (1974). *The Portage Project*. A paper presented at the Conference on Early Intervention for High Risk Infants and Young Children, N. Carolina.
Silverman, E. H. and Elfant, I. L. (1979). 'An Evaluation and Treatment Program for the Adult'. In *American Journal of Occupational Therapy* (1979) 33;6 382–392.
Steinberg, D. D. (1982). *Psycholinguistics: Language, Mind and World*. Longman.
Stuart-Smith, V. G. and Wilks, V. (1979). 'Gesture Program: A Supplement to Verbal Communication for Severely Aphasic Individuals'. In *Australian Journal of Human Communications Disorders* (1979) 7;2.
Travis, L. E. (ed.) (1971). *Handbook of Speech Pathology and Audiology*. New York, Appleton-Century-Crofts.
Wheldall, K. (1987). 'Assessing Young Children's Receptive Language Development: a revised edition of the Sentence Comprehension Test'. In *Child Language Teaching and Therapy* 3;1 (1987) 72–85.
World Health Organization (1967). *Manual of the International Statistical Classification of Diseases, Injuries and Causes of Death*, 1965 Revision. Geneva.
Wyke, M. (Ed.) (1978). *Developmental Dysphasia*. Academic Press.

Section 2

Linguistics

A

Accent. The regional variations of **pronunciation** (3) of a **language**. These variations are caused by differences in the length and type of **vowel** and **consonant** (both 3) used as well as in the phonological and **prosodic** patterns (3) produced by the speaker. It is differentiated from a **dialect**. *See Wells (1982):* 1–4.

Acceptability. An acceptable **utterance** made by one native speaker to another native speaker is one which follows the syntactic rules of that language. A linguist compares utterances with these rules and opinions from other native speakers to decide what is and what is not acceptable. Speech therapists need to know about acceptability as it will affect the content of **treatment programmes** (1) for both adults and children who suffer from **speech** and **language disorders** (all 1). *See Lyons (1968): 137–139.*

Action + Locative. See **semantics**.

Action + Object. See **semantics**.

Active voice. A syntactical construction in which an action is carried out by the actor on the patient.

(1) The dog bit the man.

In (1), 'the dog' is the actor while 'the man' is the patient. The active voice is opposed to the **passive voice**. The change in the structure of the sentence is accounted for by a rule of **transformational grammar**. *See Clark and Clark (1977): 93–94.*

Adjective. See **constituent analysis**.

Adnominal. Part of a syntactical construction which adds meaning to a noun. This may take the form of an **adjective**, **prepositional phrase**, or **possessive** (see **genitive**) marker used within the **noun phrase**. *See Lyons (1968): 295–298.*

Adverb. See **constituent analysis**.

Affix. A general term used in **morphology** to refer to the adding of **morphemes** (prefixes and suffixes) to the **base form**. *See Allerton (1979): 213–215.*

Agent. See **case**.

Agent + Action. See **semantics**.

Agent + Object. See **semantics**.

Allomorph. See **morphology**.

Anacoluthon. An **utterance** during which the speaker changes from one syntactic structure to another without finishing the first. *See Huddleston (1976): 2.*

Anaphora. A process which allows for one linguistic unit to refer back to one previously given. This may be by **deixis** or by the use of a reflective pronoun. For example:

(1) He wrote that himself.

'Himself' is the reflexive pronoun which produces an anaphoric referent. *See Huddleston (1976): 251–255.*

Animate. See **semantics**.

Applied linguistics. A part of linguistics in which **theoretical linguistics** is put into practice. This happens in speech therapy when forming **treatment programmes** (1) for patients who have **speech** and **language disorders** (1). The therapist should know about **syntax**, **semantics**, **pragmatics**, **sociolinguistics** and **psycholinguistics** to improve their treatment. *See Pit Corder (1973): passim.*

Apposition. A linguistic phenomenon which makes an implicit coordination of **constituents** without the use of a conjunction or pronoun:

(1) Fred, the baker's son, went home.

(1a) Fred who is the baker's son went home.

(1) demonstrates apposition while (1a) shows an explicit coordination with a pronoun. *See Allerton (1979): 127–129.*

Appropriateness. The type of **language** people use differs from situation to situation. For example, informal language occurs at parties and among friends while much greater care is taken in the type of language used, for example, in religious services. The native speaker knows which variety of English to use by **intuition**. This can occur in both spoken and written forms of English. *See Crystal and Davy (1969): 4–7.*

Aspect. Some forms of a verb refer to static situations while other forms may refer to continuous events.

(1) The boy went to the factory.

(2) The boy is going to the factory.

(3) The boy was going to the factory.

(1) is often referred to as a state while (2) and (3) are referred to as action or progressive aspect of verbs. *See Huddleston (1976): 65–66.*

Assign. See **constituent analysis**.

Asterisk. An asterisk which precedes a sentence in linguistic discussion means the sentence is unacceptable.

Aux. **Auxiliary** (See **verb phrase**).

Auxiliary. *See* **verb phrase**.

B

Base form. The part of a word which remains after all the **affixes** have been removed. For example, the base form of 'quickly' is 'quick' after the affix '-ly' has been removed. It is used in the **morphological** study of word formation. *See Matthews (1974): 39.*

Base word. See **base form**.

Bound form. See **bound morpheme**.

Bound morpheme. A **morpheme** which is a type of inflection in which the **affix** is already part of the word, and thus, it cannot exist on its own. For example, the affix 'de-' in a word like 'devise' is a bound morpheme as 'de-' cannot be used as a separate meaningful unit. It is opposed to **free morpheme**. *See Matthews (1974): 38, 160.*

Bracketing. A type of syntactic analysis used in **constituent analysis**. Each sentence which is either spoken or written can be analyzed into several component parts. (see example below).

Another way of showing the constituent analysis of the sentence is by **branching** in a **tree diagram**. In **phrase structure grammar**, brackets are used within the generated rules to show the units are optional to the structure. *See Lyons (1981): 119–124.*

Branching. The way of constructing a **hierarchical structure** formed by a **tree diagram**. It uses rules found in **constituent analysis**. *See Lyons (1981): 119–124.*

(	(	(THE)	(DOG)	)	(CHASED)	(	(THE)	(CAT)	)	)	)
		det	N NP		V		det	N NP VP S			

C

Case. The main component of Fillmore's **case grammar**. The categories of case which are used in an underlying structure are:

agent—the instigator, usually animate, of an action, e.g., ALLAN switched on the television;

instrument—an inanimate object which causes a state to change, e.g., Mary opened the door WITH HER KEY;

dative—an animate being affected by the meaning of the verb, e.g., Harry gave a bicycle TO JANE;

factive—the result of the effect of the verb, e.g., The artist painted A PICTURE;

locative—the place where the effect of the verb takes place, e.g., Jack put the letters IN THE LETTER BOX;

objective—a noun, the meaning of which is represented by the meaning of the verb itself, e.g., the boy put THE CUP on the shelf. *See Steinberg (1982): 54–58.*

Case grammar. This grammatical theory was proposed by Charles Fillmore in 1968. He described an underlying **semantic** system to **language** which is represented in some languages by a particular word order and inflection endings, e.g., endings to verbs in French: je donne, tu donnes, il donne, nous donnons, vous donnez, ils donnent. Other **cases**

represent agent, instrument, locative, beneficiary, object, etc. *See Steinberg (1982): 54–58.*

Case relations. See **case** and **case grammar**.

Category. Grammatical units which make up a phrase or sentence. In general, a **noun**, **verb**, **pronoun**, etc., can all be described as being different categories in a sentence. However, it would be more exact to state that a category refers to the actual properties of the noun, verb, pronoun, etc. in the sentence. Thus, category can refer to: 1. number and gender of nouns; 2. tense, voice and aspect of the verb. These are just two examples of **grammatical categories**. *See Lyons (1968): 270–274; Huddleston (1976): 40–41.*

Catenative. Verb forms which link one verb to an infinitive, e.g., he WANTED TO GO home.

Central embedding. See **embedding**.

Chomskyan linguistics. Since 1957 to the present day, Noam Chomsky has led a revolution in modern linguistics. Although his theories received wide acclaim when proposed, in recent years they have lost support. In 1957 he published his first major linguistic work, *Syntactic Structures*, in which he proposed three theories of grammar. The first two theories, he concluded, were not sufficient to deal with the structures found in English syntax, while the third, he believed, solved many of the difficulties in English. The three theories were **finite state grammar**, **phrase structure grammar** and **transformational grammar**. As the years progressed, he has developed transformational grammar to cope with the criticisms levelled at it. *See Lepschy (1982): ch. 8.*

Clause. Part of a **sentence** used mainly in **traditional grammar**. The clause fits into other traditional terms used to describe the structure of an utterance, e.g., sentence, phrase, word, morpheme. A clause can be either a main clause or a subordinate clause:

(1) The cat which was black sat on the mat.

In (1), 'the cat sat on the mat' is the main clause while 'which is black' is the subordinate clause. Some grammatical theories analyze clauses in more detail by finding out the function of the subordinate clause, e.g., object, adverbial, etc. The **linguistic profiles** (1) examine the units of the clause such as 'subject, verb, object' (SVO), 'subject, verb, complement, object' (SVCO), etc. In **gen-erative grammar**, the clause is referred to as an **embedded** sentence which is acted on by various **transformations**. *See Allerton (1979): 183–184, 204–205.*

Clinical linguistics. A particular application of **theoretical linguistics** to the treatment of patients with **speech** and **language disorders** (1). The areas of linguistics used in clinical linguistics include **psycholinguistics**, **neurolinguistics** and **language acquisition**. *See Crystal (1981): passim.*

Cocktail party phenomenon. The process of picking out what is said in a crowded room, setting aside all other linguistic information. This is known as selective listening. *See Clark and Clark (1977): 216.*

Competence. The person's ability to use **language**. It refers to the person's knowledge of vocabulary and syntactic rules, so that the person can produce **acceptable** language. It has an opposite in **performance**. Both terms were proposed by Chomsky. He believed too much emphasis had been placed on explaining performance but more explanation was required for the underlying competence of the speaker. Both terms are similar to de **Saussure's** terms of **langue** and **parole** respectively. *See Lyons (1968): 51.*

Complement. An obligatory clause in the structure of the sentence. A complement exists in the formation of a **copula** while it also exists to mark the time and place of an action, e.g., the play is in the theatre; on Monday, John was at work. In the two examples, '*the play is' and '*on Monday, John was' do not exist in English. Thus, the complement is obligatory. *See Lyons (1968): 345–349.*

Concord. The grammatical phenomenon in which the subject of a sentence agrees with the verb.

(1) The dog runs away.
(2) The dogs run away.
(3) The dog ran away.
(4) The dogs ran away.

In (1), the singular form of the verb has the **affix** (-s) while in (2), the plural form of the verb is the **base form** of 'run'. However, in the past tense, there are no verb markers to show concord either with the singular or plural nouns. *See Lyons (1968): 239–247.*

Constituent. See **constituent analysis**.

Constituent analysis. A type of analysis of both spoken and written utterances. There are certain rules which have to be followed for the analysis to be successful:

S → NP + VP

NP → (det) + (adj) + N
VP → (NP) + V
PrepP → Prep + NP

These rules follow a hierarchical structure of a sentence structure. The symbols and abbreviations represent the constituents:

S = **sentence**
NP = **noun phrase**
VP = **verb phrase**
PrepP = **prepositional phrase**
det = **determiner**
adj = **adjective**
N = **noun**
V = **verb**
→ = 'consists of'
( ) = units in brackets are optional.

The first rule means a 'sentence consists of a noun phrase plus a verb phrase'. These rules are often called **rewrite rules** as the left-hand side of the formula can be rewritten in the formula on the right-hand side. There may be only one symbol on the left while any number of symbols can appear on the right. The ' + ' symbol is an ordering symbol, so in the first rule, the verb phrase can only follow a noun phrase to make up a sentence. Constituent analysis results in a **generative grammar** as the rules can generate their own grammar, thus a sentence which is generated from these rules is ipso facto grammatical. This type of analysis can be shown graphically by use of **branching** in the form of a **tree diagram** or by **bracketing**. *See Brown and Miller (1980): ch. 6.*

Copula. A sentence constructed by the verb 'to be' and a **complement**, e.g., the men are tall. *See Lyons (1968): 322.*

Count nouns. Nouns which can show number, e.g., one boy—two boys; one book—two books, etc, as opposed to **mass noun**. *See Palmer (1976): 124.*

D

Dative. See **case**.

Declarative sentence. A sentence which makes a statement about an action or state of the subject, e.g., the man went into town. It is opposed to a sentence which contains a question.

Deep structure. See **case grammar**; **transformational grammar**.

Deictic. See **deixis**.

Deixis. A linguistic process for referring to the position of an object or person or a time for carrying out some activity. Deictic words include: here/there, now/then, I/you, etc. Deixis can also be used to express an order of events, e.g., the former, the latter, etc. *See Lyons (1968): 275–281.*

Demonstrative + entity. See **semantics**.

Demonstrative pronouns. **Deictic** words which refer the person reading or hearing them to a specific object or person near to or removed from the speaker. Such pronouns include 'this/that'. *See Lyons (1968): 278–279.*

Dependent clause. See **subordinate clause**.

Derived sentence. See **transformational grammar**.

Descriptive linguistics. A form of linguistic study which uses **theoretical linguistics** to describe systems and units in language. All languages are reduced to similar descriptions, so they can be described in comparison to each other and each specific language can be described on its own. Such a study is often called the **synchronic** study of language. *See Palmer (1978): 25, passim.*

Det. Determiner.

Determiner. See **constituent analysis**; **noun phrase**.

Developmental linguistics. The use of **theoretical linguistics** to describe the stages used by the child during **language acquisition** (1). Such an explanation has to take into account the child's background, cognitive skills, medical history, etc. Thus, **psychology** (4) and **medicine** (5) are also involved in an explanation of the development of language. *See Clark and Clark (1977): chs 8–10.*

Diachronic. One of the types of **descriptive linguistics** proposed by **de Saussure** in 1913. It studies the historical changes in language over time. Thus, a linguist studying language using this procedure would look at the progression of English from Old English to Middle English to Modern English. This is also known as historical linguistics. It is opposed to **synchronic linguistics**. *See Lyons (1968): 45–48.*

Dialect. Language variations used in particular areas of a country. It may include a lot of regular usage but it will also contain elements which are peculiar to that region of the country. For example, in Aberdeenshire (Scotland), all **Wh-words** begin with /f/. Thus, 'what' becomes /fit/. Other differences in this dialect include the words for 'boy' and 'girl' which become 'loon' and 'quine' respectively. Dialect is different from **accent** although the two phenomena may occur together. *See Lyons (1968): 34–35.*

Diglossia. A phenomenon found in **sociolinguistics** and proposed by Ferguson. It refers to a situation in which two varieties of a language co-occur. However, both variations have different uses. Usually, one is used for formal occasions while the other is used for speaking to friends, in the media and group discussions. *See Trudgill (1974): 117ff.*

Direct object. In **constituent analysis**, this is often referred to as NP2 as it is the second **noun phrase** in an **utterance**. It is the noun which stands directly after the verb. In **case grammar**, it is referred to as the **objective case** (see **case**).

Discourse analysis. An analysis of conversational patterns. A normal conversation is the logical sequencing of **utterances** so that what person *A* says will be followed by an utterance from person *B* which will either be an answer or extension of what person *A* has said:

A: Good morning!
B: Good morning, how are you?
A: I am very well and you?
B: Fine, thank you. What are you going to do?
A: I'm going to Spain tomorrow!

Discourse is also known as **pragmatics** as it shows the way in which language is used meaningfully. If discourse breaks down, the child or adult may require a period of **speech therapy** (1). Such a **discourse disorder** or **pragmatic disorder** has been produced by McTear:

A: which race would you like to be in?
C: I like to be in X at the Sports Day.
A: in X?
C: yes
A: what do you mean?
C: I mean something
A: is there a Sports Day in X?
C: there is not, there is a Sports Day in Y (Note: Y = name of school)
A: then what's X got to do with it?
C: nothing
A: then why did you mention it?
C: indeed I did mention it
A: why did you mention it?
C: I don't know

See McTear (1985).

Domination. See **tree diagram**.

E

Ellipsis. A process in language whereby the speaker can omit part of the utterance. However, the missing part can be understood from the context of the utterance, e.g., 'What have you been doing?', 'WATCHING TELEVISION'. The elliptic sentence is in upper case and in its full form should read, 'I have been watching the television.' Many children use this form of sentence and so during assessment of **language delay** or **language disorder**, (both 1) it is uncertain if the child is using ellipsis and knows the omitted part or has produced an elliptic sentence because he has not reached the stage of **language acquisition** (1) to be able to produce complex sentences. *See Lyons (1968): 174–175.*

Embedding. **Clauses** which are placed within an **utterance**, are embedded sentences. The basic sentence is known as the **matrix** sentence. If a relative clause is placed within the utterance it is central embedding.

(1) The car which he bought was a Rolls Royce.

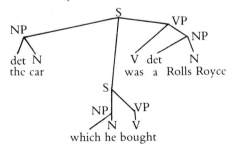

See Huddleston (1976): ch. 7.
Entity + attributive. See **semantics**.
Entity + locative. See **semantics**.

Exophora.   A reference to a person who is not in the immediate proximity to the speaker. Thus, an exophoric reference occurs when the speaker refers to a person in the distance or someone he has just met. *See Allerton (1979): 267–268.*

Exophoric.   See **Exophora**.

Expansion.   The **rewrite rules** used in constituent analysis are also known as expansion rules since one constituent is expanded into a description of several constituents, e.g.,   NP → (det) + (adj) + N.

Extended standard theory.   See **transformational grammar**.

F

Felicity conditions.   Four ways of making indirect requests proposed by Austin (1962) and Searle (1969, 1975):

   1. Ability—'you can make the cake'
   2. Desire—'I want you to make a cake'
   3. Future action—'you are going to make me a cake'
   4. Reason—'you should make me a cake because I'm hungry'.

By making indirect requests in this manner, the speaker adheres to the normal social conventions of conversation. *See Clark and Clark (1977): 125–126.*

Field.   A group of words which can be classified semantically together. Within each field there are different classes, e.g., in the field of 'Mammals' there are classes of 'dog', 'lion', 'tiger', etc. It is also possible to compare fields between languages. For example, in English in the field of 'wall' there are two classes 'wall' and 'parapet', while in French there are five 'mur' (outside wall), 'paroi' (inside wall), 'remparts' (parapet), 'muraille' (high wall) and 'enceinte' (defensive wall). It is often possible to make a **hierarchical structure** of the items in a field. *See Palmer (1976): 71–73.*

Finite state grammar.   A syntactic theory discussed by Noam Chomsky in *Syntactic Structures* in 1957. It provides an analysis of a sentence starting at a point X following a path which diverges for a choice of verb and uses a loop for any adjective encountered. Such an analysis looks like:

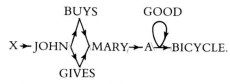

However, difficulties of using such an analysis are encountered when **verb particles** are used.

(1) John put the curtains up.

This type of grammar cannot account for the particle 'up' and so this syntactic theory is not sufficient to account for English sentences. *See Lyons (1977): ch. 5.*

Form.   In its most general sense, form refers to the structures which occur in linguistic structures, e.g., sentence, clause, word, morpheme, etc. It can be contrasted to the **function** of these structures. *See Lyons (1968): 196, passim.*

Function.   The role which each word has in a sentence. These roles depend usually on the **syntactic rules** used to form sentences. It can be contrasted to **form**. *See Lyons (1968): 194, passim.*

Function words.   Non-information-carrying words put into a sentence to account for the syntactic structure of a sentence. Such words include articles, prepositions and conjunctions. *See Palmer (1976): 114–115.*

Functor.   See **function word**.

G

Generative grammar.   A grammar which is produced by rules which generate syntactic structures. Chomsky discussed three types of generative grammar: **finite state grammar, phrase structure grammar** and **transformational grammar**. The rules which generate any of these grammars can be completely understood by the speaker without any pre-knowledge of the language. *See Huddleston (1976):* 16–17, *172–175.*

Generative semantics. A theory proposed to generate grammatical structures in opposition to Chomsky's **extended standard theory**. In the 1970s, linguists such as Lakoff, Postal and Ross proposed that **deep structure** is **semantic** rather than **syntactic** as suggested by Chomsky. The semantic level is sufficient to produce **acceptable** (see **acceptability**) sentences in **surface structure**. Thus, there is little emphasis on syntactic rules providing such acceptable sentences. *See Huddleston (1976): 257–260.*

Genitive. The **form** of a **word** which represents possession. There are two forms for possession, the use of **affix**'s and the use of the word 'of'.
  (1) The man's car is brown.
  (2) The car of the man is brown.
See Lyons (1968): 290ff.

H

Hesitation. Periods of silence or **filled pauses** (3) while the speaker either thinks of more information or reiterates and amplifies what has been said. Certain positions have been found in an **utterance** where hesitation occurs. These are at certain appropriate places in the grammar of the utterance, after other **constituents** and at the beginning of an utterance before the speaker has decided finally how to continue the utterance. *See Clark and Clark (1977): 267–268.*

Hierarchy. A structure which starts with one unit at the top and branches linking it to lower units. A **tree diagram** is a type of hierarchical structure. The units above other units are called superordinate terms while the units below other units in the structure are subordinate terms. In the tree diagram, 'sentence' is superordinate to **noun phrase** and **verb phrase**, while **determiner, adjective, noun** are subordinate to **noun phrase**. *See Lyons (1968): 164ff.*

Historical linguistics. See **diachronic linguistics**.

Homonymic clash. See **homonymy**.

Homonymy. A phenomenon in **semantic** theory in which one word can have the same spelling, pronounced the same way but have two different meanings. Such words are homonyms. In the word 'bear', there are the two meanings of 'animal' and 'carry'. It occurs in both speech and writing. If there is an ambiguity between homonyms, there is a homonymic clash. *See Palmer (1976): 65–71.*

Homophony. A phenomenon in **semantic** theory in which two words pronounced the same have a different meaning. Such words are called homophones. Such examples are 'sun/son', 'boy/buoy', etc. This is a form of **homonymy**. *See Palmer (1976): 68.*

I

IA. Item and arrangement (see **morphology**).

Icon. There are arbitrary conventions in semiotics. However, icons are fixed **signs** such as onomatopoeic words 'splash', 'crack' and 'bang'. The **forms** of these words can never change. *See Robins (1971): ch. 1.*

Idiolect. A type of **dialect** which is particular to each person. There are regional dialects which have different variations of the spoken language. However, there are also differences of dialect between people in that they have particular ways of producing **utterances** which are different from other people. Idiolect continues to develop after the child has fully acquired language as the child picks up modifications from the language of his family and friends. Haas (1963) writes of a child's

phonological disorder (1) as being 'a language of his own' or 'idiolect'. In an important passage, he writes why speech therapists need to know about idiolect: 'It would seem that speech therapy stands to gain in efficiency, if, to a greater extent than has been usual, it could take account of the underlying and interfering "idiolect" of the treated child' (Haas, W., 1963; 246). *See Trudgill (1974): 37.*

Idiom. A phrase which has an unchangeable structure with a particular meaning. Some idioms in English occur in different languages, usually French or Latin, e.g., de rigueur, in media res. Other idioms are of the form 'it's raining cats and dogs'. *See Lyons (1968): 177.*

Ill-formed. A description of badly constructed phrases or sentences. Thus, when a non-syntactical sentence is written or spoken, it is said to be ill-formed. It is found in a discussion of **generative grammar**. If a sentence cannot be generated by the rules of a grammar, it is ill-formed. It is opposed to well-formed. *See Huddleston (1976): 12–15.*

Imitation. A process which has been proposed to explain the child's language acquisition by imitating the sounds, words and sentences used by adults in his immediate environment. However, after much experimenting some doubt has been placed on such a theory of lan-guage acquisition (1). Imitation is one of the therapeutic techniques used by speech therapists. *See Clark and Clark (1977): 344–335.*

Inflection. See **morphology**.

Insertion. See **transformational grammar**.

Intuition. Beliefs used by non-linguists as to the **acceptability** or otherwise of a speaker's **utterance**. The linguist analyzes language from a theoretical point of view while the native speaker (non-linguist) examines language from what sounds correct in syntactic constructions or interrelations of meanings. *See Lyons (1968): 154.*

IP. **Item and process**.

Irregular. The **form** of words, phrases and sentences which do not follow the normal rules for these constructions. A very common example can be found in the use of plurals in English. The **allomorphs** used to show plurality in English are /s/, /z/ and /Iz/, e.g., dogs, trees, buses, while there are irregular plural forms in such plurals as 'mice', 'children', 'oxen'. *See Matthews (1974).*

Item. The different **forms** used in a language.

Item and arrangement. See **morphology**.

Item and process. See **morphology**.

J

Juncture. The **phonetic** (3) or syntactic boundaries between **words**, **phrases** and **sentences**. These boundaries are often marked by silence although they can also be marked by changes in the **intonation** and **stress** patterns (3). *See Clark and Clark (1977): 267.*

L

Label. The names given to **constituents** in a **constituent analysis** when represented by a **tree diagram** or by **bracketing**. This occurs in **generative grammar**. *See Lyons (1968): 217.*

Language. A system of linguistic units, which, when put in the correct order provide spoken or written utterances. This is the **performance** or **parole** aspect of language. The underlying knowledge of a language is often referred to as the native speaker's **competence** or **langue**. **Dialects** are regional variations of an established language while an **idiolect** is a personal variation of language. *See Lyons (1968): ch. 1.*

Langue. The grammatical system which each person has in his or her mind after having learned the **language**. It was proposed by de **Saussure** and is opposed to **parole**. *See Lyons (1968); 51–52.*

Learnability. The supposed ease with which children acquire any language when given the chance.

Linguistic competence. See **competence**.

Linguistic performance. See **performance**.

Linguistic variation. See **accent, dialect, idiolect**.

M

Mass noun. A noun which cannot be counted. An example of such a noun is 'butter' as '*one butter', '*two butter' cannot occur. *See Palmer (1976): 124–125.*

Matrix sentence. The sentence which exists before **embedding** takes place or after the embedded sentences have been removed.
(1) The car which the man bought was a Rolls Royce.
In (1), the matrix sentence is 'the car was a Rolls Royce' while the embedded sentence is 'which the man bought'. *See Allerton (1979): 192–193.*

Morph. See **morphology**.

Morpheme. See **morphology**.

Morphology. The study in linguistics which states rules for the formation of the number, tense, voice and **aspect** affixes. For example, in English, the verb 'play' has three **forms** 'play, plays, played' showing the different tense affixes. These affixes are called morphemes—the smallest meaningful unit in any **language**. The realizations of morphemes, e.g., /s/, /z/, /Iz/ for the plural morpheme, are called allomorphs. Each individual unit, i.e., each of the allomorphs in the last example, is called a morph. There are two types of morpheme:
1. A bound morpheme is an affix which can be attached to a word to represent number and tense, etc;
2. A free morpheme is a whole word which stands on its own without affixes. An example of both of these types of morpheme is the word: 'anti-dis-establish-ment-arian-ism'. The bound

morphemes are 'anti, dis, ment, arian, ism' while 'establish' is the free morpheme. Item and arrangement is a model in the study of morphology. It examines word structure and syntactic structures which follow particular, logical sequences in a linear way:
(1) The men played cricket.
The example in (1) is analyzed in the form:
   det + MAN + plural
   + PLAY + past + CRICKET.
Difficulties for explaining some morphological phenomena occur, such as 'mice' in the form 'MOUSE + pl'. Item and process was proposed to take account of the problems found in the **IA** model. A process is a derivational procedure which accounts for the form 'mice' as a vowel change from 'mouse'. Word and paradigm is a morphological model which takes the root of a word and fits it into a paradigm. The resulting words and structures are formed by rules such as the verb declensions which appear in Latin, e.g., amo, amas, amat, amamus, amatis, amant. *See Matthews (1974): chs 4, 5, 226–227.*

Morphophonemics. See **morphophonology**.

Morphophonology. A theory in **morphology** in which the linguist attempts to provide rules for which **affix** or allomorph is placed at the end of the **base form**. For example, in the plural **form** of /busIz/, there has to be an /I/ separating the two consonants at the end of the word. *See Matthews (1974): 198ff.*

N

Negation. The process of denial of the whole or part of an **utterance**. It is represented by the negative units 'no, n't, not'. Negative **affixes** can also be used such as 'un-' and 'non-'. *See Huddleston (1976): 77–80, 85–87.*

Neurolinguistics. The study of neurological programming for the production of language and attempts to work out why there is some breakdown in language or articulation. Research has come from **clinical linguistics**, to try to establish reasons for language breakdown in **aphasia, stammering, dysarthria**, etc. (all 1) and hypotheses can be found to show how the **brain** (5) can organize language. *See Clark and Clark (1977): ch. 6.*

Node. See **tree diagram**.

Noun. In **traditional grammar**, a noun was said to be the name of a person, place or object. However, this definition was not precise enough for modern linguists, who preferred to think of nouns as units onto which **affixes** can be placed, units which have a syntactic function, e.g., object, subject, etc., and units which can only be placed in particular positions in the sentence. *See Lyons (1968): passim.*

Noun phrase. A noun phrase is a **constituent** in **generative grammar** and is generated by a **noun** on its own plus either a **determiner** or an **adjective** or both although neither is obligatory. However, there must be a noun. *See Lyons (1968): 213–215.*

Number. A syntactic **category** which represents plurality in **nouns** and **pronouns**. The markers for plurality are the allomorphs (see **morphology**) /s/, /z/, /ɪz/. In pronouns, plurality is shown by a change in the form of the pronoun, e.g., he/they. *See Lyons (1968): 243ff.*

O

Object. A **noun** which is not the subject of a sentence. In syntactic analysis, it can be referred to as the second **noun phrase** (NP2). It is the noun against which the action of the verb is carried out. For example, John gives a BICYCLE to Mary. *See Lyons (1968): 148.*

Objective. See **case**.

P

Paradigm. A **base form** of a word from which other **forms** are made by the addition of **affixes**. *See Matthews (1974): 154ff.*

Paradigmatic. Relationships between units between sentences. They refer to subgroups of linguistic units, the subgroups being **determiners, adjectives, nouns**, etc. For example:

DET	N.	V.	PREP	DET	N.
His	mouse	lay	in	the	cage
That	dog	barked	from	his	kennel
My	friend	sat	on	the	seat

The sentence analyzed in this way is seen as a number of slots. Each slot can only be filled once by one of the units. A sentence such as:

DET	N.	V.	PREP	DET	N.
my	the	book	is	on	the	table

is unacceptable as there are two units in the determiner slot. The opposite analysis is **syntagmatic**. *See Lyons (1968): 70–80.*

Parole. The act of using the internalized **langue** which everyone has in their mind. It was proposed as a linguistic description by de **Saussure** in 1913. *See Lyons (1968): 51–52.*

Passive voice. A syntactical construction which traditional grammarians would describe as an action carried out by the patient on the actor. However, modern linguists describe the passive as a change of syntactic structure by adding the appropriate part of the verb 'to be' and exchanging NP1 to the position of NP2 and NP2 taking the position of NP1. Chomsky proposed a **passive trans-formation**. The **deep structure** was the **active** sentence and the **surface struc-ture**, after the transformation has taken place, is the passive sentence. *See Lyons (1968): 257ff.*

Performance. The use of the speaker's **competence** in producing **utterances**. It is opposed to **competence**. Both have been proposed by Chomsky in his book, *Aspects of the Theory of Syntax* (1965). *See Lyons (1968): 51.*

Performative. Specific **speech acts** per-formed by the speaker. Austen believed every speech act was used for a particular reason. These reasons can be given in the following sentences:

(1) I hereby name this ship H.M.S. Fortress.
(2) (the bank) promise to pay the bearer on demand... (on British pound notes).
(3) I apologize for the delay in this reply.
(4) I congratulate you on your recent success.

All the verbs used in (1)–(4) and other verbs which can be used in a similar way e.g., advise, order, thank, announce, etc., are performative verbs. Huddleston (1976) writes: 'A performative verb identifies a particular kind of speech act that can be performed by virtue of utter-ing a sentence containing the verb...' (Huddleston, 1976; 134). *See Clark and Clark (1977): 26–27.*

Phrase. See **constituent analysis**.

Phrase structure grammar. A gram-matical model discussed by Chomsky in *Syntactic Structures* in 1957. The basis of the model is a **constituent analysis** using **rewrite rules**. However, Chomsky did not believe it was strong enough to explain the structure of all sentences in the **language** nor could it explain Chomsky's belief in the **innateness** (4) of the child's language development. *See Huddleston (1976): ch. 3.*

Pragmatics. The analysis of conversation by studying **speech acts**, e.g., **perform-atives**, **felicity conditions**, etc., See *Van Dijk (1980).*

Preposition. A **constituent** (see **constit-uent analysis**) which is used to precede a **noun phrase**, **nouns** or **pronouns**. It can function as a marker for possession, destination, direction, etc. while syntac-tically it has a particular place in an **utterance**. *See Lyons (1968): 302ff.*

Prepositional phrase. A phrase found in **constituent analysis** which can be expanded into a **preposition** plus a **noun phrase**, e.g., the man went INTO THE SHOPS. *See Huddleston (1976): 232–233.*

Pronoun. A set of **words** which can be used to replace **nouns** or **noun phrases**. There are several types of pronoun:

1. Personal pronoun—I, you, he, etc.;
2. Reflexive pronoun—myself, your-self, himself, herself, etc.;
3. Possessive pronoun—mine, yours, his, etc.;
4. Demonstrative pronoun—this, that;
5. Indefinite pronoun—anyone, any-body, etc.;
6. Relative pronouns—who, which, whom, etc.

These pronouns are usually discussed in other areas of linguistics and will be found under sections such as **deixis** (4), **embedding** (6), **anaphora** (2). *See Lyons (1968): 275, 283.*

Psycholinguistics. A subdivision of linguistics in which **theoretical linguis-tics** come together with psychological theories to show the behaviour of child-ren during the **acquisition** (1) of lan-guage, how people are going to decide on what they are going to say, how they will produce it and how the listener under-stands it. *See Clark and Clark (1977): chs. 5–10.*

R

Reference. See **referent**.

Referent. A process found in philosoph-ical linguistics. A referent describes what a linguistic unit refers to in the outside world. For example, the word 'book' refers to the object 'book'. However, not all linguistic units have obvious referents, e.g., the, a, and, is, etc., while some linguistic units can be expressed differently but with similar meaning by using synonymy. *See Lyons (1981): 168–170.*

Reflexive pronoun. See **pronoun.**

Relative pronoun. See **pronoun.**

Reversal. A phenomenon used in **psycholinguistics**. Traditionally, such problems are referred to as Spoonerisms or metathesis. A very famous example is one of the many found by William Spooner himself: 'You have hissed all my mystery lectures' for 'You have missed all my history lessons.' The phonemes /m/ and /h/ have been reversed in the mistaken **utterance**. *See Clark and Clark (1977): 274.*

Rewrite rules. See **constituent analysis**.

S

Saussure. Ferdinand de Saussure is said to be the founding father of modern linguistics. His theories on the study of linguistics were written in his *Cours de Linguistique Generale* in 1913. In fact, this work was written posthumously from his student's notes and other notes made by Saussure himself. He moved linguistics from the study of **language** through time, i.e., **diachronic linguistics**, to the study of language at the present time, i.e., **synchronic linguistics**. He introduced the distinction between '**langue**' and '**parole**'. He viewed language as a system of signs which were arbitrary. For example, the signifier (or idea) represented by 'dog' is the sequence of sounds to make up the word. However, in another system the sequence of sounds could be 'lod', 'tet' or 'bloop', etc. but still refer to the signifier 'dog' as long as the 'langue' has been accepted into the parole of that speaking community. He also proposed the relationship between **syntagmatic** and **paradigmatic analyses** of a **sentence**. *See Lepschy (1982): 42–52.*

Semantics. The study of meaning. It is one of the three levels of **linguistics**, the other two being **syntax** and **phonology** (3). Words with a similar meaning can be classified together and form semantic **fields**. Semantic features are used to describe the **nouns** used in spoken and written **utterances**. They are shown using the following notation: [+/– ANIMATE], [+/– COUNT], etc. Children who reach the two-word **utterance** stage in language acquisition use utterances which show semantic relations. Such relations were proposed by Brown (1973):

Agent + Action	e.g., man put
Action + Object	e.g., kick ball
Agent + Object	e.g., mummy shoe
Action + Locative	e.g., go home
Entity + Locative	e.g., book table
Possessor + Possessed	e.g., daddy car
Entity + Attributive	e.g., cup blue
Demonstrative + Entity	e.g., that book

See Lyons (1981): ch. 5.

Semi-sentence. A sentence for which it is difficult to claim it is unacceptable or syntactically sound but, because of its context, could be accepted. Such a situation could arise in the writing of poetry to satisfy the rhythm or rhyme used in the poem.

Sentence. A string of **units** which are placed in a particular formation. The way a sentence is formed is by **syntactic rules**. Lyons has called it 'the largest unit of grammatical description' (Lyons, 1968; 172). The sentence is made up of **constituents** which are formed into **phrases**. Traditionally, a sentence was said to be a grammatical structure of subject, verb, object but this was imprecise for modern linguists. *See Lyons (1968): 172–180.*

Signifier. See **Saussure**.

Signs. See **Saussure**.

Sociolinguistics. The study of **accents** and **dialects** used in different regions of a country. It studies the different varieties used in its social context and the role of the linguistic minorities in a multi-racial society. An important area of this branch in linguistics is the study of the different styles used within the same language. This is known as **diglossia**. *See Trudgill (1974).*

Speech acts. Speech acts express the intention of the speaker. They may take the form of promising to do something, thanking someone for doing something, i.e., **performative utterances**, or making indirect requests, i.e., **felicity**

conditions. Searle has stated, 'speech acts are the basic or minimal units of linguistic communication' (Searle, 1969: 16). *See Clark and Clark (1977): 25–26; Searle (1969): passim.*

Spoonerisms. See **reversal**.

Standard theory. An early form of **transformational grammar** proposed by Chomsky (1965). In it he proposed a **deep structure** from which, by a series of **transformations**, a **surface structure** would appear. It is this surface structure of **sentences** which is spoken or written. The theory has been changed to take into account criticisms of it and so Chomsky has produced the **extended standard theory** and the **revised extended standard theory**. *See Huddleston (1976): ch. 4, 248–260.*

Suffix. An allomorphic unit which is placed at the end of a **word**. It is subsumed into the term **affix**. *See Matthews (1974): 124.*

Surface structure. See **transformational grammar**.

Synchronic linguistics. The study of **language** at the present time. It is opposed to the historical study of language, **diachronic linguistics**. *See Lyons (1968); 48–50.*

Syntagmatic relations. The linear description of **sentences**. Rules exist which result in units taking up certain positions in the sentence. In a simple sentence:

The boy hit the dog

there is a specific order of words which is unalterable. It must follow the sequence:

NP1 V NP2

See Lyons (1968): 70–81.

Syntactic. A description of any rule or structure formed from the **syntax** of the **language**.

Syntactic rule. See **syntax**.

Syntax. The process for forming spoken and written **utterances**. Each language has its own syntax, i.e., its own formation of words into phrases and sentences. The structure of a language is formed by syntactic rules which have been formed by various people. Before modern linguists, grammatical rules were made by grammarians. **Traditional grammar** was found to be too weak and, at times, illogical for modern linguists. So, they looked at grammar as a system which had to be explained logically, rather like a science. Thus, several theories arose such as **generative grammar**, **case grammar**, relational grammar and many others beyond the scope of this book. *See Lyons (1968); 133ff.*

T

Tag question. A structure placed at the end of a statement to produce a question. It will require a positive or negative answer depending on the form of the structure which, in English, is variable. The structure is formed by an **auxiliary verb** and a **pronoun**. If a **personal pronoun** (see **pronoun**) is used, it must agree, i.e., **concord**, with the subject in the statement.

(1) It's raining, isn't it?
(2) It isn't raining, is it?

(1) requires a positive answer while (2) requires a negative answer. The type of answer given depends a lot on the **prosodic features** (3) used to ask the question. In (1) and (2), the tags varied; however, in some languages, they do not vary. For example, the tag question in French is formed by the phrase 'n'est-ce pas'. *See Brown and Miller (1980): 132–133.*

TG. **Transformational grammar**.

Theoretical linguistics. A study of pure linguistics opposed to **applied linguistics**. It includes all the theories used to describe **syntax**, **semantics**, and **speech acts**. *See Lyons (1968): passim.*

Traditional grammar. See **syntax**.

Transformation. See **transformational grammar**.

Transformational grammar. A theory of **syntax** proposed by Chomsky in 1957 after he had set aside the other two theories of **finite state grammar** and **phrase structure grammar**. His initial description of such a grammar was: 'a grammatical transformation T operates on a given string...with a given constituent structure and converts it into a new string with a new derived constituent structure' (Chomsky, 1957: 44). In 1965, he put forward the **standard theory** of **TG**. The transformations which he proposed to operate between the deep and surface structures were designed to

Delete, Substitute, Insert, Move and Raise strings so that he would arrive at the spoken or written **utterance**. Chomsky believed the most important study for linguists was the syntactic component of language, and to arrive at the correct syntactical structures it was necessary to deal with the semantic component. Both surface and deep structures represent how the **phonetic** (3) and semantic components are interpreted in language. Chomsky went so far as to claim **syntax** was 'autonomous' and had nothing to do with semantics.

Chomsky found he had to revise the **standard theory** and so he proposed the Extended Standard Theory (EST). In this theory, Chomsky begins to accept the role of semantics in the surface structure. This apparent change was caused by the failure of the previous theory to account for the use of **stress** (3). In such sentences, the meaning change depends on which word is stressed. Chomsky's problem was: do such sentences all have the same deep structure or different deep structures?

(1) Is Bill coming on TUESDAY?
(2) Is BILL coming on Tuesday?
(3) IS Bill coming on Tuesday?

In the standard theory, Chomsky would have had to give all these sentences the same deep structure because transformational rules could not change the meaning of the sentence between the deep and surface structures. To overcome this problem, he proposed transformational rules which allowed for markers to be placed in the deep and surface structures, so that both structures would affect the semantics of the sentence. This is sometimes called Interpretive Semantics Grammar.

In 1973, Chomsky revised EST to the Revised Extended Standard Theory. This theory removed the relationship of the deep structure to the semantic component as in EST, so that all semantic information could be read off from the surface structure. To accomplish this, he instituted the Trace Theory. A trace ('t') is an empty **node** left behind after a **noun phrase** has been removed. Thus the **passive** transformation becomes as shown below.

(1') shows the trace from where the NP 'John' has been removed to the beginning of the sentence. Thus, traces are like chains in that when linked together, the NP can be traced back to its original position. *See Steinberg (1982): ch. 2.*

Tree diagram. A **hierarchical** structure which is used to analyze **constituents**. The **constituents** are all linked by **branches** and the points where the branches meet are **nodes**:

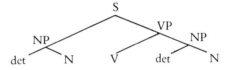

The 'S' (sentence) is said to dominate the NP and VP which are said to dominate their respective constituents. They are known also as phrase markers. *See Huddleston (1976): 38–42.*

Turn. A **sociolinguistic** phenomenon. Turn-taking in conversation is crucial for a conversation to take place. If this breaks down (see **discourse**), then speech therapy will be required. *See Clark and Clark (1977): ch. 6.*

---

deep structure　　(1)　Mary kissed John
surface structure　(1')　JOHN was kissed t (by Mary)
　　　　　　　　　　　　　i　　　　　　　i

U

Unit. Any item in a **syntactic** (see **syntax**), **phonetic** (3), **semantic** (see **semantics**) or **morphological** (see **morphology**) description. A unit in any of these areas of linguistics describes the focus for discussion. *See Lyons (1968): ch. 5.*

Utterance. An utterance is the production of a native speaker who uses the syntactic (see **syntax**) and **semantic** (see **semantics**) rules of the language. In other words, having the **competence**, he makes the **performance**. An utterance is different from a **sentence** as the former could just be a **word**, a **hesitation**, a **phrase** or an unfinished sentence. Of course, it could also be a sentence but not necessarily. *See Lyons (1968): 171–172.*

V

Verb particle. A small **unit** which is placed after a verb. It is usually a **preposition**. If it is used as a particle, it can be moved after the following **noun** or **noun phrase**, if it is an ordinary preposition which follows the verb, this cannot happen:

(1) John hung up the curtains.
(1′) John hung the curtains up.
(1″) John hung them up.

(2) John went to town.
(2′) *John went town to.

In all three versions of (1), 'up' can be said to be a verb particle while in (2), 'to' is not a verb particle. It should be noted in (1″) that the placing of the particle at the end is obligatory (* John hung up them). *See Crystal et al. (1976).*

VP.   **Verb phrase**.

Verb phrase.   See **constituent analysis**.

W

Wh- questions.   Question words which begin with 'wh-' (i.e., why, what, when, which, where). 'How' is also included in this classification as it behaves in a similar way to the other Wh- words. This type of question is opposed to **yes/no questions**.

Wh- words.   See **Wh- questions**.

Word.   A **unit** of grammar used in the construction of **phrases** and **sentences**. It is recognized **intuitively** (see **intuition**) by a native speaker but when examined more scientifically by linguists, 'what is a word?' becomes a more complex problem. Such complexities involve the relative values of words. For example, does the word 'not' have the same value as the word 'book'? Or is a unit which is made up of contractions, such as 'haven't', one word or two? Several theories have, therefore, been proposed to try to settle these matters. A word when written is represented by being separated from other words in the sentence by gaps, while in spoken language such separation is often hard to recognize until a phenomenon like **juncture** is used for an analysis. With **morphological units** (see **morphology**) such as '-ing', '-ed', etc., more

difficulties arise in their definitions. Are they words in their own right or how does one describe verbs of the **form** 'run, runs, running,' etc., when the real word is the **base form** 'run'. Thus, the notion of lexical units or lexemes was proposed. These are units which underlie its other variants. Another theory proposed a **hierarchical** structure for the word:

sentence → clause → phrase → word (→ morpheme)

(based on Allerton, 1979; 183). This means a sentence is made up of a clause which consists of phrases which, in turn, are made up of words which may have morphological modifications. *See Lyons (1968): 194–206.*

Word and paradigm.   See **morphology**.

Word-order.   The sequence of words used to construct **phrases** and **sentences**. In English, the word order is fixed (see **syntagmatic relations**) while in German, it is more variable with adverbial phrases and verbs floating around the sentence as long as the verb remains the second idea, not necessarily the second word, of the sentence. *See Lyons (1968): 203.*

WP.   **Word and paradigm**.

Y

Yes/no questions.   The type of question which will require the answer 'yes' or

'no'. In general, these questions are formed by inversion of the verb and

subject:
(1) He can play football.
(1') Can he play football?

Yes/no questions can be contrasted with **Wh- questions**. *See Clark and Clark (1977): 100–113.*

Z

Zero. The description of a non-existent **unit**. For example, in describing a **noun phrase** such as 'the ball', the **adjective** part of the NP is described as a zero because it does not exist. It is often represented by a zero with an oblique line through it. With those **nouns** which do not overtly show a plural **morph** (see **morphology**) e.g., fish, sheep, etc., the plural marker can be called a zero-morph. *See Lyons (1968): 193, 237.*

Zero morph. *See* **zero**. *See Matthews (1974): 116–118.*

REFERENCES

Allerton, D. J. (1979). *Essentials of Grammatical Theory: A Consensus of Syntax and Morphology.* Routledge and Kegan Paul.

Brown, E. K. and Miller, J. E. (1980). *Syntax: A Linguistic Introduction to Sentence Structure.* Hutchinson.

Chomsky, N. (1957). *Syntactic Structures,* Mouton.

Chomsky, N. (1965). *Aspects of the Theory of Syntax.* MIT Press.

Chomsky, N. (1972). *Language and Mind.* Harcourt, Brace, Jovanovich.

Clark, H. H. and Clark. E. V. (1977). *Psychology and Language: An Introduction to Psycholinguistics.* Harcourt, Brace, Jovanovich.

Crystal, D. (1981) *Clinical Linguistics.* Springer-Verlag kg.

Crystal, D. and Davy, D. (1969) *Investigating English Style.* Longman.

Crystal, D., Fletcher, P. and Garman, M. (1976) *The Grammatical Analysis of Language Disability: A Procedure for Assessment and Remediation.,* Edward Arnold.

Hornstein, N. and Lightfoot, D. (Eds) (1981). *Explanation in Linguistics: The Logical Problem of Language Acquisition.* Longman.

Huddleston, R. (1976). *An Introduction to English Transformational Syntax.* Longman.

Lepschy, G. C. (1982). *A Survey of Structural Linguistics.* Andre Deutsch.

Lyons, J. (1968). *Introduction to Theoretical Linguistics.* Cambridge University Press.

Lyons, J. (1977). *Chomsky.* Fontana/Collins.

Lyons, J. (1981). *Language and Linguistics.* Cambridge University Press.

McTear, M. F. (1985) 'Pragmatic Disorders: A Case of Conversational Disability? In *The British Journal of Disorders of Communication* 20; 2 (1985) 129–142.

Matthews. P. H. (1974). *Morphology: An Introduction to the Theory of Word-Structure.* Cambridge University Press.

Palmer F. R. (1976). *Semantics: A New Outline.* Cambridge University Press.

Palmer, L. R. (1978). *Descriptive and Comparative Linguistics: A Critical Introduction.* Faber.

Pit Corder, S. (1973). *Introducing Applied Linguistics.* Penguin.

Robins, R. H. (1971). *General Linguistics: An Introductory Survey.* Longman.

Robins, R. H. (1979). *A Short History of Linguistics.* Longman.

Searle, J. R. (1969). *Speech Acts: An Essay in the Philosophy of Language.* Cambridge University Press.

Steinberg, D. D. (1982). *Psycholinguistics: Language, Mind and Word.* Longman.

Stockwell, R. P. (1977). *Foundations of Syntactic Theory.* Prentice-Hall.

Trudgill, P. (1974). *Sociolinguistics: An Introduction.* Pelican.

van Dijk, T. A. (1980). *Text and Context: Explorations in the Semantics and Pragmatics of Discourse.* Longman.

Wells, J. C. (1982). *Accents of English 1: An Introduction.* Cambridge University Press.

Section 3
Phonetics/Phonology

A

Abrupt release. During the **production** of **plosives** (see **articulation**), there is a sudden release of built-up pressure in the **mouth** (5). It is opposed to **delayed release**. *See Gimson (1970): 150.*

Accent. The part of a word, phrase or sentence which is given increased loudness as well as a change to the **intonation** pattern. In English, the accent is regular in that the main accent is always on a specific syllable of each word. *See Gimson (1970): ch. 9.*

Acoustic feature. See **acoustic phonetics**.

Acoustic phonetics. The physiological study of the ways in which sounds are produced. Acoustic phonetics is the procedure used to carry out such a study. The three main acoustic features which describe the ways in which sounds are produced are:
1. Frequency
2. Intensity
3. Quality.

Frequency is the number of times in which the **vocal cords** open and close when a sound is produced. The unit used to measure frequency is the Hertz (Hz). A hertz is the number of cycles per second used in producing a sound, i.e., the number of times the cords open and close. So, if a sound causes the cords to open and close 550 times, the frequency of the sound will be 550 Hz. The increases in the fundamental frequency are known as harmonics. If a sound has a fundamental frequency (i.e. 100 cycles per second) and a frequency of 300 cycles per second, this is the third harmonic of the sound. Intensity is the measure of how loud the sound is which a person produces. The unit used to measure intensity is the decibel (dB). Quality of a sound changes in relation to the change in frequencies between sounds. Thus, there is a difference in the quality of the vowels /i/ and /u/. *See Ladefoged (1975): ch. 8.*

Active articulators. See **articulation**.

Acute. A **distinctive feature** used by Jakobson and Halle to distinguish sounds made towards the front of the **mouth** (5) and produced using the high **frequencies** (see **acoustic phonetics**) such as alveolar, dental, palatal (see **articulation**) consonants from the **vowels** (see **cardinal vowel systems**) made at a similar position. These are denoted as [+ ACUTE]. *See Hyman (1975): ch. 2.*

Affricate. See **articulation**.

Airstreams. When a sound is produced, air leaves the lungs and, depending on the type of sound required, is modified as it goes along the **vocal tract**. There are four types of airstream which can be used.

1. Pulmonic Egressive Airstream
The commonest airstream used in all varieties of English. The speaker uses **abdominal-diaphragmatic respiration** or **clavicular breathing** (5) although the length of message which can be produced in the former will be more than that produced in the latter. Thus, if the speaker takes in a deep breath, lets the air leave the **lungs** (5) and produces a **fricative**, (see **articulation**) e.g., /f/, he will produce a very long, uninterrupted sound until the end of his breath. No other airstream allows the speaker such a long uninterrupted flow for producing speech.

2. Pulmonic Ingressive Airstream
This airstream works in the opposite way to (1). The lungs are emptied of air followed by the speaker producing speech while drawing air into the lungs. If a similar **fricative** (see **articulation**) is produced as in (1), the sound will not be sustained for very long. A person's speech becomes very distorted using this airstream.

3. Glottalic Airstream
An airstream produced by a movement of the **larynx** (5) with glottal closure. An upward movement of the larynx produces a glottalic egressive airstream or **ejectives** while a downward movement of the larynx produces a glottalic ingressive airstream or **implosives**.

4. Velaric Airstream
An airstream which produces **velaric ingressive stops** or **clicks** (both, see **velaric airstream**).

In speech therapy, knowledge of airstreams is important, especially the pulmonic egressive airstream as patients suffering from **dysarthria** or **dysphonia** (both 1) may have breathing problems or have acquired another type of airstream. Therapy is designed to allow the patient to produce a normal pulmonic egressive airstream. *See Ladefoged (1975):* 113–121.

Allophone. See **phonology**.

Alveolar. See **articulation**.

Anterior. A **distinctive feature** proposed by Chomsky and Halle. It is used to produce a distinction of sounds produced towards the front of the **mouth** (5). The sounds, which are denoted as [+ ANTERIOR], are **dentals** and **labials** (both, see **articulation**). *See Hyman (1975): ch. 2.*

Anticipatory. See **assimilation**.

Apex. A description of the very tip of the tongue which is used, for example, to produce some **alveolar** sounds, known as apico-alveolar. *See Catford (1977): ch. 8.*

Apico-. See **apex**.

Archiphoneme. See **phonology**.

Articulation. The production of **vowels** and **consonants** by the active and passive articulators in the **mouth** (5). The active articulators are the moving parts in the mouth which can produce sounds while the passive articulators are the non-moving parts of the mouth against which the active articulators come into contact. There are three descriptions of the articulation of a sound:

1. Place of articulation
The different places in the mouth used to produce **consonants** are:
   a) Bilabial—both lips are used, e.g., /p,b/;
   b) Alveolar—the **tongue** (5) comes either into direct contact with the **alveolar ridge** (see **mouth**: 5), e.g., /t,d/, or close to it, e.g., /s,z/;
   c) Interdental—the only time the tongue is placed between the teeth, e.g., /θ,ð/;
   d) Palatal—the tongue may come into direct contact with the **hard palate** (5) or come close to it, e.g., /c,ʃ/.
   e) Retroflex—the **blade** of the tongue is turned back to touch the hard palate, e.g., /ʂ,ʐ/,/ʈ,d/;
   f) Palato-alveolar—the sound is made in two places, both at the alveolar ridge and hard palate, e.g., /ʃ,ʒ/;
   g) Labio-dental—the top teeth are placed over the bottom lip, e.g., /f,v/;
   h) Labio-velar—the lips come together and at the same time there is a slight closure at the **velum** e.g., /w/;
   i) Velar—the back of the tongue comes into contact with the **soft palate** (5), e.g., /k,g/;
   j) Uvular—the back of the tongue is pushed right back against the back wall of the mouth (French /R/);

2. Manner of articulation
The different ways in which the articulators are moved in the mouth:
   a) Plosive—the articulators are brought firmly together, pressure is built up behind the closure followed by **abrupt release**, e.g., /p,b,t,d,k,g/;
   b) Fricatives—the articulators are brought close together without meeting and the **airstream** is allowed to pass through producing a hissing quality to the sound, e.g., /s,z,ʃ,ʒ,f,v/;
   c) Affricates—a combination of (a) and (b) which occurs in quick sequencing, e.g., /tʃ/,/dʒ/;
   d) Lateral—the sides of the tongue are lowered while making a closure in the centre of the mouth, e.g., /l/;
   e) Vibrant—the tongue is made to vibrate (trill or roll) or touch (tap) or come close to the alveolar ridge, e.g., /r/,/ɾ/,/ɽ/;
   f) Nasal—the **mouth** (5) is closed by the soft palate and the airstream passes into the **nasal cavities** (see **nose**, 5), e.g., /n,g,m/;
   g) Approximant—the articulators are brought lightly together and there is no **abrupt release**, e.g., /w,j/.

3. Voicing
Sounds are either voiced or voiceless. In other words, the vocal cords are made to vibrate for voiced sounds but do not vibrate for voiceless sounds. Some voiced sounds are /b,d,g,v,.../ while some of the devoiced sounds are /p,t,k,f,.../.

(1)–(3) are used to describe consonants. The **cardinal vowel system** is used to describe the production of **vowels**. **Consonants** can be described as:
/p/ is a voiceless bilabial plosive
/d/ is a voiced alveolar plosive
/v/ is a voiced labio-dental fricative.
Such descriptions are important for speech therapists as they deal with **articulation delay/disorder** and **phonological delay/disorder** (all 1). *See Ladefoged (1975): ch. 1, passim.*

Articulatory phonetics. A study within **phonetics** of the way in which **articulation** of sounds takes place. For this study, instruments such as electromyography, spirometry and palatography are used. These devices seek to find out how the vocal organs produce speech sounds such as those described under **articulation**. *See Catford (1977): chs. 2, 7, 8, 12.*

Aspiration. An audible escape of air which is released with a sound. It often occurs with a **bilabial plosive** (see **articulation**). It is marked with a **diacritic** 'h' placed above the sound with which it is made. *See Ladefoged (1975): 43–44.*

Assimilation. The process whereby one sound is changed because of the influence of another sound near to it. For example, [n] becomes [n̪] because of [ð] in the phrase 'in the' (based on Ladefoged (1975): 92). There are three types of assimilation:

1. Anticipatory (or Regressive) where the sound is influenced by the next sound. This is the commonest form of assimilation in English;

2. Progressive where the sound is influenced by the preceding sound;

3. Coalescent where two or more sounds can come together to form one sound. For example, 'got you' becomes /gɔtʃa/ where the 't' and 'y' sounds come together to form /tʃ/. Knowledge of assimilation is necessary for speech therapists as children can produce this process as a symptom of **phonological delay/disorder** (1). *See Gimson (1970): 290.*

Auditory phonetics. The study of how people perceive sounds. The two main components of this study are:

1. Pitch—this feature describes the way in which the listener works out the difference between a high and a low pitched sound. Pitch is the equivalent of the **acoustic feature** of **frequency** (see **acoustic phonetics**).

2. Loudness—this feature describes the amount of air pressure in the speaker's voice which is required for the listener to hear the message. Loudness is the equivalent of the **acoustic feature** of **intensity** (see **acoustic phonetics**). Sound reaches our **ears** (6) by the movement of air particles hitting each other. The stage where the particles come together is called compression which is followed by them spreading out, known as rarefaction. The compression and rarefaction are shown in the form of a sine wave where compression is at the highest positive value while rarefaction is the lowest negative value on the sine curve. Normal atmospheric pressure is represented by the horizontal axis, known as equilibrium. Sound waves spread around from the sound source. *See Gimson (1970): ch. 3.*

B

Back. See **cardinal vowel systems**.

Bilabial. See **articulation**.

Binary feature. See **distinctive features**.

Blade. The part of the **tongue** (5) behind the **apex** or tip which is used to produce **alveolar** (see **articulation**) sounds such as /t,d,s,z/.

Breath groups. The length of **utterance** (2) which a person can produce in one breath. Knowing about breath groups is important as poor breathing may affect the syntactic, phonological and semantic content of what is said. In speech therapy, breath groups can be introduced into **treatment programmes** (1) for patients suffering from **dysarthria** or **dysphonia** (all 1). The patient is trained to reduce the number of words used in one breath to a

level which allows the patient to communicate a message meaningfully. *See Brosnahan and Malmberg (1976): 31, 145.*

Broad transcription. See **transcription systems**.

Bunching. A description of the **tongue** (5) when it is pushed to the back of the **mouth** (5) to produce **back vowels** (see **cardinal vowel systems**) and **palato-alveolar fricatives** /ʃ,ʒ/ (see **articulation**). *See Catford (1977): ch. 7.*

Burst. A phenomenon found in **acoustic phonetics** when there is a sudden peak showing a burst of energy when an **abrupt release** occurs in **plosive** (see **articulation**) sounds. *See Ladefoged (1975): ch. 8.*

C

Cardinal vowel systems. A system, devised by Daniel Jones in about 1914, which describes the way in which vowels are produced. The system has eight primary cardinal vowels which act as reference points of tongue and lip positions. The diagram for primary cardinal vowels is:

front	back
i	u
e	o
ɛ	ɔ
ae	a

In the primary vowel system, the front vowels are unrounded, i.e., the lips are spread, while the back vowels are rounded, i.e., the lips are pouted. As the tongue moves from /i/, the tongue moves down and back for the production of the other vowels and is **bunched** at the back of the mouth for the back vowels. There are four classifications of vertical tongue positions used in this system. Close refers to the highest position of the tongue, i.e., /i/, /u/, which allows the vowel to be produced without audible friction, while half-close refers to the next level, i.e., /e/, /o/, half-open to the next level, i.e., /ɛ/, /ʌ/ and open to the lowest level, i.e., /ae/, /a/ where the tongue is at its furthest point from the roof of the mouth. The secondary cardinal vowels are produced by reversing the lip positions which results in the front vowels becoming rounded while the back vowels are unrounded. The diagram for secondary cardinal vowels is:

front	back
y	ɯ
ø	ɣ
oe	ʌ
a	ɒ

All vowels and **diphthongs** can be described within the framework of either primary cardinal vowels or secondary cardinal vowels. *See Ladefoged (1975): 194–199.*

Centre. The part of the tongue between the blade and its back. It is used to produce palatal sounds and in part of the **articulation** of **palato-alveolar** (see **articulation**) sounds as it comes into contact with the **hard palate** (5). A description of any vowel which appears in the middle of the **cardinal vowel systems**. The most central vowel is the shwa [ə]. To produce such a **vowel** the **tongue** (5) takes up a central position in the **mouth** (5). *See Ladefoged (1975): 199.*

Close vowel. See **cardinal vowel systems**.

Cluster reduction. See **phonological processes**.

Coarticulation. An **articulation** which occurs almost simultaneously with another articulation. For example, in words such as 'eighth' and 'width', the [t] and [d] become dentalized as the speaker approaches the **interdental** (see **articulation**) sound [θ]. Thus, these two words would be pronounced [etθ] and [widθ]. Anticipatory coarticulation occurs where the **articulators** (see **articulation**) for both sounds move to the **place of articulation** (see **articulation**) of the second sound. For example, the word 'shoe' is pronounced with lip-rounding and even the /ʃ/ is rounded. *See Ladefoged (1975): 48–52, 80–81.*

Compact. A **distinctive feature** proposed by Jakobson and Halle for marking **open vowels**. They are denoted by [+ COMPACT] while other vowels are [– COMPACT]. The opposite is **diffuse**. Chomsky and Halle described these vowels as **low**. *See Hyman (1975): ch. 2.*

Complementary distribution. A type of **phonological** (see **phonology**) analysis. When two sounds are found in different environments, complementary distribution occurs. In other words, there is no overlap between the distribution of the sounds, i.e., no overlap in the set of contexts in which the sound is found. When the analysis has been completed, the result is shown in the formula:

$$/c/ \rightarrow \begin{cases} [a] / & \begin{matrix} x\_\_\_y \\ d\_\_\_e \end{matrix} \\ [b] / & \begin{matrix} g\_\_\_h \\ e\_\_\_\# \end{matrix} \\ [c] / & \text{elsewhere} \end{cases}$$

This is a totally hypothetical formula and does not relate to any existing language. The formula reads: The **phoneme** /c/ (see **phonology**) has three **allophones** [a], [b], [c] (see **phonology**), all of which appear in the given contexts following the oblique line. Since none of the contexts overlaps and the allophone [c] does not have any specific contexts, these three allophones are members of the phoneme /c/ and are in complementary distribution. *See Hyman (1975): ch. 3.*

Connected speech. A particular type of analysis of a person's speech. It is used to analyze conversation and the ways **utterances** (2) are put together. It is opposed to analyzing single words and phrases which can function differently in general conversation. **Prosodic features** (see **prosody**) used in flowing speech are especially analyzed. *See Gimson (1970): ch. 10.*

Consonant. A sound which is not a **vowel** (see **cordinal vowel systems**). Such sounds have specific descriptions for the way they are articulated. They are described in terms of their **voicing, place of articulation** (see **articulation**) and **manner of articulation** (see **articulation**).

Consonantal. A description of any sound or movement in the **vocal tract** which produces a **consonant**-like sound. A **distinctive feature** used to differentiate sounds into two groups: [+ consonantal] sounds are produced with an obstruction in the airstream when it reaches the **mouth** (5) and are produced with low acoustic energy; [– consonantal] sounds are produced with little or no obstruction and high acoustic energy. *See Hyman (1975): ch. 2.*

Consonant cluster. The structure which occurs when two or more **consonants** come together **word-initially** (e.g., 'step'), **word-medially** (e.g., 'birthday') or **word-finally** (e.g., 'damp').

Constriction. The description of what occurs when there is a narrowing in the **vocal tract**. This is used when making **implosive** and **ejective** sounds. *See Catford (1977): 70.*

Continuant. A **distinctive feature** proposed by Chomsky and Halle to distinguish sounds produced with friction [+ CONT] from those produced without [– CONT]. This **phonological** description is equivalent to the **articulatory** (see **articulation**) description of a **fricative** (see **articulation**) and a **vowel** (see **cardinal vowel systems**). *See Hyman (1975): ch. 2.*

Contour. See **intonation**.

Contrastive analysis. A **phonological** (see **phonology**) analysis of a person's **sound system** (see **phonology**) which involves the comparison of one sound system with another. The sound system of a young child can be compared with that of an adult so as to find out what sounds(s) the child is lacking. In the same way, it can be used with children whose sound system is disordered to some extent. By comparing the child's disordered sound system to a normal sound system, it is possible to find out what sounds the child has in his system and those he fails to use. However, Cruttenden (1972) believes that this analysis is inappropriate, if not impossible to use because the child's acquisition of sounds is so erratic. He states: 'Child language is so unfixed, so constantly changing that it is doubtful whether the term is appropriate'. If this type of analysis is used by the clinician, the variation in the child's acquisition of sounds should be taken into account. By using this form of analysis, it is possible to find out if there is a regular error pattern since the therapist can work out in which part of the word(s) the sound substitution, omission, distortion or addition takes place. *See Grunwell (1982).*

Coronal. A **distinctive feature** proposed by Chomsky and Halle to distinguish sounds produced with the tip of the tongue [+ COR] from those which are not [– COR]. This **phonological** description is similar to the **articulatory** (see **articulation**) description of **alveolar, dental** and **palato-alveolar consonants** (see **articulation**). *See Hyman (1975): ch. 2.*

Creaky voice. A description of a person's voice which contains very low pitch. This occurs usually in males. The **arytenoid cartilages** (5) hold one end of the cords tightly closed, so vibration can only occur at one end. It may also be called laryngealized. *See Ladefoged (1975): 123–124.*

CV, CVC. See **phonotactics**.

D

Decibels. See **acoustic phonetics**.

Delayed release. A **distinctive feature** proposed by Chomsky and Halle. It distinguishes sounds produced by gradual release as in the case of the **fricative** part of **affricates** (see **articulation**) which are all described as [**+ delayed release**]. It is opposed to **abrupt release**. *See Hyman (1975): ch. 2.*

Dental. See **articulation**.

Devoiced. Sounds which are devoiced are those which are usually **voiced** but because of their environment lose some of their voicing. This often occurs with the voiced plosives /b,d,g/ when used **word-finally**, e.g., big, bad, etc. In narrow transcription, this process is represented by the **diacritic** [₀] placed under the affected sound. *See Gimson (1970): 152, 153, 179.*

Diacritic. In **narrow transcription**, markings have to be placed above or below the sound to show any particular features which are used in its production. For example, [ʰ] is the diacritic placed above and in the gap between the sounds to show **aspiration**, e.g., /pʰɪn/. Diacritics are used in **suprasegmental phonetics**. These diacritics show **intonation contours** and mark **stress** (see **prosody**) in a word or sentence. In transcribing the speech of either children with **phonological delay/disorder** or patients suffering from **dysarthria** (both 1), the speech therapist will have to know the diacritics used to mark the characteristics of these patients' speech. *See Ladefoged (1975): 37; Abercrombie (1967): 125–127.*

Diffuse. A **distinctive feature** proposed by Jakobson and Halle for marking **close vowels** [+ DIFFUSE] (see **cardinal vowel systems**). It is opposed to **compact**. Chomsky and Halle changed it to **high**. *See Hyman (1975): ch. 2.*

Digraph. Two sounds which come together and are pronounced as one sound unit. It occurs usually with **vowels**. When children learn to read, vowel digraphs can cause difficulty, especially when using Scottish-English. Such words are 'eat', 'feet', 'break', etc. In RP, these vowel sounds would be produced with a **diphthong** but in Scottish-English, the two vowels together are produced as a single **pure vowel**.

Diphthong. A description of the production of **vowels**. Two sounds are produced, but unlike **digraphs**, both are produced separately, not as a single unit. In **RP** (see **received pronunciation**), there are many diphthongs, e.g., /meɪk/, /tʃeð/, /kaep/, whereas in Scottish-English such diphthongs are produced as **pure vowels**. However, they do have diphthongs in common such as /naɪn/ ('nine'), /haʌs/ ('house'), /naɪf/ ('knife'),

etc. The production of **diphthongs** can be explained using the **cardinal vowel system**. The **phonetician** can start at one sound (e.g., /a/) and show the glide to another, e.g., /ɪ/, to produce /aɪ/. *See Catford (1977): 215–217.*

Discontinuous. A **distinctive feature** proposed by Jakobson and Halle to distinguish sounds which are made with a complete closure in the **vocal tract** [+ DISCONTINUOUS] from those which are not, i.e., **fricatives** (see **articulation**), **vowels** (see **cardinal vowel system**), etc. *See Hyman (1975): ch. 2.*

Dissimilation. A process in which a neighbouring sound influences another sound but, unlike **assimilation**, the influence changes the sound. This occurs in **diachronic** linguistics (2) to show phonetic changes in **language** (2). *See Brosnahan and Malmberg (1976): 134–135.*

Distinctive feature. **Phonological** descriptions of the way in which sounds are produced. The terms, placed in square brackets, are in **binary** notation which shows two polar ends, e.g., [+ continuant], [– continuant]. Jakobson and Halle (1956) and Chomsky and Halle (1968) proposed many such features. Jakobson and Halle's distinctive features were **acoustic** in formation:

acute	grave
compact	plain
diffuse	sharp
flat	checked
lax	unchecked
mellow	tense
discontinuous	

Chomsky and Halle's distinctives features follow the **articulatory** positions for producing sounds:

coronal	high
continuant	low
anterior	back
strident	nasal
voice	lateral
sonorant	round
delayed release	distributed

See Hyman (1975): ch. 2.

Distributed. A **distinctive feature** proposed by Chomsky and Halle to distinguish sounds produced with a **stricture** such as **bilabial** and **palato-alveolar fricatives** [+ DISTRIBUTED] (see **articulation**) from those which are not made at this **place of articulation** [– DISTRIBUTED] (see **articulation**). *See Hyman (1975): ch. 2.*

Disyllable. Two syllables which make up a phonetic unit. It is contrasted to mono-syllable, etc. *See Catford (1977): 89–91.*

Dorsum. The back of the tongue which

produces sounds such as **velars** and **palatals** (see **articulation**) by coming into contact with the **hard** and **soft palates** (see **mouth**, 5). *See Catford (1977): 158–160.*

E

Egressive airstream. See **airstream**.

Ejective. A sound which is produced by a glottalic egressive airstream. The sequence of movements required for producing an ejective is:
1. close the glottis (cf. lifting a heavy weight);
2. make a **bilabial** (see **articulation**) closure, e.g., /p/;
3. move the **larynx** (5) up (feel the air compressed in the mouth);
4. release the closure;
5. a voiceless ejective /p'/ is produced.
See Catford (1977): 70.

Elicitation. The process of obtaining

Duration. The length of time, in milliseconds, used to produce sounds in **connected speech**. The time taken to carry this out depends on **tempo, voice onset time**, etc. *See Catford (1977): 195–199.*

data, e.g., words, syllables, phrases, sentences, to find out how the person uses particular phenomena. In speech therapy, elicitation takes the form of **formal** and **informal assessments** (see **assessments**, 1).

Elision. A process by which some words in certain contexts can lose a sound or syllable in certain environments (e.g., 'ladies an' gentlemen'). This occurs especially in colloquial speech spoken at fast **rates**. *See Gimson (1970): 297–299.*

Epenthesis. A sound which is inserted in the middle of a word as a form of **intrusion**.

F

Feedback. A monitoring process for speakers. It can either be self-monitoring, i.e., they hear what they themselves have said by internal feedback, or monitoring the effect of what they have said by the reactions from the listener. Many **communication disorders** (1) are a result of poor monitoring by the speaker. Such disorders can include **stammering, dysphonia, phonological disorder** (all 1) and learning problems such as those encountered by children learning to read using the phonic approach. **Delayed auditory feedback** (7) is used with those who speak at a very fast **rate** to try and slow their speech down in such conditions as **stammering** (1). *See Brosnahan and Malmberg (1976): 182–183.*

Filled pause. A gap between **utterances** (2) which has been filled by a hesitation, e.g., 'em, ur, eh', etc. Otherwise these gaps would remain silent. *See Clark and Clark (1977): 262.*

Filter. An electronic method of producing part of an acoustic analysis. It reduces the **amplitude** of a **frequency** (see

acoustic phonetics) but at the same time allows others to pass through with little or no reduction in their amplitude. The frequencies which do pass through are called the bandwidth of the filter. *See Fry (1979): 57–60.*

Flap. See **articulation**.

Flat. A **distinctive feature** proposed by Jakobson and Halle to distinguish sounds produced with **lip-rounding** (see **cardinal vowel systems**) [+ FLAT] from those which are produced with spread lips [– FLAT]. *See Hyman (1975): ch. 2.*

Formant. See **spectography**.

Fortis. A description of sounds which are produced with a strong **egressive airstream** (see **airstream**). They require also more muscle power to produce the sound. It is usually the voiceless **consonants** which are fortis, e.g., /f/, while voiced ones are described as **lenis** (e.g., /v/). *See Gimson (1970): 32.*

Free variation. A **phonological** description of the distribution of sounds or **phonemes** (see **phonology**). It occurs when two sounds appear in the same position of a word without changing its meaning. For example, the 'r'-sounds found in some varieties of English are freely interchangeable in the word 'burns', which can either be [bʌrnz] or [bʌrhz]. In a **phonological delay/ disorder** (1), the child can produce a sound in the same position of many of the words he uses. Such a sound is said to be in free variation in this child's **sound system** (see **phonology**). *See Grunwell (1982): 30–31, passim.*

Fricative. See **articulation**.

Friction. The type of sound produced for **fricatives**.

Fronting. In **articulatory phonetics**, sounds which are produced at the front of the mouth. This includes the front **vowels** in the **cardinal vowel system** and the **consonants** made by the tip and blade of the tongue. In **generative phonology** terms these sounds are described as [+ anterior] or [+ coronal]. It describes also a **phonological process** proposed in **natural phonology** by David Stampe. *See Ladefoged (1975): 11–12, 68–69; Grunwell (1982): 177.*

Fundamental frequency. See **acoustic phonetics**.

G

Generative phonology. A **phonological** theory in which phonological changes are used to describe sound changes in particular contexts or environments of the word. For example, the rule which allows for **vowels** to be nasalized before nasal consonants would appear thus:

$$\begin{bmatrix} + \text{voc} \\ - \text{cons} \end{bmatrix} \dashrightarrow [\, + \text{nas}\,] \Big/ - \begin{bmatrix} + \text{cons} \\ + \text{nas} \end{bmatrix}$$

(Grunwell, 1982: 135)

The terms used in square brackets are **distinctive features**. An explanation of the above rule is: 'a sound which is voiced but is not a consonant (i.e., a vowel) becomes nasalized in the context preceding a nasal consonant.' Such rules could be useful to speech therapists in that the child's representation of a sound can be compared to the adult **target** sound by working out the differences of the features used by the child compared to the adult. The input side of the rule has the child's pronunciation described in the form of distinctive features while the output of the rule shows the adult pronunciation, i.e., the one regarded as the **norm** (4), and if the rule is context-sensitive, i.e., the error occurs in the same position of the word consistently, the therapist can find out if the child is making a consistent error in a particular part of the word. Grunwell gives an example where /f/ is pronounced as a **homorganic affricate** (see **articulation**) in **word-initial** position:

'feet'	[pɸit]
'fence'	[pɸeş]
'fish'	[pɸɪ̣ş]

The rule describing this error is:

$$\begin{bmatrix} + \text{cont} \\ + \text{ant} \\ - \text{cor} \\ + \text{strid} \\ - \text{voice} \end{bmatrix} \rightarrow \begin{bmatrix} - \text{cont]} \\ + \text{del rel} \end{bmatrix} \Big/ \begin{bmatrix} + \text{voc} \\ - \text{cons} \end{bmatrix}$$

(Grunwell, 1982: 138)

An explanation of this rule is: a sound which is fricative-type ([+ cont]), made towards the front of the mouth ([+ ant]), not made with the tongue tip ([– cor]), a strong sound ([+ strid]) and unvoiced ([– voice]) becomes a non-fricative sound ([– cont]) and has a longer release time than a single consonant ([+ del rel]) in the context of coming before a vowel. Generative phonology is quite widely used in analyzing child speech and its application to omissions, substitutions, distortions and transposition is:

— change feature specifications (i.e., change segments)
— delete segments; cf. omission
— insert segments; cf. additions
— interchange (reorder or permute) segments (i.e., metathesis) cf. transpositions
— coalesce segments

(Grunwell, 1982: 142)

These phonological rules describe patterns of errors. Thus, if the therapist decides to use rule-based therapy, then the generative framework for analyzing a child's speech may well be useful. *See Grunwell (1982): ch. 6.*

Glide. When two sounds are produced together, and the speaker moves from the first and glides to the second. This often occurs with **diphthongs** which are also known as gliding vowels. The reason for this name can be seen easily by looking at diagrams of the **cardinal vowel system** (Ladefoged, 1975: 194). *See Gimson (1970): 39, 126.*

Glottal constrictions. A narrowing of the **glottis** (5) for producing **ejectives** and **implosives**. It is a **distinctive feature** to mark **place of articulation** (see **articulation**) proposed by Chomsky and Halle. *See Ladefoged (1975): ch. 6.*

Glottal stop. This sound occurs when the cords come tightly together and are opened suddenly during a period of silence. It is represented by /ʔ/. In some varieties of Scottish-English, a glottal stop is very prevalent. In Glasgow, it appears in words such as 'butter', /bʌʔə/ and 'bottle', /bʔ l/, etc. *See Ladefoged (1975): 46.*

Glottalic airstream. See **implosives** and **ejectives**.

Grave. A **distinctive feature** proposed by Jakobson and Halle to distinguish sounds made at the **back** of the mouth such as back vowels, **velars** and **labials** [+ GRAVE] (see **articulation**) from those made at the front of the mouth [– GRAVE]. It is opposed to **acute**. *See Hyman (1975): ch. 2.*

Groove. A description of the tongue when it has a groove along the central longitudinal line of the tongue. It is used for some **fricatives** (see **articulation**) such as /s, z, ʃ, ʒ/. It is opposed to **slit**. *See Catford (1977): 127, 153, 154.*

H

Harmonic. See **acoustic phonetics**.

Hertz. See **acoustic phonetics**.

High. A **distinctive feature** proposed by Chomsky and Halle to distinguish sounds produced with the tongue in a raised position of the mouth [+ HIGH] from those produced with the tongue in a low position [– HIGH]. *See Hyman (1975): ch. 2.*

Homorganic. A phenomenon where two **articulations** are made by the same **articulators** (see **articulation**). Thus, /p/ and /b/ can be described as homorganic sounds in that they are both produced by two lips. *See Ladefoged (1975): 47–48.*

Hz. **Hertz**.

I

Implosive. A glottalic ingressive voiced **stop**. It is very difficult to produce **voice** with an **ejective** stop while devoicing is difficult with implosives. The sequence of movements for producing an implosive is:
  1. close the **glottis** (5);
  2. make a closure of the lips, e.g., /b/;
  3. move the **larynx** (5) downward (cf. taking a gulp);
  4. release the closure;
  5. a voiced implosive /ɓ/ is produced.
See Catford (1977): 73.

Ingressive. See **airstreams**.

Interdental. See **articulation**.

International Phonetic Alphabet. A system of symbols used in transcribing a person's speech. It was devised by the International Phonetic Association which was inaugurated in 1886 by a small group of language teachers in France who found phonetics useful in their work. The Association has produced the IPA chart (1951; rev. 1979) which divides up the sounds into **place** and **manner of articulation** (see **articulation**) for **consonants**. It also shows the **cardinal vowel systems** as well as a list of the **diacritics** which can be used in **narrow transcriptions** (see **transcrip-**

tion systems). *See Abercrombie (1967): 123–124.*

Intervocalic. A consonantal sound which appears between two **vowels**, (see **cardinal vowel systems**) e.g., /t/ in 'butter' where the /t/ sound is intervocalic.

Intonation. See **suprasegmental phonetics**.

Intrusion. Sounds which do not appear in the written form of a language but do appear in some **accents** (2). A very common intrusive sound in English is the intrusive /r/ as in such phrases /lɔr aen ɔrdə/. The first /r/ is intrusive as it does not appear when 'law and order' is written out. *See Gimson (1970): 97, 209–210.*

Inventory. A gathering together of data concerning the sounds people use in different situations. There is no structure to this list. When an inventory, for example, of sounds has been collected, it is called that person's sound inventory.

IPA. International Phonetic Alphabet.

L

Labial. See **articulation**.

Labio-dental. See **articulation**.

Labio-velar. See **articulation**.

Laminal. A description of sounds made with the **blade** or lamina of the tongue. These include the **alveolar** (see **articulation**) sounds /t,d,s,z/. *See Catford (1977): 152ff.*

Lateral. See **articulation**.

Lax. A **distinctive feature** proposed by Jakobson and Halle to distinguish sounds made with little muscular effort [+ LAX] from those which are produced with a stronger muscular effort [– LAX]. It is opposed to **tense**. *See Hyman (1975): ch. 2.*

Length. The period of time used to produce a sound or syllable. Length modifies the articulation and makes a difference between sounds. It is also known as duration and **quality**. *See Catford (1977): 195–199.*

Lenis. A sound which has little air pressure in the **airstream** to produce the sound. There is also a reduction in muscle power required. It is opposed to **fortis**. *See Gimson (1970): 32.*

Linking. A sound which appears in the spoken language but does not appear in the orthographic form of the language. An example is the linking-/r/. *See Gimson (1970): 112, 116, passim.*

Lip rounding. See **cardinal vowel systems**.

Liquid. A description of sounds sometimes used to refer to **apico-alveolar** (see **apex**) sounds such as /l/ and /r/. *See Ladefoged (1975): 79.*

Loudness. See **auditory phonetics**.

Low. A **distinctive feature** proposed by Chomsky and Halle to distinguish sounds made lowering the tongue in the mouth [+ LOW] to produce **open vowels** (see **cardinal vowel systems**) from those made with the tongue raised in the mouth [– LOW]. It is opposed to **high**. *See Hyman (1975): ch. 2.*

M

Major class feature. A major grouping of Chomsky and Halle's **distinctive features**. This group distinguishes sounds which are made with different degrees of openness in the **vocal tract**. This produces the distinctive features of **sonorant/non-sonorant, vocalic/non-vocalic** and **consonantal/non-consonantal**. *See Ladefoged (1975): ch. 11.*

Manner of articulation. See **articulation**.

Mellow. A **distinctive feature** proposed by Jakobson and Halle to distinguish sounds which are made with a low frequency such as **plosives** and **nasals** [+ MELLOW] from those made with a higher frequency such as **fricatives** [– MELLOW] (see **articulation**). It is opposed to **strident**. *See Hyman (1975): ch. 2.*

Minimal pairs. A phonological analysis in which two words are said to have a different meaning if they differ by one sound in the same environment of the word. For example, 'pin' and 'bin' are minimal pairs since they differ by one sound, i.e., /p/ vs /b/, and thus change in meaning. A minimal pair can only exist if there is one difference in the sounds which occur in the same place in either word. This is also known as variation in sound. Minimal pairs have an important role in speech therapy since they mark the fundamental difference between **treatment programmes** for **phonological** and **articulation delay/disorder** (all 1). In the former the therapist teaches

the child individual sounds, while in the latter the therapist teaches the sounds with which the child is confused. Thus if the child shows difficulty in producing /k/ and, instead, produces a /t/ **word-initially** (e.g., /tuk∂r/---- [kuk∂r]), the therapist would give the child lists of words in which the meaning changes by the changing of the /k/ or /t/ in this position of the word. In most cases, the child can say the sound correctly in other positions of the word. *See Grunwell (1982): 29–30.*

N

Narrow transcription. See **transcription systems**.

Nasal. See **articulation**.

Natural phonology. A **phonological** theory proposed by David Stampe in the late 1970s. In essence, he believes a child will simplify sounds which cause difficulty. These simplifications are called **phonological processes**. The thrust of his theory is that as these processes are **innate** (4), those sounds which are found difficult by the child will automatically be simplified by young children as they acquire speech and language. Thus, natural phonology becomes a suitable means for analyzing children's speech as it is based on simplifying **sound systems** (see **phonology**). By treating the child's simplifications the therapist is showing the complexity of sound production to the child and the sounds for which he is aiming. *See Grunwell (1982): ch. 7.*

Neutral. A **vowel** sound which is described as being produced not at the front or back of the mouth or high or low but in a central position. This is

shown clearly in the diagram of the **cardinal vowel systems**. The vowel in question is known as a shwa, or schwa /∂/. *See Gimson (1970): 124.*

Neutralization. A phenomenon which describes sounds which can be interchanged in certain contexts with other sounds because they lose their distinction. For example, /p,t,k/ and /b,d,g/ can be distinguished from each other by the opposition of **voicing** (see **articulation**) and **aspiration**. In the former set of sounds, aspiration is present, e.g., 'pin/bin', 'pit/bit', etc., while in the second set of sounds there is no aspiration present. However, when they follow an /s/, e.g., skate, spate, steak, they do not require this distinction because /b,d,g/ in similar positions do not exist, e.g., *sgate, *sbate, *sdeak. Thus, the distinction between these two lots of **phonemes** (see **phonology**) is lost in the context of following /s/, i.e., s_v; 'v' = vowel. *See Gimson (1970): 48–49.*

Nucleus. See **suprasegmental phonetics**.

O

Obstruent. A sound which is produced by an obstruction in the **mouth** (5) made by the **articulators** such as **plosives**, **fricatives** and **affricates** (see **articulation**). It is also a **distinctive feature** proposed by Chomsky and Halle to distinguish such sounds from those

produced without such an obstruction. It is opposed to **sonorant**. *See Ladefoged (1975): 53.*

Off-/on- glide. A description of movements of **articulators** (see **articulation**) which occur in the production of contiguous sounds. An off-glide occurs after the production of one sound and the articulators are beginning to take up the position for the next sound while an on-glide occurs as the articulators are taking up the position for the intended sound from a previous sound or from rest. *See Gimson (1970): 150.*

Open. See **cardinal vowel systems.**

Opposition. See **distinctive features.**

Oral. Sounds which have no **nasal** (see **articulation**) quality in their production. As suggested by the name, these sounds are produced in the **oral cavity** (see **mouth,** 5) which produces the difference between them and nasal sounds made in the nasal cavities. *See Ladefoged (1975): 8.*

Overlapping. A description in **phonology** of sounds which are mutually exclusive. In other words, if the sound [k] is to exist by itself and not be realized as [f] from time to time, there must be certain contexts in which [k] appears and not [f] and vice versa. If this were not the case, the two sounds would overlap and lose their contrasting qualities. Such contrasts are sometimes lost in **phonological delay/disorder** (1) and the making-up of rules becomes almost impossible. *See Grunwell (1982): 76–78.*

P

Palatal. See **articulation.**

Palatalization. The process where a sound which is not a **palatal** per se becomes affected by the **hard palate** (see **mouth,** 5). This occurs often in **secondary articulation.** It occurs also in **phonological delay/disorder** (1) when a child produces a non-palatal sound with a palatal **quality.**

Palato-alveolar. See **articulation.**

Paralanguage. See **suprasegmental linguistics.**

Phonation. **Voicing** (see **articulation**) which occurs when the **vocal cords** are activated. The two main types of phonation are breathy and **creaky voice.** Patients who suffer from **dysarthria** and **dysphonia** (both 1) can have problems with phonation. *See Catford (1977): ch. 16.*

Phone. See **phonology.**

Phoneme. See **phonology.**

Phonemic structure. See **phonology.**

Phonemic system. See **phonology.**

Phonemic transcription. See **transcription systems.**

Phonetician. See **phonetics.**

Phonetics. The study of the articulatory mechanism producing sounds. Starting from the **lungs** (5), a **pulmonic egressive airstream** (see **airstreams**) is produced and forces the air through the **vocal tract,** into the **mouth** (5) where the **articulators** (see **articulation**) move in particular sequences to produce the desired sound. The phonetician who makes this study describes **consonants** in terms of **place** and **manner of articulation** (see **articulation**) and **voicing** (see **articulation**) and **vowels** in terms of the openness and rounding of the lips. Such descriptions of sounds can be used in describing virtually all the languages of the world. *See Ladefoged (1975): 23.*

Phonological processes. Rules which are used in **natural phonology** to describe the simplifications made by a child. These processes include:

1. Weak Syllable Deletion. Children omit one or more unstressed syllables

'banana'	[nænæ]
'pyjamas'	[dæmǝd]

2. Final Consonant Deletion. Children produce open syllables by failing to finish words:

'pen'	[pɛ]	'cold'	[ko]
'bib'	[bɪ]	'zip'	[zɪ]
'bath'	[bæ]	'cat'	[kæ]

3. Reduplication. Children repeat the first syllable in the position of the second syllable.

'mummy' [mæmæ]   'kitten' [kɪkɪ]

4. Consonant Harmony. Children make consonants in the word phonetically similar. The **place of articulation** (see **articulation**) changes but the same **voicing** (see **articulation**) distinction is maintained between the **realization** and the **target** sound.

'cup'	[pʌp]	'table'	[pebl]
'duck'	[gʌk]	'kettle'	[kɛkl]
'goat'	[gok]	'cat'	[kæk]

5. Cluster Reduction. Children reduce a group of consonants which begin words:

'smoke'	[mok]	'string'	[srɪŋ]
'skid'	[kɪd]	'splash'	[plæʃ]
'christmas'	[kɪsmǝs]	'scratch'	[skætʃ]

6. Stopping. Children substitute a **stop** for a **fricative** or **affricate** (see **articulation**) and at the same **place of articulation** (see **articulation**).

'fine' [bain] 'church' [tʌt]
'size' [taid] 'jump' [dʌmp]

7. Fronting. Children produce all **velor** sounds at the fornt of the mouth, usually as **alveolar** sounds:

'cat' [taet] 'cake' [tek]/[tet]
'cow' [taʌ] 'key' [ti]

8. Gliding. Children produce the **target liquid** sounds /l,r/ as [w,j].

'lunch' [wʌnʃ] 'red' [wɛd]

9. Context-Sensitive Voicing. Children change the voicing of **obstruents**. Voiced obstruents become voiceless **word-initially** and **word-medially** while voiceless obstruents become voiced **word-finally**.

'fat' [væd] 'cat' [gæd]
'sad' [zæt] 'bid' [pɪt]

See Grunwell (1982): ch. 7.

Phonologist. See **phonology**.

Phonology. The study of the sound systems in any given language. A sound system is a framework which reveals contrasts in sounds and how such contrasts allow for different meanings in a language. The phonologist undertakes such a study. These systems are made up of phonemes, the smallest unit of sound. The phoneme is represented in speech production by the phone. Variations of the phoneme are known as allophones, e.g., the phoneme /p/ can have allophones of /pʰ/ (**aspiration**), /P'/ (**ejective**), etc. When all the allophones are put together, they form a phonemic system or phonemic structure. In English, there are about 44 phonemes. These systems change for every language. *See Hyman (1975); Ladefoged (1975): 23–24; Grunwell (1982): passim.*

Phonotactics. Rules which allow the possible combinations of sounds in any language. The basic syllable in English has the structure **CVC**, i.e., **consonant, vowel, consonant**. Rules exist for the production of two place **consonant clusters**:

(1) where C1 is /s/, C2 must be one of the following /p,t,k,m,n,l,f/

(2) where C2 is one of /w,r,l,j/, C2 may be one of a large number of conson-

ants, predominately obstruents including /p,t,k,b,d,g,f/ etc. (Grunwell, 1982: 23–24)

Phonotactics is useful in speech therapy as the therapist can show the sounds which are not contrasting and in which position of the word or cluster the errors occur:

C1		C2	
[p,b,t,d,f]		[λ]	
'pram' [pλam]		'queen' [tλin]	
'bread' [bλɛd]		'glove' [gλʌv]	
'swing' [sλɪŋ]		'straw' [dλɔ]	

(from Grunwell, 1982: 27)
See Grunwell (1982): 23–29.

Pitch. See **auditory phonetics**.

Place of articulation. See **articulation**.

Plain. A **distinctive feature** proposed by Jakobson and Halle to distinguish sounds which are produced with the mouth open and a high frequency [+ PLAIN] from those produced with the mouth more closed and a low frequency [– PLAIN]. It is opposed to **flat**. *See Hyman (1975): ch. 2.*

Plosive. See **articulation**.

Postvocalic. A description of a **consonant** which follows a **vowel**.

Production. See **articulation**.

Prosody. A general description of the phonological features of **tempo** (see **rate**), rhythm, **loudness** and **pitch**. Prosody and **suprasegmental phonology** are often thought to be the same but the latter describes **paralanguage** and not the other features already given which are the sole preserve of prosody. *See Gimson (1970): 56.*

Pure vowels. **Vowels** which have not been made into **diphthongs**. Most of the vowels in Scottish-English are pure vowels, e.g., /p t/, /m k/, etc. The Scottish-English vowel system is:

i	ɪ	u
e	ʌ	o
ɛ	a	ɔ

ai	ʌu
ʌi	
ɔi	

See Gimson (1970): 39.

Q

Quality. Sounds have a particular quality depending on the **timbre** and **resonance** used in their production. Both **vowels** and **consonants** can be described in this way. Each vowel in the **cardinal vowel** systems can be said to have a different quality. It is opposed to **quantity**. *See Ladefoged (1975): 65–72.*

Quantity. See **length**.

R

Rate. The speed at which people speak. It may also be described as tempo. An analysis of rate is made under **suprasegmental phonology**. This phenomenon can be affected by **dysarthria** (1). *See Gimson (1970): 25.*

Realization. The sounds or words produced by people. The realization is usually different from the **target** (the correct production of a sound). In **articulation delay/disorder** or **phonological delay/disorder** (all 1), it describes the difference between the child's realization and the target sound. It is this difference which is analyzed by the therapist. The aim of treatment for such disorders is to match the realization to the target so the differences disappear. *See Grunwell (1982): 139, 141.*

Received pronunciation. A non-regional **accent** (2) which is used to speak English. All accents are compared to RP. At one time, it was used by well-educated people only; however, it has now gone out of fashion even in the BBC (cf. BBC English). The symbols provided on the **IPA** chart are the pure sounds of RP. *See Gimson (1970): 85–89.*

Reciprocal assimilation. See **assimilation**.

Reduplication. See **phonological processes**.

Register. The way in which people use their **vocal cords** to change the quality of their voice. In speaking, there are different types of register such as breathy, creaky and hoarse voice while in singing there are the different voices such as soprano, tenor, falsetto, etc. These voice changes are caused by changes in the thickness, length and tightness in the vocal cords. *See Catford (1977): 101, 103, 109.*

Regressive assimilation. See **assimilation**.

Release. See **abrupt release** and **delayed release**.

Resonance. A phenomenon found in **acoustic phonetics** to describe the setting in vibration of one structure at the frequency of the other structure which starts off the vibration. This occurs in the **supraglottic** (5) part of the **vocal tract**. It occurs, in particular, when the air particles begin to vibrate in the nasal cavities. These cavities can change shape, increase loudness and frequency at the source of the sound. In disorders of **nasality** (1), the degree of resonance will be increased (**hypernasality**) or reduced (**hyponasality**) (5). *See Catford (1977): 54–56, 138.*

Resonant. A sound produced at the **glottis** (5) without any narrowing of the **vocal tract**, thus letting the sound be produced without any audible friction. Thus, **vowels** and **continuants** without friction are produced in this way. It is opposed to **sonorant**. *See Catford (1977): 121, 124, 125, 127.*

Retract. The movement made to produce **back** sounds by the tongue. This can result in **bunching** and the production of back vowels as well as **velar** (see **articulation**) sounds. *See Catford (1977): ch. 9.*

Retroflex. See **place of articulation**.

Rhythm. See **prosodics**.

Roll. See **articulation**.

Rounding. See **cardinal vowel systems**.

RP. **Received pronunciation**.

S

Schwa. See **neutral**.

Secondary articulation. A sound which is made by the **active articulators** (see **articulation**) coming into contact with the **passive articulators** (see **articulation**) at two places, not just one. The second closure is slightly less than the first. It occurs in a sound such as /w/ where the main closure is at the lips but there is also a slight closure made at the back of the mouth. Thus, /w/ is called a **labio-velar** (see **articulation**). *See Ladefoged (1975): 207–209.*

Segment. See **segmental phonology**.

Segmental phonology. A study of the interaction of **phonemes** (see **phonology**) in any given language. Phonemes are regarded as the segments under study. It is opposed to **supraseg-mental phonology**. *See Hyman (1975): ch. 1.*

Semi-vowels. The sounds subsumed under this term are also known as **approximants** (see **articulation**). They are classified as **consonants** but have a vowel-like quality in that they are produced without closure or friction. The sounds which follow this pattern in English are /j,w/. *See Ladefoged (1975): 205–207.*

Shwa. See **neutral**.

Sibilant. An acoustic description of some **fricative** (see **articulation**) sounds. The fricatives in English are /f,v,s,z,ʃ,ʒ,θ,ð/. Some fricatives are produced with greater acoustic energy and hence a higher pitch. This produces a loud, hissing noise. These fricatives, i.e., /s,z,ʃ,ʒ,/, are sibilants and opposed to the non-sibilants, i.e., /f,v,θ,ð,/. *See Ladefoged (1975): 146.*

Slit. A description of the tongue for producing **fricatives** (see **articulation**). The tongue is flat for the fricatives /f,v,θ,ð,/ while it is **grooved** for the fricatives /s,z/ etc. *See Catford (1977): 127.*

Sonorant. A **major class feature** proposed by Chomsky and Halle to distinguish sounds produced without any blocking of the **vocal tract** [+ SONOR-ANT], i.e., **liquids**, **nasals** (see **articulation**) and **laterals** (see **articulation**), from those which are produced with a block [– SONORANT]. *See Ladefoged (1975): 248.*

Sonority. A phenomenon in **auditory phonetics** which examines **loudness** relative to **pitch**, **stress** and **duration**. *See Ladefoged (1975): 219–220.*

Sound system. See **phonology**.

Source feature. A classification in Chomsky and Halle's **distinctive features**. The others are **major class feature**, cavity features, manner of articulation features and prosodic features. The feature describes the modification which happens to the **airstream** producing **voice** and **strident** sounds. *See Hyman (1975): ch. 2.*

Spectography. The acoustic measurements of sounds. The spectograph was invented in the late 1940s. Every sound consists of **frequencies** with each of these frequencies shown on the spectograph. The graph has a time scale along the horizontal axis while the frequency is measured down the vertical axis. The frequencies show up as light or dark marks depending on their **intensity**. In a typical spectograph, there are dark bands

which are called the **formants** of the sound, usually **vowels**. Each formant is numbered from the bottom of the graph to the top. The bottom formant is F1, the next one is F2 and so on. When voiced sounds are used the spectograph produces vertical lines. *See Ladefoged (1975): 168–191.*

Speech chain. The means by which a speaker transmits information to a listener. The speaker forms an **utterance** (2) by selecting the words and making-up the correct **word-order** (2) in the **brain** (5). This is the **performance** (2) part of the speech chain. These words are sent by nerve impulses along the **vocal tract** uttered by the **articulators** (see **articulation**) whereupon they are transferred into sound waves. These waves are acoustic energy which are sent across the gap between speaker and listener. The latter receives them through his **ear** (6) where they undergo a physiological change in the form of nerve impulses to the brain where they are decoded so that the listener can understand the utterance. Thus, one human can communicate through the medium of speech to another human—a feature of man's existence which raises him above other animal life. In speech therapy, the therapist has often to find out which part of this chain is broken. It may be the nerve impulses going to activate the speaker's **facial muscle** (see **cranial nerves**, 5) and muscles of the **tongue** (5) such as in **dysarthria** (1). It could also be that the patient has difficulty in formulating his utterance either by not finding the word he wants to use or not being able to put them in the correct **word-order** such as in **dysphasia** (both 1) or it may be his feedback system which does not function such as in **hearing loss** (6). When this broken link is found by **assessment**, a **treatment programme** (both 1) can begin to repair it. *See Denes and Pinson (1973): passim.*

Spread. See **cardinal vowel systems**.

Stop. A type of sound which includes **plosives**, **nasals** and **laterals** plus their **allophonic** variations. *See Catford (1977): 213–214.*

Stress. See **suprasegmental phonology**.

Strident. A **distinctive feature** proposed by Chomsky and Halle to distinguish sounds produced with a high **frequency** and **intensity** (see **acoustic phonetics**) as in /f,s,ʃ,ʒ/ [+ STRIDENT] from those produced with low frequency and intensity [– STRIDENT]. It is opposed to non-strident. *See Hyman (1975): ch. 2.*

Suction. A **distinctive feature** proposed by Chomsky and Halle to describe sounds made in a specific way in the **glottis** and **velum** (both 5) such as in **clicks** (see **velaric airstreams**) and **implosives** [+ SUCTION]. *See Hyman (1975): ch. 2.*

Supplementary movements. A classification for **distinctive features** proposed by Chomsky and Halle. They are used to distinguish **manner of articulations** (see **articulation**). The two distinctive features subsumed by this term are **suction** and **pressure** which describe such sounds as **ejectives**, **implosives** and **clicks**. *See Hyman (1975): ch. 2.*

Suprasegmental. See **suprasegmental phonology**.

Suprasegmental phonology. The study of stress and intonation. Stress often marks the difference between verbs and nouns, e.g., re'cord/'record; (') is a stress mark. A speaker's intonation contours are usually described in terms of pitch direction (e.g., fall-rise) and these tones give a contrastive element to the **utterance** (2). The speaker can also vary his pitch range when using these tones. The pitch range could be higher or lower than his average range or widened or narrowed until it becomes a monotone. A tone group is the part of the sentence which contains such changes. In the tone group, there is normally one single syllable which receives a major pitch change—the tonic syllable or nuclear syllable. The direction change of the tonic syllable, also known as the nucleus, is most important in understanding speech since it usually gives information concerning the attitudes of the speaker:

ỳes (falling)	— the answer is 'yes'
ýes (high-rise)	— did you say 'yes'
ⱱes (low-rise)	— please go on I'm listening?
῀yes (fall-rise)	— I'm doubtful
῀yes (rise-fall)	— I'm certain

(based on Ladefoged, 1975: 97). Such tone changes are known as paralanguage. It shows changes in voice depending on the speaker's attitudes or social status or some other language meaning context. Some patients who suffer from **dysarthria** (1) have lost the distinctions used in stress and intonation patterns and so cannot make changes in meaning as in the examples given above. *See Ladefoged (1975): 14–15, 93–103.*

Syllable. A unit of a **word** (2). Each unit can be pronounced as single units as in 'pic-ture'. A syllable has been described as an increase in the speaker's lungs and as being more **sonorous** than other parts of a word. In **phonology**, the syllable is described in terms of **phonotactics**. *See Ladefoged (1975): 217–222.*

T

Tamber. See **timbre**.

Target. A description of the correct production of a sound. It is opposed to **realization**.

Tempo. See **rate**.

Timbre. The ability on the part of the listener to distinguish different characteristics of sound even if the **loudness**, **pitch** and **length** (see **auditory phonetics**) are the same. It is often referred to as quality or tamber. *See Abercrombie (1967): 10–11.*

Timing. The process of moving the **articulators** (see **articulation**) into the correct sequences for producing sounds and making them into words. This can produce important features in **rhythm** (see **prosody**) and other **prosodic features**. *See Clark and Clark (1977): 288–291.*

Tip. See **apex**.

Tone. See **suprasegmental phonology**.

Tone group. See **suprasegmental phonology**.

Tonic syllable. See **suprasegmental phonology**.

Tonicity. See **suprasegmental phonology**.

Transcription systems. Ways in which a person's speech can be represented usually by the symbols on the **IPA** chart. When it is carried out by a speech therapist, it shows which sounds have changed and to what they have changed. There are three types of transcription:

1. Phonemic Transcription, also known as broad transcription, is the easiest of the three systems to use since every sound produced is represented by one symbol. Each symbol represents all

allophonic (see **phonology**) variations.

2. Allophonic Transcription, also known as narrow transcription, is more technical as it requires the representation of all allophonic variations of each **phoneme** (see **phonology**) produced. **Diacritics** should also be used to make the transcription as accurate as possible.

3. Impressionistic Transcription is used for languages which are unknown to the transcriber and he has had to use all his knowledge and skill to represent sounds and devise new ones if the ones on the **IPA** chart are not sufficient for his needs. In speech therapy, (1) and (2) are the most commonly used to transcribe the speech of children suffering from **articulation delay/disorder** or **phonological delay/disorder** (all 1). *See Abercrombie (1967): 127–130.*

Trill. See **articulation**.

U

Uvular. See **articulation**.

V

Velar. See **articulation**.

Velaric airstream. An **airstream** used to produce clicks which are also described as velaric ingressive stops. The sequence of movements for this sound is:

1. raise the back of the tongue to the **velum** (see **velopharyngeal**, 5);

2. press the **tip** (see **apex**) of the tongue hard against the **alveolar ridge** (see **mouth**, 5);

3. pull the tip of the tongue away like a suction pad creating a vacuum and causing air to rush in.

By using this procedure the following clicks are made:

a. tongue-tip click—/7/

b. lateral click—/ʃ/ (as in the 'gee-up' sound for horses)

c. retroflex click—/C/.

In English, clicks are only used to express the speaker's feelings and not linguistically as in such languages as Hottentot in which all three types of clicks are used to produce linguistic meaning. *See Ladefoged (1975): 118–120.*

Vocal cords. The ligaments which vibrate while a person is speaking. It is this vibration which produces the **voice quality** (see **register**) in speech. They are found in the **larynx** (5). The process of producing voice is called **phonation**. They may also be called vocal folds. Any growths or structural damage to the cords can produce **dysphonia**. *See Catford (1977): 20.*

Vocal folds. See **vocal cords**.

Vocal tract. The whole system through which sounds are produced. It begins with an expulsion of air from the **lungs** which moves up through the **trachea** and **larynx** (all 5) in which the **vocal cords** are located. From this point, the air reaches the **mouth** (5) where it is modified by the muscles of the face and **tongue** (5) to produce the required sounds. *See Catford (1977): ch. 1.*

Vocalic. A **major class feature** set up in the **distinctive feature** theory of **phonology**. It distinguishes sounds which are made with a free passage for air through the **vocal tract**. In a **spectograph**, there is a distinct **formant** structure [+ VOCALIC]. *See Hyman (1975): ch. 2.*

Voice onset time. A phenomenon found in the **production** of **bilabial plosive** (see **articulation**) sounds. There is a period of time between the **articulators** (see **articulation**) coming together and then releasing to make the sound. This delay occurs in all plosives except for fully voiced **stops**. Such a gap can be seen in **spectography**. *See Ladefoged (1975): 124–127.*

Voicing. See **articulation**.

Voice quality. See **register**.

VOT.   **Voice onset time**.
Vowel.   See **cardinal vowel systems**.
Vowel system.   Different languages have different vowel systems as have different **dialects** (2) of the same language. For example, in English, there are two major varieties: Scottish-English and **received**

pronunciation. The vowel system for the former can be seen under **pure vowels**. The system used in **RP**, however, is a jumbled mass of **pure vowels** and **diphthongs**. *See Ladefoged (1975)*: *68–70*.

W

Word-initial.   The description of a sound which occurs at the beginning of a word. For example, in the word /bɪn/('bin') the sound /b/ is said to appear word-initially.
Word-medial.   The description of a sound occurring in the middle of the word. For example, in the word /bʌtər/

('butter'), the sound /t/ is said to appear word-medially.
Word-final.   The description of a sound which occurs at the end of a word. For example, in the word /buk/ ('book'), the sound /k/ is said to appear word-finally.

REFERENCES

Abercrombie, D. (1967). *Elements of General Phonetics*. Edinburgh University Press.
Brosnahan, L. F. and Malmberg, B. (1976). *Introduction to Phonetics*. Cambridge University Press.
Catford, J. C. (1977). *Fundamental Problems in Phonetics*. Edinburgh University Press.
Clark, H. H. and Clark, E. V. (1977). *Psychology and Language: An Introduction to Psycholinguistics*. Harcourt, Brace, Jovanovich.
Cruttenden, A. (1972). 'Phonological Procedures for Child Language'. In *The British Journal of Disorders of Communication*, 7, pp. 30–37.
Denes, P. B. and Pinson, E. N. (1973). *The Speech Chain: The Physics and Biology of Spoken Language*. Anchor.
Fry, D. B. (1979). *The Physics of Speech*. Cambridge University Press.
Gimson, A. C. (1970). *An Introduction to the Pronunciation of English*. Edward Arnold.
Grunwell, P. (1982). *Clinical Phonology*. Croom Helm.
Hyman, L. M. (1975). *Phonology, Theory and Analysis*. Holt, Rinehart and Winston.
Ladefoged, P. (1962). *Elements of Acoustic Phonetics*. Chicago University Press.
Ladefoged, P. (1975). *A Course in Phonetics*. Harcourt, Brace, Jovanovich.

Section 4
Psychology/Psychiatry

A

Aberrant. A description of behaviour which is found to be **abnormal**.

Ability. See **intelligence**.

Ability tests. See **intelligence tests**.

Abnormal behaviour. Behaviour which can also be described as being **aberrant**. Such behaviour is found in those suffering from conditions such as **schizophrenia**, **affective disorders**, **anxiety disorders**, **personality disorders** and drug dependency. Treatment is usually provided by **behaviour therapy** and **psychoanalysis** although some disorders can be improved through drug therapy. *See Atkinson et al. (1983): ch. 15.*

Abreaction. See **psychoanalysis**.

Accommodation. See **assimilation**.

Adaptation. See **assimilation**.

Affective disorders. A group of disorders which produce abnormal moods in a patient (e.g., **depression** and **manic-depression**). *See Atkinson et al. (1983): 463–470.*

Age equivalent scores. Scores which are obtained after working out the results of **assessments** (1) by looking up tables in the manuals of the assessments concerned. Such tests have undergone **standardization** and so these scores can be compared to the **chronological age** of the patient.

Ageing. A description of changes which take place as a person becomes older.

1. Physical changes

The skeleton shrinks, voluntary muscles lose their elasticity, bones become brittle and the skin becomes wrinkled. There are problems in taking food as well as problems found in excreting it. Perception becomes less efficient with visual and **hearing losses** (6) appearing. Problems occur in breathing and there is poor blood circulation.

2. Psychological changes

Changes occur in the intellectual capacities of the person although this is difficult to show. Verbal scores, vocabulary and reasoning do not decrease. Terminal drop occurs in a period before death when physical and psychological functions drop off suddenly. Thus, towards death decline is sudden rather than gradual.

3. Memory changes

Those suffering from **senile dementia** (see **Alzheimer's disease**) have a definite memory loss. In general, however, problems occur more with material which requires organization and material requiring full attention to retain it.

Research has shown ageing producing different reactions among people. Neugarten *et al.* (1963) in Bromley (1974) have shown the following:

1. Reorganizer—one who substitutes other activities for lost activities;

2. Focused—one who is selective in choosing new activities;

3. Disengaged—one who withdraws voluntarily from former activities;

4. Holding-on—one who is trying to put aside anxiety about old age;

5. Constricted—one who avoids any threats from outside but withdraws increasingly from the world;

6. Individual—one who is prepared to be looked after in all aspects of daily life;

7. Apathetic—one who has become disengaged from life although probably was like this for most of his life. He has little ability to cope;

8. Disorganized—one who is low in activity and poor on general psychological functioning.

In a study of 87 old men, Reichard (1962) in Bromley (1974) produced five different categories:

1. Mature man—accepting of old age having no regrets concerning the past or present;

2. Rocking chair man—may have been passive during life but following retirement is happy to see life pass by;

3. Armoured man—rejects ageing, so takes up several activities to retain interest in life;

4. Angry man—feels he has failed in what he set out to do in life and blames this failure on society. Thus, becoming old is the last straw;

5. Self-hater—turns his anger of becoming old in on himself and belongs to the group most likely to suffer from **depression**.

Davison and Neale summed up growing old as: '...the greatest challenge of old people is to cope with reality, the gradual loss of loved ones and friends, the deterioration of physical and psychological capacities, the low regard in which they are held by the culture at large' (Davison and Neale, 1982: ch. 17). *See Bromley (1974).*

Aggression. The reaction of some to particular life situations (e.g., frustration). This phenomenon may result from learned behaviour from their in-born personality or surrounding environment. *See Atkinson et al. (1983): 427–428.*

Alternate hypothesis. This hypothesis must be proved by statistical analysis if the experiment is to be worthwhile. This hypothesis states that a significant difference between scores does exist if it is proven by carrying out a **parametric** or non-**parametric test**. The alternate hypothesis will be proved if the **null hypothesis** is rejected. Both hypotheses are used in **inferential statistics**. The alternate hypothesis is also known as the **experimental hypothesis**. *See Miller (1975): 58–59.*

Alzheimer's disease. In general, occurring after the age of 65 years it is more commonly called senile dementia, but it is called Alzheimer's disease before 65 years of age. Both are regarded as having similar symptoms. These consist of a gradual loss of **short-term memory** which becomes worse while **long-term memory** (for both see **memory**) is retained intact until the later stages of the dementia. A change in **personality** also occurs, e.g., quiet people become aggressive with outbursts of rage, etc, as do transient **hemiplegias** (5). Women are affected twice as frequently as men and death can occur two to five years after the original onset. *See Stafford-Clark and Smith (1983): 72–73.*

Amitriptyline. The commonest used **antidepressant** drug. Its side-effects are dry mouth, palpitation, tachycardia, postural hypotension, dizziness, constipation, vomiting, glaucoma, loss of accommodation (i.e., eye problem with focusing) and urinary problems. *See Stafford-Clark and Smith (1983): 117.*

Anal stage. See **psychosexual stages of development**.

Antidepressant drugs. Tricyclic drugs given to treat those who suffer from **endogenous depression** (see **depression**). The depressive illness begins to improve after ten days to two weeks but it may take ten to twelve weeks for the drugs to be most effective.

The anti-depressant drugs used are:

Amitriptyline	Protryptiline
Imipramine	Dothiepin
Clomipramine	Trimipramine
Noritryptiline	Doxepin

The side-effects are similar to those of **amitriptyline**. *See Stafford-Clark and Smith (1983): 117–118.*

Anxiety. A neurotic disorder (see **neurosis**). Abnormal anxiety is caused by acute fear which is often irrational and produces feelings of panic in the patient. A sufferer of such irrational anxieties may show some of the following features. In some patients, anxiety may dominate their mental condition, some may have physical symptoms such as tachycardia, i.e., abnormal rhythm of the **heart** (5), restlessness, sleeplessness and sweating, etc. while others are so overcome with anxiety and fear they may suffer from choking, suffocation and near collapse. **Hypochondriasis** is quite common. Treatment is given by **psychotherapy**, relaxation, drugs (see **anxiety drug treatment**), **behaviour therapy**, **occupational therapy** (5) and through self-help groups. Acute anxiety can be treated successfully by these methods unless the patient produces secondary symptoms of **depression** and **hysteria**. *See Stafford-Clark and Smith (1983): 128–138.*

Anxiety disorders. A group of disorders which produces **abnormal behaviour**. The main symptom is **anxiety** or anxiety-producing **phobias** or **obsessive-compulsive behaviours**. *See Atkinson et al. (1983): ch. 15.*

Anxiety drug treatment. The main drug used is Benzodiazepine. It acts partly on the **brain** (5) and partly by decreasing the activity of the spinal reflex centres. The drugs which take a long time to act are:

Diazepam	Chlordiazpoxide
Meduzepam	Clorazepate
Oxazepam	

The main side-effect of these drugs is drowsiness. They should not be taken with alcohol or when driving. The drugs which take a short time to act are:

Lorazepam
Temazepam
Triazolan

These drugs are used with old people and can produce problems with the kidneys. The drug is taken at night so that the patient can be fully aware of what is happening during the day. The only problem with such drugs is a growing dependence on them and so the patient will become unreceptive to other non-medication forms of therapy. Other drugs used in the treatment of anxiety are **monoamine oxidase inhibitors** and tricyclic **antidepressant drugs**. Beta-blocking drugs can also be given to reduce an abnormally fast heartbeat and for sedation during the night. *See Stafford-Clark and Smith (1983): 135–136.*

Anxiety hierarchy. See **systematic desensitization**.

Apathy. A reaction of certain people to various situations (e.g., frustration). They withdraw and become indifferent to certain situations while others react with **aggression** to similar situations. It is uncertain why this should happen but it may be learned behaviour or their in-born personality or due to their surrounding environment. *See Atkinson et al. (1983): 428–429.*

Assertive training. A form of treatment given during **social skills** training. It exists for those who allow themselves to be dominated either, in the case of children, by younger children, or, in the case of older people, by those with less authority. Such people are placed in situations in which they have to assert themselves either gradually, by giving step-by-step training or very quickly by placing the person in the situation and not allowing them to leave the situation until they show themselves to be sufficiently assertive. *See Trower et al. (1978): 82–85.*

Assimilation. A phenomenon proposed by **Piaget** to explain the development of the child's ability to 'understand'. He introduced the notion of schema or schemata which are 'well-defined sequences of actions...their chief characteristic, whatever their nature or complexity, is that they are organised wholes which are frequently repeated and which can be recognised easily among other diverse and varying behaviours' (Beard, 1969: 3). Assimilation occurs when the child brings new experiences into schemas which already exist. Accommodation occurs when a child has to work out a response to a new experience which allows him to modify his schema continually. Eventually the child can organize all this information into a whole and so one schema can be subordinated to another. Piaget called assimilation, accommodation and organization invariant functions. There are three types of assimilation:

1. Reproductive—the child assimilates an experience to a schema but cannot fit it into an organization, so keeps assimilating the experience getting nowhere.

2. Generalization—the child begins to extend the range of objects or experiences to a schema.

3. Recognitory—as the child generalizes his range of objects into a schema, he realizes he has to accommodate certain actions to the object, e.g., there is only one way to hold a cup. *See Beard (1969): 3–7.*

Attachment. The way in which children bond with their parents, usually their mother or the person who provides the initial care and security. Thus, children tend to explore unknown environments when this person is with them. It has been suggested that a failure to develop such bonding may lead to the failure of making close personal relationships in later life. Erikson (1963) suggested eight stages of psychosocial development which people go through from birth to old age. He believed a person's psychological development depended on the kinds of social relations made at various times in life but each relationship had problems which had to be faced. His stages were:

1. trust vs mistrust (1 year old) affecting the relationship between mother or the primary caregiver. If the relationship is successful the child will have trust in the person.

2. autonomy vs doubt (2 year old) affecting the relationship with his parents. The child tries to do things himself (i.e., 'me do it') in safety. If this relationship is successfully formed, the child will have gained in self-control.

3. initiative vs guilt (3–5 years) affecting the relationship with the family unit. The child initiates various activities but the reaction of the parents can lead to feelings of guilt especially if they deprecate what the child has done as being shameful.

4. industry vs inferiority (6 years-puberty) affecting the relationship with the environment (i.e., peer group, neighbours, school, etc). The child sets out to socialize in different situations but can be made to feel inferior if such efforts fail.

5. identity vs confusion (adolescence) when the child tries to form his own identity. This can involve the growing away from the authority of the parents and doing what they think is best. Actions become dictated by the peer group rather than the parents. At times, this conflict can produce confusion.

6. intimacy vs isolation (early adulthood) is a stage in which the person

forms a close personal relationship which may lead to marriage. Those who cannot make such a relationship will be isolated and less happy than those who can form an intimate relationship.

7. generativity vs self-absorption (middle adulthood) is a stage in which the person takes pleasure in preparing teenagers for adulthood. If the person cannot do this, he becomes introverted and does not care about others.

8. integrity vs despair (after 65 years) is a stage during which the person looks back at his past life. If he is happy with the way in which he has coped with life's problems he can face the future with integrity, while if he regrets what has happened in his life, he will face the future in despair. *See Atkinson et al.* (1983): 74–80, 96–99.

Autism. A **childhood psychosis**. It is a syndrome characterized by a severe failure to develop social relationships, language retardation with **echolalia** (1), lack of **comprehension** (1) and various ritualistic and stereotyped phenomena. Most of these characteristics develop before 2½ years of age. It affects two in 10,000 children, three-quarters of whom require **special education**.

1. Poor social relationships
Children suffering from autism do not cling to their mothers in strange situations as unaffected children do; they treat people like objects and other children like toys; they have little warmth and behave in strange ways; they fail to make personal friendships; they spend very little time playing and behave with a lack of social propriety toward their peers.

2. Speech and language problems
These include 'I/you reversal', robotic voice and **flattening of affect**; **language delay/disorder** (1) (only about half the children suffering from autism acquire language normally); lack of **imitation** (2); **delayed echolalia** (1); use of platitudes; understanding only concrete instructions and having extreme idiosyncrasy in their language.

3. Ritualistic and stereotyped phenomena.
Stereotypical play is found quite commonly, e.g., twirling things around. They are fascinated by what most people find peripheral, and use a facsimile of normal speech while insisting on doing things as they have always done them.

There is uncertainty as to the cause of autism. It may arise from some difficulty in forming a relationship with the natural mother. Young autistic children are more sluggish at sucking, tend not to smile, may not respond to the human voice and are undemanding. While not completely rejecting environmental causes, investigations are being made into organic causes of autism. Researchers are looking for possible brain pathologies such as **encephalitis** (5) in early years, complications from **rubella** (5) passed to the child by the mother during pregnancy, **tuberose sclerosis** (5), untreated **phenylketonuria** (5), infantile spasms (severe epileptic attacks during first year) and complications in the **perinatal stage** (5). These causes have been found in one-third of children suffering from autism. Another possible cause could be linked to the site of lesion in the **brain** (5), but no conclusive evidence has been provided although sites such as the **dominant** hemisphere (see **dominance**, 5), **reticular system** (5), **basal ganglia** (5) have been proposed. Finally, the reasons for the difference in psychological behaviour of the autistic and non-autistic child may lead to a possible cause being discovered. However, the most likely outcome of all this research will be to provide a group of interrelated causes and not just one cause for autism.

Treatment is aimed at improving the child's socialization and providing him with socially acceptable behaviour. Such treatment is aimed at removing the child's 'self-encapsulation in an isolated world' (Jaspers, K., 1963 in Wolff, S., 1981). *See Wolff (1981): 174–178; Wing (1980)*.

Autonomy vs doubt. See **attachment**.

B

Bar chart. See **histogram**.
Beck's cognitive therapy. An approach to producing acceptable behaviour by

treating the person's thought processes. Beck provided therapy which was aimed at making patients aware of their thinking processes, teaching them to recognize maladaptive thoughts in various situations, producing more normal thought patterns for such situations and, having accomplished this, the therapist gives praise and reinforcement to cognitive and behaviour changes during therapy. *See Rachman and Wilson (1980): 220–223.*

Behaviour modification. See **behaviour therapy**.

Behaviour therapy. Aims at the modification of **abnormal** patterns of behaviour which have not a medical origin. It is sometimes called the two-factor model of learning as it consists of two learning procedures—**classical conditioning** and **operant conditioning**. In the former several behaviour therapies have been evolved such as **systematic desensitization, flooding, modelling** and **assertive training**, while in the latter the behaviour therapies of **individual conditioning paradigms** and **token economies** have evolved. Behaviour therapy occurs also in the form of cognitive behaviour therapies such as **rational emotive therapy** (Ellis), **self-instructional training** (Meichenbaum) and **Beck's cognitive therapy**. Sjode *et al.* described the most important aspect of behaviour therapy as: 'being task-specific rather than based on personality the therapist has respect for the client as a learning, striving and a coping person who is not sick but will benefit from guided experiences in dealing with particular specified situations' (Sjode *et al.,* 1979). *See Atkinson et al. (1983): ch. 7.*

Binet. Alfred Binet (1857–1911) believed a child who was slow in learning was similar to a 'normal' child except for some retardation in his mental development. The French Government in 1881 passed a law that all children should go to school including those with learning difficulties. Binet was approached to provide a test to find out the children who required **special education**. Thus, the first of the **Stanford-Binet intelligence scales** was produced. *See Atkinson et al. (1983): 356.*

Bipolar disorder. See **depression**.

British Ability Scales. An extensive battery of tests for assessing general cognitive abilities. It produces **IQ** scores and a detailed profile of the child's cognitive abilities in 23 areas of cognitive development. These 23 areas are organized into six major process areas:

1. speed of information processing
2. reasoning
3. spatial imagery
4. perceptual matching
5. short-term memory
6. retrieval and application of knowledge.

The test can be administered in separate parts to children in the age range 2½–17½ years. *See British Ability Scales test manuals.*

C

CA. Chronological age.

Capgras syndrome. A **neurotic** syndrome. The patient suffers from a **delusion** that a close relative has been replaced by his/her double. It is usually part of **schizophrenia**.

Carbon monoxide poisoning. See **Wernicke-Korsakoff syndrome**.

Central tendency. A method of finding out the distribution of scores received from experiments. There are three such measures:

1. Mean—the sum of scores of each person tested, divided by the number of people who took part in the experiment;

2. Mode—the most frequently occurring score in the experiment;

3. Median—the middle score after all the scores have been put in order.

If all these measures are the same, i.e.,

mean = mode = median, it is called a symmetrical or **normal distribution** of scores and can be shown as such on a graph. If the scores diverge they are said to be **skewed** and again can be shown in graph form. *See Miller (1975): 36–40.*

Chi square. Chi square (χ^2) is one of several tests which can be carried out on the data obtained from single subjects. The data are set out in the form of a contingency table. The test allows the experimenter to discover if there is a relationship between the subject variable and the response variable. In speech therapy, this test could be useful when analyzing the results of an **assessment** (1) statistically. For example, if the child suffers from **mental handicap**, the effect of his expressive and/or comprehension disability could be compared to the scores from observation. So, chi square assesses the differences between the observed distribution of scores and the expected distribution of scores. *See Miller (1975): 85–90.*

Childhood onset pervasive developmental disorder. A new name given in the United States to try and avoid confusion with **childhood schizophrenia**. It was put forward in the *Diagnostic and Statistical Manual of Mental Disorders*, 3rd edition (abbreviated to DSM-III), and is supported by many mental health professionals in the US. The condition differs from schizophrenia as it does not include **delusions**, **hallucinations** or **thought disorders** as symptoms. However, children who are diagnosed as suffering from it show difficulties in forming social relationships and produce odd facets to their behaviour. *See Davison and Neale (1982): 509.*

Childhood psychoses. A group of different disorders with a prevalence of 0.04 per cent. The commonest form of childhood psychosis is **autism**. Less common childhood psychoses are childhood schizophrenia (cf. **childhood onset pervasive developmental disorder**) which produces **auditory hallucinations** (see **hallucinations**) and confusion with accompanying mood disturbances, **flattening of affect**, mannerisms and grimacing while the child's **IQ** is usually within normal limits; disintegrative psychoses in which the child develops normally until 3–4 years of age after which there is a sudden loss of skills as well as of **expressive language** (1) and their behaviour regresses; **manic-depressive psychoses** which are very rare before puberty. *See Davison and Neale (1982): 73–74, 509.*

Childhood schizophrenia. See **childhood psychoses**.

Chlorpromazine. A drug for treating **manic-depression** (see also **phenothiazines**).

Chronological age. The natural age of a child or adult. It is used in assessments carried out by speech therapists and psychologists. The child's **CA** can be compared to the **age equivalent score** obtained in any of these assessments. **CA** is also used by psychologists in the formula to work out an **IQ**.

Classical conditioning. A learning procedure used in **behaviour therapy**. It is based on the theory first proposed by Pavlov in his experiments with dogs. He found the dogs could learn a conditioned response (**CR**). He based his theory on the fact that people can learn certain reactions by giving an unconditioned response (**UR**) to an unconditioned stimulus (**US**). His experiments were aimed at finding out if a conditioned response (**CR**) could be learnt from a conditioned stimulus (**CS**). For example, Pavlov found that dogs salivated (**UR**) when they smelled or tasted meat (**US**). Pavlov switched on a light when the dogs were given the meat (**CS**—dogs learn light is only on when given meat) and the dogs salivated (**UR**). However, he found that if the light were switched on, the dogs still salivated (**CR**—as they had been conditioned to salivate at the meat when the lights were on).

There are three stages in learning a conditioned response to a conditioned stimulus starting from an unconditioned stimulus:

1. Simultaneous conditioning occurs when both the light (**CS**) and the meat (**US**) are presented together, thus making the dogs salivate (**UR**);

2. Delayed conditioning occurs when the light (**CS**) is switched on for a few seconds before the meat (**US**) is given to the dogs and is left switched on until the dogs salivate;

3. Trace conditioning occurs when the light (**US**) is switched on, then switched off before the meat (**US**) is given so that only a 'memory trace' of the light remains for the conditioning process to take place. By repetition of placing the **CS** next to the **US**, the association of the two is reinforced. If reinforcement does not take place, extinction of the **CR** may take place. *See Atkinson et al. (1983): 194–199.*

Clinical psychology. A clinical psychologist assesses and treats **emotional** and **behaviour disorders** which occur among the mentally and physically handicapped, juvenile delinquents, drug addicts and in families where relationships have broken down. Such psychologists work in hospitals with inpatients and in out-patient clinics and prisons. *See MacKay (1975): 60–80.*

Cognitive behaviour therapy. See **behaviour therapy**.

Compulsion neurosis. See **obsessive-compulsion neurosis**.

Compulsive rituals. See **autism**.

Concrete operations. The third stage of **Piaget's** theory of the child's cognitive development during the 7–11 year period, having overcome the difficulties found during the **pre-operational stage**. The child's thought processes are now becoming more logical but he can still only understand relationships directly perceived by him (i.e., the child cannot yet think abstractly). During this stage the child can work out **hierarchies** (2) of classes and subclasses and the child can also place shapes in order by size without measuring them. *See Beard (1969): ch. 5.*

Conditioned response. See **classical conditioning**.

Conditioned stimulus. See **classical conditioning**.

Conduct disorder. Persistent socially disapproved behaviour associated with social impairment. The prevalence is 3–9 per cent of school age children. Conduct disorders are commoner in boys 4:1, they can result in reading difficulties and most children thus affected come from social classes IV and V. The causes arise from the child's experience of life, family factors, e.g., persistent conflict, divorce, etc., social factors, e.g., poor housing, educational factors, e.g., one-third of these children have learning difficulties, especially with reading, and temperament, e.g., unpredictable, irritable children. The commonest symptoms include fighting and bullying, aggression and temper tantrums, defiance and disobedience, destructiveness, lying, stealing, truancy, fire setting and arson. The major types of conduct disorders include:

1. Socialized conduct disorder which affects children who have failed to acquire socially approved standards of behaviour. However, within the family they can often form warm relationships and are described as 'likeable rogues'.

2. Unsocialized conduct disorder is more severe as these children form poor peer relationships, they are frequently self-destructive, aggressive and seem keen to be punished. Family life is always discordant, discipline harsh and little affection is shown to the children who thus experience rejection.

3. Mixed conduct and emotional disorder is recognized in children who are indifferent to distress, resulting in abnormal behaviour. Many children with a conduct disorder are restless and overactive for a short period of time but a small number are extremely and persistently overactive. Such children have problems from an early age. All **psychotherapies** can be used to treat this condition. *See Rutter (1975): ch. 7.*

Conservation. See **pre-operational stage**.

Control condition. See **control group**.

Control group. When an experiment is carried out, there have to be at least two groups of subjects—the **experimental group** and the control group. The latter is regarded as the group of 'normal' subjects against which the performance of the experimental group will be compared. Control groups and experimental groups are used in **independent group designs**. This is also called the control condition. *See Miller (1975): 27.*

Conversion reaction. The sudden impairment of muscular and sensory functions associated with psychological factors. The arms and legs can become weak, blindness can occur and those affected no longer feel pain although they are physiologically normal as well as **dysphonia** (1). The effects of a stress-provoking situation produce these symptoms or a nervous reaction following a long period of excitement which suddenly ends. *See Davison and Neale (1982): 179–180; Fawcus (1986) (for conversion reaction and dysphonia).*

Correlation. The statistical relationship of two variables. It has the symbol 'r' to show the correlation. The range of correlation is from 0 to 1. The nearer to the value of '1', the nearer is the correlation between the two variables. *See Miller (1975): 102–107.*

Counterbalancing. A process used in the **repeated measures design** in which the two groups are tested under the same conditions. If the two groups were to carry out both conditions in the same order, the results could be affected by their feelings of tiredness, etc. Thus, the subjects are split in half and each carries out both conditions separately and then they change over.

CR. Conditioned response.

CS. Conditioned stimulus.

Cushing's disease. See **depression**.

D

Death instinct. See **psychoanalysis**.
Degrees of freedom. See **T-test**.

Delayed conditioning. See **classical conditioning**.

Delusion. False, unreasonable beliefs which the patient holds and will not waver from under any amount of reasoned argument. Of course, what is deemed to be reasonable and unreasonable depends on the culture in which the patient lives. These are often called primary delusions. When suffering from secondary delusions, the patients follow a similar pattern but they try to find a reasonable explanation for other abnormal experiences such as **hallucinations**, **illusions**, etc. *See Stafford-Clark and Smith (1983): 29–30.*

Dementia. The global loss of intellectual function affecting **intelligence**, learning, **memory**, motor skills and **social skills**. Its progress is slow but inexorable. The prevalence of dementia is 5 per cent of people by 65 years of age and 15–20 per cent of people by the age of 80 years. It can occur in children though rarely. The main types of dementia are **Alzheimer's disease/senile dementia**, **multi-infarct dementia**, **Pick's disease**, **Huntington's chorea**, **Jacob-Creuzfelt disease**, **normal pressure hydrocephalus** and **Wernicke-Korsakoff syndrome**. (See also 1 and 5.) *See Stafford-Clark and Smith (1983): 71–81.*

Depression. An **affective disorder**. Its precise cause is unknown but it is thought it could be a combination of factors with one or two being more prominent than the others including genetic, sex, life stress, biochemical as well as cognitive problems. It affects three areas —mood, response to stimulation and functioning of the **autonomic nervous system** (5). These problems have all been summed up succinctly by Stafford-Clark: 'Unable to sleep, to eat, to work efficiently, to hope or to enjoy any of the simple pleasures of life, he may all too often despair of this plight, to die may then seem to him to be all that is left' (Stafford-Clark, 1983: 107). There are three types of depression:

1. Simple/minor depression taking the form of a general slowing down in activity with people feeling sad, miserable, and worried resulting in a loss of interest in everyday activities. It does not appear as a medical problem.

2. Endogenous/major depression is much more serious. Sufferers have a permanently depressed mood, have feelings of hopelessness, helplessness, worthlessness, poor sleep and appetite regimes due to **anxiety**.

3. Psychotic depression characterized mainly by **delusions** plus a severely depressed mood, severe weight loss and a high risk of suicide. It is a very treatable condition. Psychotic depression has as a contributory factor Cushing's disease which is a disorder of the adrenal glands producing an abnormal amount of cortisol. Depression in itself is a unipolar disorder while **manic-depression** is a bipolar disorder. Depression can be treated by tricyclic **antidepressant drugs, monoamine oxidase inhibitors, ECT, psychosurgery, lithium** and **psychotherapy**. *See Stafford-Clark and Smith (1983): 101–113, 116–122.*

Descriptive statistics. A part of **statistics** which analyzes the scores obtained from experiments using bar charts, **histograms, measures of central tendency, standard deviation, percentile scores** and **Z scores**. *See Miller (1975): 27–53.*

Deviation. See **abnormal behaviour**. See **standard deviation**.

E

ECT. **Electroconvulsive therapy**.

Educational psychology. An educational psychologist assesses and treats children in school who suffer from learning difficulties (e.g., reading problems, **developmental dyslexia** (1) or **emotional disorders** (e.g., **elective mutism, autism**, etc.) or **conduct disorders**. They are also involved in **special education**. They counsel parents and teachers as well as other professionals about the causes of the child's problems at school. *See Atkinson et al. (1983): 17.*

Ego. See **personality**.

Egocentricity. See **pre-operational stage**.

Egocentric speech. See **pre-operational stage**.

Elective mutism. A condition in which a child chooses not to speak in certain situations, most commonly at school. However, although he may not speak at school, he will probably speak at home. He may also speak to members of his class outside school but refuse to speak to the same children in school. In very severe cases, the child refuses to speak at all, at home, school and elsewhere. The incidence is 8 : 10,000 children with the sexes being equally affected. There are several possible causes for this condition including **separation anxiety, sibling rivalry**, overprotective mothers, family history of mental disease, and severe **neurosis** or **depression**. It may also be because of an **articulation** or **phonological** problem (1), for which the child has been teased and mocked since he first spoke at school. Such behaviour by other children may force the child to decide to stop trying to speak in school. Reinforcement can occur if other children or parents speak about the condition in front of the child to the teacher or therapist. It is an **emotional disorder** which, for some children, takes the form of shyness when the child starts school. The child requires time to adapt to school life and after a few weeks this shyness will disappear. For other children, the problem is more severe and can become a lasting disorder revealing an **abnormal** temperament which appears as **apathetic** (see **apathy**), morose, unprepossessing, withdrawn, timid, anxious or fearful. Since it results in a **communication disorder** (1), it can be treated by a speech therapist as long as it is recognized that there may very probably be underlying psychological factors. **Psychotherapy** in the form of **behaviour therapy** or **psychoanalysis** has been successful with such children. *See Rutter (1975): 224–227.*

Electroconvulsive therapy. Used with patients suffering from **depression**. Most patients are given a low electrical current to the non-dominant **cerebral hemisphere** (5) (see also **dominance**, 5) which is intended to relieve any confused state after the treatment is finished. It is just as effective if given unilaterally or bilaterally. During the treatment, some of the muscles, e.g., facial muscles, give a slight tremor but there are no other physical movements or effects during therapy. The patient is anaesthetized intravenously by succinyl choline or suxamethonium. After the session has ended, the patient's normal breathing has been restored and he has regained full consciousness, he cannot remember anything of the treatment although his memory of what occurred prior to treatment is intact. Treatments are usually in the frequency of once or twice per week. The number of treatments for severe **depression** is six to twelve if **ECT** is provided bilaterally and increases to up to 20 treatments if provided unilaterally. **ECT** is not sufficient in itself to help the patient recover from depression. Psychotherapy is also required. In fact, it has been found that both forms of treatment working at the same time provide the most beneficial treatment programme for such a patient. *See Stafford-Clark and Smith (1983): 120–123.*

Emotional disorders. Found in children suffering from **depression** or **anxiety**. Both these factors have **obsessional** (see **obsessive-compulsive disorders**), **phobic** (see **phobias**) and **psychosomatic** symptoms. The prevalence rate is $2\frac{1}{2} - 5\frac{1}{2}$ per cent of all children with an equal incidence between the sexes although as children grow older there is a gradual increase in the number of female children affected. It is unlikely that there is one sole cause for emotional disorders but rather several intermingled such as **separation anxiety**, developmental **fears and phobias** (see **fears and phobias in pre-school children**), developmental rituals (see **autism**), etc., life events producing **stress**, e.g., loss, overwhelming traumatic events; family influences involving unconscious conflict and the use of defence mechanisms, e.g., **id** vs **ego, sibling rivalry, Oedipal conflict**, etc. **Psychotherapy** has been shown to be useful in treating these disorders. *See Rutter (1975): ch. 6.*

Encounter groups. A form of **sensitivity training** used with those who lack **social skills**. The members of the group pair-off and spend about one minute telling each other the most important facts about themselves, followed by two things of which they are proud and two things of which they are ashamed. *See Trower et al. (1978): 92–93.*

Endogenous depression. See **depression**.

Experimental hypothesis. See **alternate hypothesis**.

Extinction. See **classical conditioning**.

F

Factor analysis. See **trait approach**.

Fears and phobias in pre-school children. Causes of **emotional disorder** which can affect young children. At the age of 2 years, children can be afraid of ghosts, witches and the supernatural which they hear about in fairy stories; at about 3 years of age, they have a fear of small animals which may turn into a fear of any size of animal or anything furry, while at the age of 4 years, they become often self-conscious and have feelings which make them frightened. They may also have the fear of losing someone close to them, e.g., a parent, especially after the death of one parent or close relative, or they may even fear that they themselves may die. Similarly, after a divorce in the family, they may become very frightened that the other parent will disappear. If the family has to move house, the child may have a fear of leaving his friends and having to make new friends. All such fears become phobias when they become extreme and begin to interfere with the everyday life of the child. For example, a phobia of the dark may arise because the child has been shut in a cupboard either accidentally or intentionally. As the child is so vulnerable at this age to such events, his most fearful symptom, i.e., in this case fear of the dark, becomes a phobia. Such phobias may even be reinforced by parents who agree with the phobia because they are frightened by the same stimulus. Thus, children learn to be phobic because the parent is phobic about similar things, e.g., mice. Children do have their own devices for dealing with fears and phobias. Some follow ritualistic routines, e.g., walking on the lines of the pavement, so that they will not be harmed, or they have favourite toys or objects, e.g., safety blanket, they believe will keep them safe. **Behaviour therapy** has been successfully used with such a disorder. *See Rutter (1975): 219–227.*

Fear thermometer. See **systematic desensitization**.

Flattening of affect. A phenomenon found in **schizophrenia** in which the patient fails to produce an emotional response to almost any stimulus. The patient stares into empty space and there is weakness in facial muscles. The voice shows no **prosodic features** (see **prosody**, 3). *See Davison and Neale (1982): 402.*

Flooding. A therapeutic technique devised by Stomfl and Lewis (1967) used in **behaviour therapy**. The patient is placed in his most feared situation. It is opposed to **systematic desensitization**. Some patients recover faster under flooding although it can be highly traumatic for the client. *See Purser (1982): 291.*

Formal operations. The final stage of cognitive development as proposed by **Piaget**. It begins about 11 years of age, when the child can understand abstract relationships and may begin to think in terms of possibilities. He will use hypothetico-deductive reasoning for working out these possibilities. This is probably the least controversial part of Piaget's theory as it is a familiar thought process for most people in everyday life. *See Beard (1969): ch. 6.*

Free association. A part of **psychoanalysis**. The patient is encouraged to say everything which is in his mind however irrelevant, shameful or stupid it may seem. If the patient stops or hesitates, it is assumed by the therapist that the client is hiding some sensitive information which is worth further investigation. It was first used by Freud. *See Atkinson et al. (1983): 497–498.*

Freud. See **psychoanalysis** and **personality**.

Functional analysis. See **operant conditioning**.

G

Generativity vs **self-absorption.** See **attachment**.

Genital stage. See **psychosexual stages of development**.

Gilles de la Tourette syndrome. A particularly rare **neurotic syndrome**. It takes the form of obscene language, violent vocalizations and motor **tics**. These symptoms usually appear altogether. The condition begins before 12 years of age (75 per cent of cases) or before 20 years (96 per cent of cases). The incidence is 2 : 1 in favour of males. It can be a life-long illness although antipsychotic drugs, e.g., haloperidol, can suppress the obscene language and odd motor tics. *See Davison and Neale (1982): 481–482.*

Group design. A design used for experiments. It is opposed to **single case studies** where statistical analysis attempts to show the effects of variables on single people. On the other hand, the group design is aimed at showing the effects of variables on groups of subjects which are either put into **independent group designs, repeated measures** and **matched subjects design.** *See Miller (1975): 17–22.*

H

Hallucination. The person believes by using his senses there is something there when there is nothing there. It has a quality of reality for him. Auditory hallucination occurs when the person believes he hears a sound when none exists. Hallucinations occur in **schizophrenia** when patients believe they sense audible thoughts, voices arguing and commenting. *See Davison and Neale (1982): 402–403.*

Histogram. A type of graph used in **descriptive statistics** to analyze the results of an experiment. It shows the frequency distribution of scores. It is also known as a bar chart. *See Miller (1975): 34.*

Huntington's chorea. A rare **autosomal dominant** (see **chromosomes,** 5) disease producing **dementia.** The onset of the disease occurs in middle age. The person's **personality** becomes psychopathic, violent and a dependence on alcoholism begins. The patient shows a tremor at the distal parts of the muscles and **athetotic** (see **cerebral palsy,** 5) movement begins. Although there is no treatment available for this condition, **L-dopa** (5) is given to stop the tremor. It is caused by problems in the **caudate nucleus** (5) and **basal ganglia** (5). *See Stafford-Clark and Smith (1983): 72–73.*

Hypochondriasis. A **neurosis** in which a person's life becomes tortured by fears of having contracted some serious disease. In most cases, such people have ordinary illnesses which can be as minor as an irregular heartbeat, sweating, minor cough, etc. Men tend to suffer more from this condition than women. It is very difficult to reassure them that their illness is not as serious as they believe. The condition can be a symptom of **depression.** *See Stafford-Clark and Smith (1983): 196–198.*

Hysteria. A **neurosis** in which stress becomes so overwhelming that, unconsciously, the person presents, and may even experience, symptoms of physical illness. Stress can also be shown by severe mental illness, e.g., **depression, schizophrenia.** Minor hysteria causes a loss in or interference with the person's normal or sensory function. Such problems take the form of blindness, **deafness** (6), anaesthesia, **paraphasia** (1) and paralysis or disturbance of motor activity. The symptoms must be primarily physical. Treatment involves the removal of the underlying stress and/or depression. **Psychotherapy** or hypnosis have also been used successfully to remove such symptoms. *See Stafford-Clark and Smith (1983): 139–152.*

I

Id. See **personality.**
Ideal self. See **phenomenological approach.**

Identity vs confusion. See **attachment.**
Imitation. A form of therapy given to those suffering from poor **social skills.** It

is a difficult form of therapy as the instructor has to provide almost impeccable social skills for the client to try to copy exactly. *See Trower et al.* (*1978*): *181.*

Independent group design. An experimental design which uses two groups, each randomly selected. One group is a **control group** while the other is the **experimental group**. *See Miller* (*1975*): *20–22.*

Individual conditioning paradigms. See **operant conditioning**.

Industrial psychologist. See **psychology**.

Industry vs inferiority. See **attachment**.

Inference making. See **pre-operational stage**.

Inferential statistics. A study of **statistics** in which statistical tests are used to show whether or not a significant difference exists between the **control** and **experimental groups**. It also allows the experimenter to generalize the result of one small group to other groups of people. The tests which can be used are divided into **parametric** and non-**parametric tests**. *See Miller* (*1975*): *54–68.*

Initial interview. The first session which a therapist or any other professional has with a patient. This session is important for setting up a rapport with the patient and any accompanying relatives who might have accompanied the patient to the clinic and for taking a sufficient **case history** (1). The initial interview usually has six stages:

1. Introduction which is often called 'meeting, greeting and seating' (Nelson-Jones, 1982). It is important to make the patient feel as comfortable as possible at this stage since therapy of any kind can be seen as a threat. There can also be a stigma attached to coming for therapy. On the other hand, some patients have their hopes raised too high and expect therapists to be miracle workers.

2. Assessment of the presenting disorder. This can be either a **formal assessment** or an **informal assessment** (see **assessments**: 1) to find out what the patient can and cannot do. This should be explained to the patient as some of the subtests will be very easy while others will be very difficult.

3. Exploration of presenting disorder. This is really the case history, finding out how the disorder occurred and how it affects family life and the relationships within the home.

4. Reconnaissance where the therapist tries to find out how the patient views

him/herself since the onset of the disorder and examines the history of the disorder.

5. Contracting takes place when the therapist and patient come to an agreement on the type of therapy which the patient will begin to receive regularly.

6. Termination is the final stage where the therapist clears up any confusions which may have arisen from this initial interview and, most importantly, another appointment is made.

During these six stages the therapist should have in mind the following four interrelated objectives:

1. Creating a 'working alliance', i.e., a good rapport, with the patient;

2. Forming a 'working model' of the patient, i.e., patient's feelings concerning change in lifestyle and aspirations for the future;

3. Forming 'working goals', i.e., **treatment programme**: (1);

4. Deciding which therapy method to use.

The initial interview is often the most important session the therapist will have with the patient since much of the information which the therapist obtains then will determine how to proceed with therapy, and possibly indicate what other agencies may be required to help the patient and family, e.g., social services, **physiotherapy, occupational therapy**, (5) etc. *See Nelson-Jones* (*1982*): *275–297.*

Initiative vs guilt. See **attachment**.

Innate. See **innateness**.

Innateness. A theory to explain how people learn. Noam Chomsky used this theory to explain the **language acquisition** (1) of children. He believes humans are born with several different areas in their **brains** (5) for specific functions. Language is one of these areas. This innate knowledge of language has become known as the **language acquisition device** (1). It is **LAD** which sparks off the hypothetical language area in the child's **brain** (5). *See Steinberg* (*1982*): *94–100.*

Insight. See **psychoanalysis**.

Integrity vs despair. See **attachment**.

Intelligence. The **ability** to learn skills necessary for normal living. Steinberg (1981, 1982) put forward four components which go to make up intelligence:

1. Ability to learn and profit from experience

2. Ability to think or reason abstractly

3. Ability to adapt to the vagaries of a changing and uncertain world

4. Ability to motivate oneself to

accomplish expeditiously the tasks one needs to accomplish (Steinberg in Atkinson *et al.*, 1983: 370).

A person's intelligence is measured by **intelligence tests**. *See Atkinson et al.* (*1983*): *ch. 12.*

Intelligence quotient. The score obtained from carrying out an **intelligence test**. It is calculated using the formula:

$$IQ = MA/CA \times 100$$

This reads, 'the patient's IQ is his **mental age** (**MA**) divided by his chronological age (**CA**) multiplied by 100', to bring the result to a whole number. *See Atkinson et al.* (*1983*): *358.*

Intelligence tests. **Psychological** tests are aimed at finding out the **ability** of the child or adult to carry out various tasks presented to him usually without reference to previously learned material. Psychological testing tends to be controversial but there are safeguards built into most tests to make as sure as possible that the scores obtained are **reliable** and **valid** (see **validity**). The controversy surrounding the tests arises from a number of misconceptions. Some believe **intelligence tests** measure **innate** intelligence and that **IQ**s are fixed and cannot be changed; they measure all one needs to know about a person's intelligence; **IQ**s obtained from several tests are interchangeable and a battery of tests

tells the **psychologist** all he needs to know to enable him to make judgements about a person's competence. All such beliefs can be countered by arguing that test results should not be taken strictly at face value but any interpretation put on them must take into account other factors such as **case history** (1) information as well as any behaviour disorder from which the patient may suffer, his temperament, e.g., fatigue, stress, anxiety, or medical problems, e.g., brain damage, **speech** and **language disorders** (1), etc., at the time of testing. In certain parts of the country, it will be necessary also to take into account the child's cultural background. It is therefore important to note that the **IQ** obtained is dependent on the child's emotional state at the time of testing and the appropriateness of the test used. Intelligence tests which are most frequently used include the **Stanford-Binet intelligence scale**, **British Ability Scales**, **Wechsler Intelligence Scale for Children** (revised), **Wechsler Adult Intelligence Scale, Merrill-Palmer pre-school performance scale** and **Ravens progressive matrices** (1) and Vocabulary Scales. *See Atkinson et al.* (*1983*): *ch. 12.*

Interpretation. See **psychoanalysis**.
Intimacy vs isolation. See **attachment**.
Invariant functions. See **assimilation**.
IQ. **Intelligence Quotient**.

J

Jacob-Creuzfelt disease. A disease which produces **dementia**. It affects people between the ages of 35 and 63 years and is found worldwide. It lasts for about six months to three years. The symptoms include a loss of **short-term memory** (see **memory**), **aphasia** (1) and

hallucinations. The patient may also suffer from cortical blindness, **ataxia** (see **cerebral palsy**, 5) and **myoclonus** (5). There is a fast decline to dementia. There is no effective treatment. *See Gilroy et al.* (*1982*): *254–255.*

L

Latency stage. See **psychosexual stages of development**.
Learning. See **classical conditioning, operant conditioning, innateness**.
Life instinct. See **psychoanalysis**.
Lithium. A drug treatment technique used in **depression** and **mania**. The level

of the drug rises in the body and as it is only effective in this manner, it will take a few days after therapy begins for it to take effect. It is used mainly for the maintenance of recovery from mania and depression. *See Stafford-Clark and Smith* (*1983*): *124–125.*

M

MA. **Mental age**.

Major depression. See **depression**.

Maladaptive behaviour. See **abnormal behaviour**.

Manic-depression. Mania always appears with **depression** to create a bipolar disorder compared to depression itself which is a unipolar disorder. Those who suffer from attacks of mania appear in a happy and euphoric mood. While in this mood, sufferers become overtalkative, overactive, suffer from sleeplessness, become very distractable, have sudden flights of ideas and can begin punning and rhyming. A severe case of mania causes personal physical collapse, incoherent thought processes and superficial moods. The treatment is by tricyclic **antidepressant drugs**, **monoamine oxidase inhibitors**, **lithium**, chlorpromazine (see **phenothiazines**) and three to four sessions of **ECT**. *See Stafford-Clark and Smith (1983): 114–116, 124–125.*

Mann-Whitney test. A non-**parametric test** used in **inferential statistics**. It is used in experiments using the **independent group design** and has its equivalent **parametric test**, the **independent t-test** (see **T-tests**). It is used for data which are arranged on a scale which makes no assumptions concerning the shape of the population distribution. For example, two independent groups of subjects who are taught to read by different methods and subsequently rated on a scale of reading fluency from 1 to 10. The ratings are put on an ordinal scale and so the results of the experiment in this example could be ranked in order of fluency. Such scales do not allow for the calculations of mean score and so the Mann-Whitney test cannot show differences of means between subjects. 'By finding the sum of the ranks of one of the samples, this test allows the tester to determine the probability that a given difference between the ranks of the two samples could have arisen by chance' (Miller, 1975: 82). *See Miller (1975): 82–85.*

MAOI. **Monoamine oxidase inhibitors**.

Matched subjects design. A design used in preparing to carry out an experiment. so that the results will be reliable. In this approach, there are two groups but unlike the **independent group design**, they have different people in each group. The subjects are matched according to their similarity in relation to the variables which will be the subject of the experiment. *See Miller (1975): 19–20.*

Mean. See **central tendency**.

Median. See **central tendency**.

Memory. There are two types of memory—short-term memory (STM) and long-term memory (LTM) called dual memory theory. It is believed that these two areas of memory are linked. When STM receives input, it is rehearsed so that it will be remembered and can be transferred to the LTM area. When information is displaced from memory, it never reaches LTM but comes out of STM. STM has a storage capacity of $7 + / - 2$ chunks of information whereas the storage capacity of LTM is limitless. When information is retrieved from STM there are few errors, while it is more likely errors will occur in information retrieved from LTM. *See Atkinson et al. (1983): ch. 8.*

Memory trace. See **classical conditioning**.

Mental age. An age equivalent score which is obtained from **intelligence tests**. It is used in calculating an **IQ** score by comparing it to the **chronological age** to see if a child is below average, average or above average compared to other children of his own age.

Mental handicap. Those children and adults who are mentally handicapped can have difficulty in learning tasks, in **communication** (1), with motor skills and with sensory input. Such problems can be helped by therapy, but such therapy programmes as are necessary must be carefully planned because of the learning difficulties experienced by such children. Research has shown that these difficulties are complicated by additional handicaps such as attention problems, being unable to learn incidentally and so the child requires long and frequent exposure to the stimulus; such children react badly to pressure; they can process information much better auditorily than visually; memory is improved by using more than one modality; clang associations confuse them; they have difficulty generalizing what has been learnt and so concrete stimuli should be used as they are learnt better than abstract stimuli and verbalizing helps improve memory during the task. They require a structured approach and they can retain learned material taught appropriately as well as normal children. *See Shakespeare (1975): 77–78.*

Merril-Palmer pre-school performance scale. An assessment for finding out the learning abilities among children between the ages of 1½ and 5. Devised in 1931, the scale has 19 verbal and performance subtests which test motor and language skills, manual dexterity and matching skills. Most of these subtests take the form of games so that the children readily pay attention to them. The **raw scores** which are obtained can be converted to **mental age, intelligence quotients, percentile ranks** and **standard deviations**. *See test manual.*

Minor depression. See **depression**.

Mixed conduct/emotional disorder. See **conduct disorder**.

Mode. See **central tendency**.

Modelling. A therapeutic approach to **behaviour therapy** introduced by Bandura in 1969. It is known also as vicarious conditioning since its aim is to provide a model participating successfully in the patient's feared situation while being watched by the patient. After each stage the patients are encouraged to copy this behaviour. *See Atkinson et al. (1983): 502–504.*

Monoamine oxidase inhibitors. A form of drug treatment used with patients suffering from **depression**. The three main **MAOI** drugs are:

1. Phenelzine
2. Isocarboxazid
3. Tranylcypromine.

The evidence of efficacy of these drugs on depression is poor but they can act as a mild anti-**anxiety** drug. There is also a possibility they are effective in cases where **phobias** and irrational anxiety are prominent. Dizziness, dry mouth and fatigue are common side-effects in the first few weeks of starting the drugs. These drugs interact with certain foods, e.g., cheese, broad beans, yeast, producing unbearable headaches and a swing to low blood pressure. They should not be mixed with tricyclic **antidepressant drugs** or **ECT**. *See Stafford-Clark and Smith (1983): 119–120.*

Morbid jealousy. A **neurotic syndrome** which usually occurs in association with alcoholism. The patient becomes so jealous, he becomes fanatically preoccupied at finding out if his beliefs have any truth. For example, an alcoholic could have a **delusion** that his wife is having an affair. He begins to follow her everywhere and may assault anyone to whom she stops to speak. If the wife gives a false admission about any man she knows, it could lead to murder. *See Stafford-Clark and Smith (1983): 181–182.*

Mother's depression. **Abnormal** moods suffered by a mother which may affect her child. These moods are associated with low self-esteem, loss of energy, poor sleep, poor appetite or compensatory overeating, anxiety, obsessional symptoms, increased use of drugs and alcohol and a loss of sexual desire and pleasure. Maternal depression can double the chance of disturbance in the child from about 15 to 30 per cent. The moods have specific effects on the child. The mother's **apathy** produces decreased interaction and stimulation which causes **speech** and **language delay** (1) and attention-seeking behaviour in the child. If the mother's use of discipline and management is inconsistent, this may produce behaviour problems of all sorts (e.g., temper tantrums, eating and sleeping problems). If the family is socially isolated, there may be a lack of peer contact for the child which could produce a failure to develop **social skills** and possibly, speech and language problems. A mother's resentment and threats of abandonment can produce fearfulness and **separation anxiety**. Irritability in the mother may make her use excessive physical punishment against the child which produces fearfulness and/or aggressiveness between the child and his peers. The child's difficult behaviour in turn can worsen the mother's depression. When the mother comes to the clinic, she will probably present **psychosomatic** complaints or **anxiety** about the child. She may not openly admit she is suffering from depression. Depression affects 5 per cent of women and 2 per cent of men. Depression affects 30–50 per cent of working class women. **Psychotherapy** can be used in treating such conditions. *See Rutter (1975): 251.*

Multi-infarct dementia. The symptoms include lability of mood, sudden crying associated with **depression** and a mild form of the severe loss of emotional control of patients who suffer from **pseudobulbar palsy** (5). It is associated with hypertension. It can be treated by decreasing the patient's blood pressure which can arrest the progress of the dementia but not reverse it. Patients may also suffer from motor problems and **dysarthric** (see **dysarthria**: 1) characteristics of speech. *See Stafford-Clark and Smith (1983): 72–73.*

Munchausen syndrome. Named after Baron Munchausen who told very tall stories concerning how good a cavalry officer he was. It is a syndrome from which some suffer such as those who like hospital operations, but, when discharged, because their symptoms do not require surgery, they appear at another hospital sometime later. There was a patient recently who appeared for speech therapy (see 1) under similar circumstances.

Mutism. A severe form of **elective mutism**.

Myxoedema. A **neurotic** syndrome caused by hypothyroidism which typically occurs in middle-aged women. It is quite rare. This can produce a **flattening of affect** as well as possible **articulation/language disorders** (1). *See Davison and Neale (1982): 718.*

N

Neurosis. Neurotic disorders are those which affect emotional and intellectual functioning without losing reality. Such disorders include **anxiety, stress, obsessive-compulsive disorders, depression** and **manic-depression**. *See Stafford-Clark and Smith (1983): 16, passim.*

Neurotic. See **neurosis**.

Norm. Describes what is regarded as normal. *See Atkinson et al. (1983): 569–570.*

Normal distribution. A statistical analysis of scores which are analyzed by **central tendency**. It can be drawn in graph form as a normal distribution curve. *See Miller (1975): 46–52.*

Normal pressure hydrocephalus. The symptoms of this **dementia** are a clumsy gait, urgency of micturition and eventual incontinence. The patient's unsteadiness is due to a mixture of **ataxia**, **spasticity** (see **cerebral palsy**: 5) and dyspraxia of gait. It can be reversed by placing a **shunt** in the **ventricles** of the **brain** to drain the excess **CSF** (all 5). *See Stafford-Clark and Smith (1983): 74.*

Null hypothesis. This hypothesis must be disproved by **statistical analysis** (see **statistics**). It states that there is no significant difference between the distributions of scores. All researchers start off with the null hypothesis which, if their experiment is worthwhile, will be rejected. If they fail to reject it, there must have been something wrong with the experiment either methodologically, e.g., the wrong design was used, or theoretically, e.g., the assumptions made about the experiment were wrong, or else there was too great a variation in the variables present in the environment in which the experiment was to be carried out. If the researcher has doubts about the possibility of rejecting the hypothesis, he may use a more rigorous level of significance than 0.5 and may use 0.01 or 0.001. This could result in a type 2 error where a significant difference is said to exist but does not exist. *See Miller (1975): 58–59.*

O

Object permanence. A theory developed by **Piaget** on the cognitive development of children. Piaget argued that if a child is presented with a toy with which he is allowed to play or handle and it is then hidden under a box or cloth, the child will not make any effort to find or look for that toy. This stage is present until 5–6 months of age. According to Piaget, this shows the child's egocentricity (see **pre-operational stage**), i.e., the child is only concerned by his own world and ignores external stimuli. The critics put forward the argument that perhaps it was the way in which the object was hidden that prevented the child from making the effort to look for the toy. Experiments were carried out which showed that it did make a difference how the object was made to disappear. *See Donaldson (1978): 26–28.*

Observation. An informal technique for assessing the patient's behaviour. It is important for the therapist to decide what the target behaviour to be aimed for is and the stages the patient has to go through to reach this behaviour. It is possible by observation to see changes in behaviour patterns starting from a baseline (found in initial assessment). If two therapists are observing the one patient, they must have a common language which they can both use to express their findings. There are five types of observational recordings:

1. Continuous recording in which the observer tries to record everything that happens, e.g., diary studies. However, this can be very time consuming and it is impossible to observe everything. The use of video recording can be of more help and reduce the number of problems although it is quite time consuming going through video tapes.

2. Event recording is a frequency measure of the number of times the target behaviour occurs in a given period of time.

3. Interval recording in which the observer takes a preset duration of time and divides it up into smaller units. So, the therapist may observe for ten minutes, stop for ten minutes, etc. The observer must stick to the time interval even if a behaviour occurs after the time interval has passed.

4. Duration recording in which the observer records how long the behaviour lasts.

5. Latency recording in which the observer records how long it takes for the patient to respond. *See Davison and Neale (1982): 111–112.*

Obsessive-compulsive disorders. A **neurosis** present in 0.05 per cent of the population at any one time. The patients who have obsessions or compulsions about something, e.g., keeping clean, will spend their life carrying out such activities as are required to fulfil their obsession. For example, if a person has a compulsion concerning cleanliness, there could be excessive handwashing, washing utensils several times before using them, washing sink surrounds before using them to wash in as well as keeping soap, cloths and towels in receptacles for cleanliness. Compulsive rituals are carried out a certain number of times which becomes a magical figure. If the ritual is repeated more often than the magical number of times the ritual starts all over again. Repetitive, unwelcomed and resisted thoughts become strengthened, i.e., ruminations. People's lives can be ruined by this disorder. **Psychotherapy** such as **behaviour therapy** or **psychoanalysis** can be used successfully. *See Stafford-Clark and Smith (1983): 153–159.*

Oedipus complex. The very young child forms a close bond to his mother or a substitute, e.g., foster-mother. This bonding is produced by an emotional tie between the child and the mother. Thus, the child finds difficulties in life when separated from the mother (see **separation anxiety**). The child faces another problem when he sees his father as a rival for the affection of his mother. The child is faced with a terrible dilemma: on the one hand he is jealous of his father as a rival, while on the other hand he knows he depends on his father emotionally in the family circle. Such frustrations lead to feelings of aggression against the father which the child has to suppress because of the love and respect he has for his father. As the child is so young, he cannot speak about these feelings nor can he work out what he should do about such feelings himself. He is in conflict over his emotional feelings towards his father. The Oedipus complex was first put forward by Freud, who suggested that it was a possible cause of various neuroses from which some people suffer. *See Stafford-Clark and Smith (1983): 45–46.*

One-tail test. A **statistical** (see **statistics**) interpretation of any **parametric** and non-**parametric** tests. Assumptions are made about the experiment before it is carried out. It is a rule that one of two assumptions is made. The assumption for a one-tail test is that the difference between the two distributions will be significant at 5 per cent. This is the normal level of significance for all tests. If the experimenter is uncertain about the result being significant, then he must use a two-tail test and so there is only 1 in a 2½ per cent chance of the result not being significant. The tails refer to the ends of a **normal distribution** curve. In a one-tail test only the positive tail is used, while with a two-tail test both tails of the curve are used. *See Miller (1975): 78–80.*

Operant conditioning. A learning theory used as a basis for **behaviour therapy**. It is also known as radical behaviourism and was put forward by T. B. Skinner. He developed these principles by experimenting with rats in boxes known as Skinner boxes. These boxes had a bar in them which, when pressed, released a pellet of food. Thus, the rats were conditioned to press the bar because they learnt they would receive food.

Those who undertake such behaviour modification believe the reaction of a person to his environment causes the person's maladaptive behaviour. Such therapists see all maladaptive behaviour as a learned response received through environmental reinforcement. To combat this a suitable conditioning programme has to be evolved. First of all a functional analysis is developed to provide a set of possible sources in the environment of the reinforcement of the present maladaptive behaviour. Sometimes such behaviour can be caused by the acceptance of it by others thus allowing the person to continue living in a comforting

situation and so they give the person an indirect reward. The functional analysis must detail the maladaptive behaviours of the individual, showing the number of occurrences and the particular environments in which these behaviours take place. A target behaviour pattern is then developed and various interventions decided on to try and establish a more acceptable behaviour pattern. These treatment plans are specific to each individual patient. Such therapeutic interventions are individual conditioning paradigms which attempt to identify the source of the reinforcement of the maladaptive behaviour and try to remove it either by physical removal or by aversive reinforcement. **Token economies** are also used in this form of therapy. *See Atkinson et al. (1983): 200–208.*

Oral stage. See **psychosexual stages of development**.

Organization. See **assimilation**.

P

Parametric tests. One of two types of tests which are used in **inferential statistics**. Parametric tests are perhaps the most powerful tests from a statistical point of view and are very rigorous in their assumptions which are three in number:

1. the data must fall in a **normal distribution**;
2. the **standard deviation** and variations must be relatively equal producing homogeneity of variation;
3. the data must be on an interval-ratio scale.

Two parametric tests which are used to a large extent in **statistics** are the independent t-test (see **T-tests**) with an **independent group design** and the related t-test (see **T-tests**) with a **repeated measures design**. These tests take account of all the data which are collected by the assessment or whatever method is used to gather it. If the data do not fall under a normal distribution curve, a nonparametric test must be used. These tests are less powerful and discard some of the data. Two such tests are the **Mann-Whitney test** for **independent group design** and the **Wilcoxon test** for **repeated measures design**. These tests compare the results by ranking the

results of both groups, and the experimenter can calculate if there is a significant difference in the results. Because of the ranking system of scores used in this type of test, much of the actual data is lost and thus they become less powerful than parametric tests. *See Miller (1975): 64–68.*

Pavlov. See **classical conditioning**.

Peak experience. See **phenomenological approach**.

Perceived self. See **phenomenological approach**.

Percentile score. A score or rank which shows how many subjects belonging to the **norm** fall below the **raw score** in question. For example, if a child is given a percentile score of 79, this means that there are 79 per cent of the norm group below this child's score. They are used widely in assessments of all kinds. *See Aiken (1985): 74–77.*

Personality. Freud proposed **psychoanalysis** to describe the development of personality. It consists of three parts—the id, ego and superego. The 'id' is present at birth and works at an unconscious level. The child's personality at this stage requires immediate gratification. The overriding need is pleasure and is often known as a primary process. If the child is going to develop from this stage, his 'ego' must develop. Unlike the 'id', the 'ego' works at a conscious level. It produces the reality principle which makes the child react to what is happening around him. Fantasies occur rarely as the child's personality is guided by the secondary process. Just as the 'id' produces the biological self, the 'ego' produces the psychological self. The 'superego' operates on the social and moral functioning of the person. These three parts of personality development can be summed up as: 'The id seeks pleasure, the ego tests reality and the superego strives for perfection' (Atkinson *et al.* 1983: 396). *See Atkinson et al. (1983): 395–396.*

Personality profile. See **trait approach**.

Phenothiazines. The type of drugs used in treating **schizophrenia**. The parent drug is chlorpromazine (largactyl). It can be given orally, intramuscularly or intravenously. It does have some side-effects which include drowsiness, hypotension, hypothermia, rare cholestatic jaundice (reversible when drug stopped), Parkinsonian symptoms and dyskinesias. Thioricazine (melleril) is from the same family of drugs but if given in very high doses, it can produce rare retinal damage. Trifluoperazine (stelazine) does not produce problems with blood pressure and jaundice but is more potent in producing Parkinsonian symptoms. It produces alertness rather than drowsiness. *See Stafford-Clark and Smith (1983): 96–97.*

Phallic stage. See **psychosexual stages of development**.

Phenomenological approach. An approach often thought of as a reaction against **psychoanalysis**. It was developed by Carl Rogers. The personality is viewed as a conflict within the unconscious mind. However, it is the way in which the client perceives and interprets events which is important. Some theories within this approach are termed humanistic while others are theories of the self. An important part of Rogers' self theory is how the people evaluate their self image as that may have a bearing on how they perceive the world and events happening around them. This is often called perceived self. The person is also made to think of how he/she would like to be compared with what they are. This is known as the ideal self. Self-actualization occurs when a person chooses what they want to become and progresses to this goal rather than regresses from it. A peak experience occurs when people go through periods of self-actualization. It is usually characterized by feelings of fulfilment and happiness because they have reached their goal. In general terms, this approach is a subjective approach in that the individual must examine his own experiences of the world and his reaction to them. *See Atkinson et al. (1983): 399–40.*

Phobias. A **neurosis** and a possible cause of **anxiety**. A phobia is an irrational fear which will not be dissipated by any amount of logical discussion. Such a fear-provoking behaviour may happen only in particular situations. For example, someone who has a phobia of dogs will only show this irrational fear in the presence of dogs and will produce quite normal, rational reactions to other aspects of daily life. As the person approaches a feared situation, the irrational fear may produce an acute **anxiety** state. Some phobias, like the one just cited, may not affect the person's life greatly, while other social phobias or agoraphobia, i.e., fear of crowds, enclosed spaces, etc., can cause isolation and loneliness to such a degree that the sufferer's life-style can be altered significantly. Sixty per cent of all phobias are agoraphobic by nature with an incidence of 2 : 1 in favour of males; 8 per cent of phobias are social by nature with a similar incidence in favour of males; while animal phobias account for 20 per cent of phobias with an equal sex incidence. The most popular **psychotherapy** is **behaviour therapy**. *See Stafford-Clark and Smith (1983): 128–138.*

Piaget. Jean Piaget (1896–1980), a Swiss psychologist, observed a child's cognitive behaviour from birth to about 11 years of age. He included his own child, and as a result evolved a theory of cognitive development which proceeded through several distinct stages as the child grew —**sensorimotor stage**, **pre-operational**, **concrete operations** and **formal operations**. Piaget's theory of language development is based on the empiricist view according to which a child is believed to be born with a 'tabula rasa' or 'an empty mind' and develops language only by his own experience and experimenting with what he hears in the environment around him. This is opposed to Chomsky's theory of **innateness** in language development and to the existence of a **language acquisition device** (1). *See Atkinson et al. (1983): 69–73.*

Pick's disease. A rare type of **dementia** caused by neurone degeneration. It is an **autosomal** (see **chromosomes**: 5) gene inherited disease. A major characteristic is the change of personality in later life particularly in the person's moral standards. **Aphasia** (1) can also appear. The prognosis is not good as death can occur within six to twelve months which is caused by chest problems. *See Stafford-Clark and Smith (1983):* 72.

Play. A vital component in the child's development as it allows him to develop manipulative and social skills so that he can learn to cope with his total environment. It functions also as a bridge between the child's internal world of fantasy and the external world of his environment, thus the child plays out his anxieties and fears, his jealousies and feelings of aggression. Play is often used in **psychotherapy** for treating the child's **emotional disorders** and **conduct disorders**. It can also be used in speech therapy to produce a natural setting for children to develop their communication skills, especially with those who suffer from **language delay** (1). Garvey has described play happening 'in a period of dramatically expanding knowledge of self, the physical and social world, and systems of communication' (Garvey, 1977: 7). *See Wood (1981): ch. 6.*

Play therapy. The use of **play** in treating a child's **emotional disorders**, **conduct disorders** and also **communication disorders** (1). *See Wood (1981): 189.*

Population. A grouping of people, objects or abstract material which is to be analyzed statistically. On occasion, the population will be so large that it would be impossible to test every member of the population. In such cases, the tester has to pick a random **sample** and then project the scores of this sample onto the population. For example, the organizations such as Gallup, MORI, Marplan, etc. which test the public's opinion, usually on their political views, take a random sample of the population around the country, ask their questions, and work out the results. By statistical analysis, they can work out the voting intentions of the population with varying accuracy. *See Miller (1975): 59–61.*

Pre-operational stage. The second stage of **Piaget's** theory of cognitive development. It lasts from about 2 to 7 years of age and assumes that the child can now think independently about what he perceives using his developed sense of sym-

bolization. However, he may still have difficulties within his cognitive skills. When posed with a problem, the child can only see it from his own perspective, not from anyone else's viewpoint. This is egocentricity (e.g., three mountains test in Donaldson, 1978: 19–23). Piaget introduced this theory of egocentricity into his theory of language development. He claimed a child could not understand the position of a listener in a two-way conversation and so children used collective monologues with which to communicate, not conversations. He called this egocentric speech. During this stage the child fails to make inferences about various problems he is set. If the child is told, 'A is greater than B, B is greater than C' and asked what is the relationship between A and C, he fails to respond correctly. However, Donaldson (*op. cit*: 53–56) has found children can make inferences in real situations. Failure to conserve volume, weight, number, etc. occurs during this stage. However, Donaldson (*op. cit*: 63) has shown it depends on how the conservation task is presented to the child for him to succeed. *See Beard (1969): ch. 3; Donaldson (1978): chs 4 and 5.*

Psychiatrist. See **psychiatry**.

Psychiatry. A branch of medicine which provides treatment for those suffering from **mental illness** such as **affective disorders**, **neuroses**, **psychoses** and **schizophrenia**. The psychiatrist can give treatment in the form of **psychotherapy** and drug therapy for the various disorders found under the classifications already given. *See Stafford-Clark and Smith (1983): ch. 1.*

Psychoanalysis. A **psychological** theory evolved by Sigmund Freud in 1900. The basis of this theory is that there are two basic motivators in life—sex and aggression. Freud believed people had certain instincts which guided them through life—the life instinct and the death instinct. The former, he believed, was concerned with the libido and sexual drives, while the latter was concerned with people's destructive feelings leading either to suicide or aggression against others. Both drives are found in young children but often suppressed by their parents. Thus, the drives become unconscious motives and produce **anxiety** in the child as he knows he will incur his parent's disapproval if he tries to express them.

Within the framework of psychoanalysis, Freud produced a theory for the development of one's **personality** using the unconscious motives of the id, the ego and the superego. The child's emotional development was described in terms of **psychosexual stages of development**. In **psychotherapy**, psychoanalysis also plays a role. It is based on the Freudian concepts of **free association**, abreaction, insight, interpretation, transference and working through. During abreaction the patient can release emotions in a safe environment. Following this, there is a period of insight when the patient is encouraged to discover the root cause of the conflict and how to interpret these emotions. Having discovered the cause, the patient transfers his emotional feelings to the therapist. Thus, patients begin to see the therapist in the role of person(s) with whom they have or have had difficulty in forming a relationship. It may be parents or friends with whom they are having such problems. By discussing such a transference, the patient is often helped to work through his feelings. *See Atkinson et al. (1983): 395–399, 498–499.*

Psychodrama. A therapeutic technique used in **social skills** training devised by Moreno in 1946. It can be used to produce **insight, modelling, systematic desensitization, social skills** and **assertive training**. It helps people to share their problems and to make clear their emotions in certain situations (i.e., those in which the patient has difficulty in expressing himself). It can also improve empathy in the group and defuse any **anxiety** within the group. *See Trower et al. (1978): 93–95.*

Psychologist. See **psychology**.

Psychology. A science which studies behaviour and mental functioning in animals and men. The **psychologist** uses **psychotherapy** to treat patients suffering from **abnormal behaviour, emotional disorders** and **conduct disorders**, learning difficulties and a lack of **social skills**. There are different branches of psychology to deal with such problems. The two main branches are **clinical** and **educational psychology**. However, psychologists take part also in industry with firms and companies having their own psychologist, sometimes dealing with time and motion studies and with industrial disputes and personal problems affecting inter-staff relationships. *See Atkinson et al. (1983): ch. 1.*

Psychosexual stages of development. Freud proposed five distinct stages in the development of the child's **personality**.

He believed children were more aware of different parts of their body at different ages and their manipulation satisfies the **id**. These stages are:

1. Oral stage in which children are most conscious of their mouths. The pleasures which are gratified by such manipulation are those of feeding and sucking.

2. Anal stage in which gratification comes from defecation. During this stage toilet training usually occurs.

3. Phallic stage in which the id is gratified by manipulation of the genitalia. It is at this stage that the **Oedipus complex** affects the child.

4. Latency stage which is not strictly a psychosexual stage of development as the children show no sexual behaviour as they turn away from the Oedipal conflict and begin an interest in outside friends, school, etc.

5. Genital stage during which heterosexual relationships develop.

Many critics believe these stages to be too simple to explain the development of personality. Erikson describes this development in terms of **attachment**. *See Atkinson et al. (1983): 397.*

Psychoses. Psychotic disorders are those which cause the patient to lose contact with reality. Such disorders include major **affective disorders**, e.g., **psychotic depression**, paranoia and **schizophrenia**. Such patients also suffer from **hallucinations** and **delusions**. *See Davison and Neale (1982): 73.*

Psychosomatic. A description of disorders which produce changes in the body due to emotional reactions. *See Stafford-Clark and Smith (1983): 122.*

Psychosurgery. A treatment technique used to relieve severe **depression** by cutting some of the tracts in the white matter of the **brain** (5). *See Stafford-Clark and Smith (1983): 122.*

Psychotic. See **psychoses**.

Psychotic depression. See **depression**.

Psychotherapy. Different types of therapy used by **psychologists** and **psychiatrists** for treating disorders. It includes **behaviour therapy, psychoanalysis, psychodrama**, humanistic therapy and group therapy (1). *See Atkinson et al. (1983): 497–512.*

Punch-drunk syndrome. A medical condition which can lead to **dementia**. It is caused by a subdural haematoma which can develop to affect the rest of the **brain** (5) and produce dementia. *See Stafford-Clark and Smith (1983): 74.*

R

Radical behaviourism. See **operant conditioning**.

Randomization. See **independent group design**.

Range. A measure of dispersion to show the spread of results received from an experiment. Range is calculated by subtracting the highest score from the lowest score. However, there are occasions on which this is not very useful since one of the two groups of scores could have a highest score which is atypical and thus produce an inaccurate range. The statistician would use the interquartile range in such circumstances. *See Miller (1975): 41.*

Rational emotive therapy. A cognitive behaviour therapy developed by Ellis in the early 1960s. It is aimed at analyzing the individual's distorted perception of life events, not those events in themselves. Ellis listed 12 assumptions of distorted cognition. The therapy is aimed mainly at the **neurotic** population who do not always rehearse these distorted cognitions deliberately. The onus is put on the individual to identify irrational thoughts and replace them with positive thoughts. *See Rachman and Wilson (1980): 195–208.*

Raw score. The score which a child or adult receives after an **assessment** (1) has been carried out. This score can be turned into a **standard score**, **age equivalent score** or a **percentile score**.

Reinforcement. See **operant conditioning**.

Reinforcer. See **operant conditioning**.

Reliable. See **reliability**.

Reliability. If an **assessment** (1) is to be worthwhile, it must be reliable, have **validity** and be discriminating. For an assessment to be reliable, each of the subtests must measure the same variable. For example, in **assessments of language** (1), all the subtests must be a measure of various aspects of language and not have a subtest which measures, for example, **social skills**. It must also be consistent over time, so that if a child is tested with a particular test, he should have the same score when tested six months later if no improvement has taken place. This is known as test-retest reliability. *See Purser (1982): 176–177.*

Repeated measures design. A design used for carrying out an experiment the results of which will be analyzed statistically. There are two groups but each group is made up of the same subjects. Each subject performs under all the conditions of the experiment. Thus, it is possible to find out how the two conditions affect the same subject. The subjects have to be **counterbalanced**. The commonest **parametric test** used in this design is the **related t-test** (see **T-tests**) while the commonest non-**parametric test** is the **Wilcoxon test**. *See Miller (1975): 17–19.*

Rogers. See **phenomenological approach**.

Role reversal. A therapeutic technique used commonly in training **social skills**. The patient adopts the role of the assertive person and the supervisor takes the non-assertive role. If there is a role conflict, this type of therapy is often difficult to implement. It is part of **assertive training**. *See Trower et al. (1978): 79, 83, 94.*

S

Sample. See **population**.

Schema(ta). See **assimilation**.

Schizophrenia. A syndrome or group of mental illnesses characterized by specific psychological symptoms which interfere with an individual's thinking, emoting and behaviour and with each of these in a characteristic way. The patient suffers from **thought disorders, flattening of affect** and disorders of speech and language (see **schizophrenia**: 1). There are three main types of schizophrenia:

1. Hebephrenic schizophrenia can be recognized by the disorganized features of their movements, ideas and moods.

2. Catatonic schizophrenia is usually

recognized by the odd movements caused by motor disturbances.

3. Paranoic schizophrenia is recognized by **delusions** which are often grandiose in nature.

Schizophrenia can be treated by the **phenothiazine** family of drugs. *See Davison and Neale (1982): chs 13, 14.*

Self-actualization. See **phenomenological approach**.

Self-instructional training. A cognitive behaviour therapy developed by Meichenbaum (1977). It is based on the theory that the individual's behaviour depends on what the individual says to himself about the events he encounters. Thus, **aberrant** behaviour is a result of inappropriate self-instruction or no self-instruction at all. *See Rachman and Wilson (1980): 208–220.*

Self-theory. See **phenomenological approach**.

Senile dementia. See **Alzheimer's Disease**.

Sensitivity training. A therapeutic technique used commonly in **social skills** training. It takes the form of the participants learning from their own immediate and direct experiences within the group. It is not so much a procedure for learning social skills but a way of learning sensitivity to others, improving interpersonal relationships and improving the patient's self-confidence. There are two techniques used for this end—**encounter groups** and **t-groups**. *See Trower et al. (1978): 91–93.*

Sensorimotor stage. The first of **Piaget's** four stages of cognitive development in children. This stage lasts from birth to 2 years of age and concerns the ability of the child to perceive objects but not think about them. In other words, the child can only act upon an object when it is within his vision but not if it is hidden. This is Piaget's theory of **object permanence**. The development of **imitation** (2) and **play** are important in the child's ability to symbolize objects. Towards the end of this stage, the child may use deferred imitation, i.e., the ability to act out events which the child has stored in memory, and play with objects using them to symbolize other objects. This idea of symbolization is the mainstay of Piaget's theory of language development. He believed a child could not develop language until the child had acquired the notion of symbolization. More concisely, Piaget believed language did not appear until the cognitive events underlying symbolization have been achieved and thus language develops out of cognition. *See Beard (1969): ch. 2.*

Separation anxiety. A possible cause of **emotional disorder** from which children suffer. Feelings of fear and anxiety are quite common and normal reactions in children to certain circumstances but when these feelings begin to interfere with everyday life, they become **abnormal**. During the child's early life, he is very sensitive and vulnerable to traumatic events and separation is one such event. The mother, often regarded by the child as being someone special (since she is usually the parent with whom bonding first takes place), may have to leave home suddenly, for example, to have another child or for medical reasons. If the child has been adequately prepared for this separation, he will have less of a problem accepting the situation than if the mother disappears suddenly and no preparation has been made. In the latter case, the child becomes 'lost' and suffers severe anxiety. **Psychotherapy** of all kinds has been used successfully with such children. Family therapy and/or parental counselling is also useful. *See Rutter (1975): 156–165.*

Sibling rivalry. It is common knowledge that there is almost always some degree of rivalry between or among siblings. This may take the form of play-fighting or trying to do better at school, etc. It is usually caused by just wanting to do better than the other sibling to obtain more praise from parents. However, if parents go out of their way overtly to show preference to one sibling rather than to another, the one to whom preference is not given may produce feelings of aggression either to the other sibling(s) or to parents or both. These feelings can produce both **conduct disorders** and **emotional disorders** such as **elective mutism**. For example, if the child wishes to be vindictive towards parents, he may decide not to speak at school and so make life as difficult as possible for his parents. *See Rutter (1975).*

Simple depression. See **depression**.

Simultaneous conditioning. See **classical conditioning**.

Single case study. In studies of the efficacy of certain treatment techniques, it has been found to be insufficient to use test designs such as **independent subject**, **matched pairs** and **repeated measures**. Thus, statisticians proposed the single case study. In this type of study, the subjects have to act as their own

control group. The aim is to test the subject during periods of treatment and non-treatment. The best design for such studies is the ABA design. This means that during 'A' (no treatment) the patient is tested, during 'B' treatment is provided, and the last 'A' (no treatment) the patient is retested. This is also known as the cross-over treatment design. *See Coltheart (1983)*.

Skew. See **central tendency**.

Skinner's boxes. See **operant conditioning**.

Social skills. A phenomenon in which a person produces socially acceptable behaviour and the behaviour produces the desired effect on others. Any child or adult who does not possess such skills has to be given a treatment programme to teach him/her how to cope in various situations through experience. Such treatment takes the form of **assertive training, sensitivity training** and **psychodrama**. *See Trower et al. (1978): passim*.

Socialized conduct disorder. See **conduct disorder**.

Special education. A description of the education received by children suffering from varying degrees of **mental handicap** (see also 1). The classes are often small and outside agencies such as speech therapy, physiotherapy and psychology are involved in the rehabilitation of the children.

Standard deviation. A process in **descriptive statistics** used for finding out how far from the **mean** (see **central tendency**) in a **normal distribution** a person's score is. The standard deviation is worked out as the square root of the variance of the dispersion of scores. *See Miller (1975): 44–46*.

Standard score. A score obtained in various assessments from the **raw score**. It is based on the **standard deviation**. *See Atkinson et al. (1983): 608–609*.

Standardization. See **standardized tests**.

Standardized tests. To standardize a test it must be given to a large number of the population covering the age range for which it is intended to be used. In this way, the tester can discover the most frequent or normal responses of the different age groups and, thence, be enabled to compare the scores obtained from patients with those of the norm for that age group. Following this, the **mental age** and resulting **IQ** can be calculated.

Stanford-Binet intelligence scales.

Binet published his first test in 1905 with the help of Theodore Simon (1873–1961), a French psychologist. These tests became known throughout the world and translations into English followed. The scale which became widely used had been translated and adapted by Lewis Terman of Stanford University. Terman introduced the **Intelligence Quotient** to the scales while Stern, a German psychologist, proposed the **IQ** scale. There have been three editions subsequently since 1916. The latest edition (4th edition) was published in 1985. Its age range is similar to the other editions, 2 years to adulthood. There are four areas from which the tester obtains scores—cognitive ability, verbal reasoning, quantitative reasoning, abstract/visual reasoning and short-term memory. The scale comprises 15 subtests—vocabulary, **comprehension** (1), verbal relations, absurdities, pattern analysis, matrices, paper folding and cutting, copying, quantities, number series, equation building, memory for digits, sentences, objects and beads. *See Aiken (1985): 151–153*.

Statistics. A study which makes theories into realities. **Psychology** is often said to be common sense, but the use of statistics makes it into a science. There are two types of statistics—**inferential** and **descriptive statistics**. In the former measures of **central tendency** and dispersion are used, while in the latter **parametric** and non-**parametric tests** are used to analyze the scores obtained from experiments. *See Miller (1975): passim*.

Stern. See **Stanford-Binet intelligence scales**.

Stress. See **hysteria**.

Superego. See **personality**.

Symbolization. See **sensorimotor stage**.

Systematic desensitization. A **behaviour therapy** based on **classical conditioning**. It has as its aim the gradual reduction of a learned **anxiety**. The client tells the therapist what is causing the anxiety. He is relaxed and asked to rate his fear on a fear thermometer. Thus, the therapist can construct an anxiety hierarchy. As the patient continues to relax he is asked to imagine the least feared stimulus and after it has been overcome due to the relaxation, the next most feared stimulus is treated similarly and so on. However, it is uncertain for how long fears can be extinguished. *See Atkinson et al. (1983): 500–501*.

T

T-groups. A therapeutic technique used in the **sensitivity training** approach to **social skills** training. In these groups, the patients make their own decisions as the therapist takes a backseat. The patients have to make up their minds who is going to be group leader, what their feelings for each other are, while some may fail to participate completely. If necessary, the therapist will show them how to express such feelings for each other, their reactions to each other, encourage openness and he himself may provide a model. *See Trower et al. (1978): 92.*

T-tests. There are two types of t-tests depending on whether a **parametric** or a non-**parametric test** is used. If the former is being used with an **independent subject design**, the independent t-test will be used, while if the latter is being used with a **repeated measures design**, the related t-test is used. As with other tests degrees of freedom are used so that the experimenter can find out how many scores can vary; this is usually N – 1 with N being the **mean** (see **central tendency**). *See Miller (1975): 70–81, 93–95.*

Target behaviour pattern. See **operant conditioning**.

Terman. See **Stanford-Binet intelligence scale**.

Thought disorder. A symptom of **schizophrenia** (see also 1). There are two different kinds of thought disorder—form and content.
The former consists of:
1. incoherence in conversation;
2. **neologisms** (1);
3. loose associations—while patient communicates successfully with the listener, he has difficulty sticking to the one topic;
4. clang associations—the words used are put in a certain order because of their rhyme rather than their syntax;
5. poverty of speech—either the amount of **discourse** (1) is increased or conveys little information;
6. **perseveration** (1);
7. **blocking** (1).

The latter consists of:
1. **delusions**;
2. delusional percept—a normal perception which has a special meaning for the patient and an often delusional system develops quickly;
3. somatic passivity—inability to rouse the patient by outside forces operating on his body;
4. thought insertion—thoughts, different from those of the patient, are placed in the patient's mind from an outside agent;
5. thought withdrawal—the patient believes their thoughts are being removed from their mind without warning;
6. thought broadcast—the patient believes their thoughts are being transmitted to others;
7. 'made' feeling;
8. 'made' volitional acts;
9. 'made' impulses.

See Davison and Neale (1982): 398–401.

Tic. Repeated jerky movements, usually of the face and neck. **Gilles de la Tourette's syndrome** is a grouping together of symptoms, one of which is meaningless grunting by the patient. *See Stafford-Clark and Smith (1983): 319.*

Token economy. A **behaviour therapy** technique based on the theory of **operant conditioning**. Basically, the patient will receive a reward if he overcomes the **anxiety**-provoking situation. The tokens which are given are intended to act as sufficient reinforcers to reduce the **aberrant** behaviour and promote the behaviour of the **norm**. *See Kazdin (1981).*

Trace conditioning. See **classical conditioning**.

Trait approach. An approach to **psychology** which has as its aim finding out the characteristics which make the person act the way he does. Traits are descriptions of behaviour characteristics such as aggressiveness, emotional stability, agreeableness, etc. In fact, a trait is any characteristic which differs significantly from person to person. It does not explain the person's behaviour. A method for measuring traits is factor analysis. This method allows the therapist to reduce a large number of measures to a small number of independent dimensions. Cattell developed a 16 personality factor questionnaire. The client is asked over 100 questions to which he need only reply 'yes/no', and from his replies Cattell could work out the patient's personality profile. For the trait approach to be effective, each person's profile should be compared in different situations to find out in which situation the patient's traits are most affected. *See Atkinson et al. (1983): 388–392.*

Transference. See **psychoanalysis**.

Tricyclics. See **antidepressant drugs**.

U

Unconditioned response. See **classical conditioning**.

Unconditioned stimulus. See **classical conditioning**.

Unconscious motives. See **psychoanalysis**.

Unipolar disorder. See **depression**.

Unsocialized conduct disorder. See **conduct disorder**.

UR. Unconditioned response.

US. Unconditioned stimulus.

V

Validity. If an **assessment** (1) is to be worthwhile, it must have **reliability**, validity and be discriminating. An assessment will be valid if it does measure what it claims to measure. There are several types of validity:

1. face validity occurs if the test looks as if it measures what it claims;

2. concurrent validity occurs when one and two assessments correlate closely together;

3. predictive validity occurs when the test is seen to correlate with the future performance of the patient;

4. construct validity occurs when it is possible to find out how well the test results correlate with hypothetical results which a therapist would expect from a particular patient.
See Purser (1982): 177–178.

Vicarious conditioning. See **modelling**.

W

WAIS. Wechsler Adult Intelligence Scale.

Wechsler tests. Tests produced by David Wechsler in the 1930s and 1940s. He produced the **Wechsler Intelligence Scale for Children** and the **Wechsler Adult Intelligence Scales**.

Wechsler Adult Intelligence Scale —Revised. The first version of **WAIS** was published in 1939 and revised in 1955. The latest edition was published in 1981. There are 11 subtests, five performance tests and six verbal tests. It can be used with adults in the age range of 16–74 years of age. The subtests have been designed from the easiest to the

most difficult and administration is stopped after the patient has failed a certain number of items. The test usually lasts over an hour. The **raw score** is converted into a **standard score** scale with a **mean** of 10 and a **standard deviation** of 3. When the six scaled scores of the verbal subtests and the five performance subtests are added together, as well as the scaled scores on all the 11 subtests, the three sums are converted to **IQ** scores—verbal, performance and full scale. The **IQs** have deviations with a mean of 100 and a **standard deviation** of 15. *See Aiken (1985): 154–158.*

Wechsler Intelligence Scale for Child-

ren—**Revised**. The original **WISC** was first designed in 1949. The revised version of **WISC** was published in 1974. It can be administered to children between the ages of 6 and 16 years. There are five verbal and five performance subtests with an additional two alternative subtests which are to be used with the child if one of the performance subtests is spoiled or proves difficult to administer. The test usually lasts one hour and the tester receives verbal, performance and full scale **IQ**s. *See Aiken (1985): 158–159.*

Wernicke-Korsakoff syndrome. A syndrome which can lead to **dementia**. It is produced by a vitamin deficiency in the **brain** (5). The vitamin in question is thiamine. Such deficiency of thiamine occurs in alcoholism, starvation and malnutrition. It has two stages:

1. Wernicke's encephalopathy. The person becomes disorientated in time and place, becomes drowsy, develops abnormalities of the eyes and **ataxia** (5). This is caused by the person taking drink only without anything to eat. Such a condition could be fatal unless the patient is given an injection of thiamine. If there is a delay in giving thiamine, the patient may recover but will be left with Korsakoff's syndrome.

2. Korsakoff's syndrome. During this part of the syndrome, the patient has problems with short-term **memory**. Proceeding from Wernicke's encephalopathy, the person cannot remember what he has been doing. He cannot find his way to places, and if he does, he cannot get back. Patients have difficulty forming new memories and they make up stories as they go along. The patient should be put on adequate diet with vitamin supplementation and should abstain from alcohol. Some people suffering from this syndrome commit suicide with the use of carbon-monoxide poisoning. *See Stafford-Clark and Smith (1983): 204.*

Wilcoxon test. A non-**parametric test** used with the **repeated measures design** for statistical analysis. It is the equivalent of the related t-test (see **T-tests**). The scores should be ranked in an interval ranking scale. *See Miller (1975): 96–98.*

WISC. **Wechsler Intelligence Scale for Children**.

Working through. See **psychoanalysis**.

Z

Z scores. A score or rank which shows how many of the **norm** group are above the patient's **raw score**. For example, if the person receives a Z score of 21 per cent, this means there are 79 per cent of the norm group above this score. It is part of **descriptive statistics**. *See Miller (1975): 51.*

REFERENCES

Aiken, L. R. (1985). *Psychological Testing and Assessment*. Allyn and Bacon.

Atkinson, R. L. Atkinson, R. C. and Hilgard, E. R. (1983). *An Introduction to Psychology*. Harcourt, Brace, Jovanovich.

Beard, R. M. (1969). *An Outline of Piaget's Developmental Psychology*. Routledge and Kegan Paul.

Bromley, D. B. (1974). *The Psychology of Human Ageing*. Penguin.

Coltheart, M. (1983). 'Aphasia Therapy Research: A Single-Case Study Approach'. In Code, C. and Muller, D. J. (1983). *Aphasia Therapy*. Edward Arnold.

Davison, G. C. and Neale, J. M. (1982). *Abnormal Psychology: An Experimental Clinical Approach*. John Wiley.

Diagnostic and Statistical Manual of Mental Disorders (3rd ed.) (DSM-III) (1980) Washington DC: American Psychiatric Association.

Donaldson, M. (1978). *Children's Minds*. Fontana.

Fawcus, M. (1986). *Voice Disorders and their Management*. Croom Helm.

Garvey, C. (1977). *Play*. Fontana.
Gilroy, J. and Holliday, P. L. (1982). *Basic Neurology*. Macmillan.
Kazdin, A. (1981). 'The Token Economy'. In Davey, G. (Ed.) (1981). *Applications of Conditioning Theory*. Methuen.
MacKay, D. (1975). *Clinical Psychology: Theory and Therapy*. Methuen.
Miller, S. (1975). *Experimental Design and Statistics*. Methuen.
Nelson-Jones, R. (1982). *The Theory and Practice of Counselling Psychology*. Holt, Rinehart and Winston.
Purser, H. (1982). *Psychology for Speech Therapists*. Macmillan.
Rachman, S. J. and Wilson, G. T. (1980). *The Effects of Psychological Therapy*. Pergamon Press.
Rutter, M. (1975). *Helping Troubled Children*. Penguin.
Shakespeare, R. (1975). *The Psychology of Handicap*. Methuen.
Stafford-Clark, D. and Smith, A. C. (1983). *Psychiatry for Students*. George Allen and Unwin.
Steinberg, D. D. (1982). *Psycholinguistics: Language, Mind and World*. Longman.
Trower, P., Bryant, B. and Argyle, M. (1978). *Social Skills and Mental Health*. Methuen.
Wing, L. (1980). *Autistic Children: A Guide for Parents*. Constable.
Wolff, S. (1981). *Children under Stress*. Penguin.
Wood, M. E. (1981). *The Development of Personality and Behaviour in Children*. Harrap.

Section 5
Medicine

A

Abdomen. The lower part of the alimentary system. The walls comprise muscles and bones. The roof of the abdomen is formed by the diaphragm which controls a person's respiratory volume. This structure produces **abdominal-diaphragmatic respiration**. The anterior wall is wholly muscle while only part of the back wall is made up of muscle. *See Tortora et al (1984): 13.*

Abdominal-diaphragmatic respiration. Breathing produced by movement of the diaphragm in the **abdomen**. As a person takes in a breath, the diaphragm increases in size and pushes out the stomach wall. As the breath is let out the opposite happens. This form of breathing is regarded as being correct. It is opposed to **clavicular respiration**.

Abducens nerve. See **cranial nerves**.

Abduction. A description of how joints move away from the midline. It is opposed to **adduction**. Speech therapists require to know about abduction as **dysphonia** (1) can result from an abductor nerve paralysis (see **laryngeal nerve palsies**: 1) affecting either one or both **vocal cords** (3). *See Tortora et al. (1984): 183.*

Accessory nerve. See **cranial nerves**.

Acrocephalosyndactyly. See **Apert's syndrome**.

Acute. A description of the sudden onset of an illness or disease.

Adam's apple. The non-technical term for the **larynx**.

Adduction. A description of how a joint moves towards the midline. It is opposed to **abduction**. Speech therapists require to know about this process as **dysphonia** (1) can result from an adductor nerve paralysis (see **laryngeal nerve palsies**: 1) affecting either one or both **vocal cords** (3). *See Tortora et al (1984): 183.*

Adenoid. A piece of lymphatic tissue found in the posterior wall of the **nasopharynx** (see **pharynx**). At birth, the adenoid is small and as the child grows older, the adenoid grows until puberty when the adenoid disappears. If it becomes too large, it may block the **eustachian tube** (see **ear**: 6) causing hearing problems and/or problems in the nasal cavaties causing nasal obstruction. Such obstruction results in **mouth**

breathing and snoring. If a child does have problems caused by adenoids, he will have a particular facial appearance—adenoidal facies. The problem may become so significant that an adenoidectomy in which the adenoids are removed is necessary. *See Pracy et al. (1974): 105–106.*

Adenoidal facies. See **mouth breathing**.

Afferent. A description of how sensory nerve impulses reach the **central nervous system**. *See Taverner (1983): 132.*

AFP. **Alpha-feto protein**. See **amniocentesis**.

Aglossia. See **glossectomy** (1).

Agonist. A description of the contraction of one muscle against another which acts as an **antagonist** muscle. This muscle contraction is also known as a prime mover. *See Tortora et al (1984): 227.*

Alpha-feto protein. See **amniocentesis**.

Alveolar ridge. See **mouth/swallowing**.

Alveoli. See **lung**.

Alzheimer's Disease. It is also known as **senile dementia**. The cause is unknown but the rate of loss of neurones increases in the **CNS**. **Atrophy** occurs in both the white and grey matter of the **brain** while the **sulci** (see **sulcus**) widen and the **gyri** (see **gyrus**) narrow. See also 1 and 4. *See Gilroy et al. (1982): 170–172.*

Amniocentesis. An invasive technique to monitor the development of the fetus in utero at 14 weeks into the pregnancy. A quantity of amniotic fluid, which surrounds the fetus, is drawn off and an examination of its cells is carried out. A chromosomal analysis will show if there are the correct number of **chromosomes**, if they have the correct structure and if the sex chromosomes are present or damaged. If there is a disorder found, the child, when born, is likely to suffer from a disease caused by a chromosomal abnormality (see **chromosome**). Alpha-feto protein is also examined. This is a protein which can leak out of the placenta. If there is raised alpha-feto protein, the child will probably suffer from **spina bifida**. *See Hosking (1982): 62.*

Anatomy. A study of the structures which exist in the human body. Some of these are visible to the eye, e.g., **mouth**, face, while others cannot be seen until the body is dissected or 'cut-up' (the word 'anatomy' means 'cutting-up'). A **speech therapist** (1) should know about the anatomy of the head, **mouth** and upper body including **pharynx**, **larynx**, **oesophagus**, **bronchi** and **lungs**. *See Tortora et al (1984): 4, 21–23.*

Angiomatous meningiomas. Type of **meningioma** tumour found in the **central nervous system** which is lined by endothelial cells. See **tumours of the central nervous system** (2d). *See Gilroy et al (1982): 206.*

Angle of the mandible. See **mandible/ muscles of mastication**.

Angular gyrus. A structure found in the parietal lobe (see **cerebral hemispheres**) of the **brain**. There are two parts which form the inferior parietal lobule, the angular gyrus is one and the supramarginal **gyrus** is the other. The angular gyrus is considered important in the acts of reading and writing. A disorder in it can produce **Dejerine syndrome**. *See Barr (1979): 176.*

Ankyloglossus. Often called a **tongue-tie**, produced by the **lingual frenulum** (see **tongue**) being attached all the way along the underside of the **tongue**. Tongue movement is restricted and **articulation delay/disorder** (1) can develop. *See Travis (1971).*

Anosognosia. Failure of a patient to recognize the disabled side of the body caused by a **CVA** or **head injury** to one of the **cerebral hemispheres**. Language may remain intact.

ANS. Autonomic nervous system.

Antagonist A muscle contraction which is opposed to the contraction of the prime mover i.e., **agonist muscle** (see **agonist**). *See Tortora et al (1984): 227.*

Apert's syndrome. A condition which involves an abnormal growth of the cranium and malformed fingers and toes. The patient's face has a particular appearance with wide-set, bulging eyes, abnormally small **maxillae**, crowded **teeth** and a protruding **mandible**. Usually, **intelligence** (4) is within normal limits although there can be a degree of **mental handicap** (1 and 4). It

is known as Acrocephalosyndactyly. *See Hosking (1982): 205–206.*

Apgar score. Devised by Virginia Apgar, it is a test given to newly born babies. If the test scores remain low for a considerable time, the prognosis for the baby's life and possible neurological sequelae are poor. It examines the baby's heart rate, respiratory effort, reflex irritability, muscle tone and colour. *See Illingworth (1983): 27, 89.*

Arcuate fasciculus. A band of fibres which links Broca's area to Wernicke's area (see **cerebral hemispheres**). A disturbance in this area of the **brain** produces **conduction aphasia** (1). Sometimes called the superior longitudinal fasciculus. *See Barr (1979): 197–198.*

Arnold-Chiari malformation. See **hydrocephalus**.

Articular disc. See **muscles of mastication**.

Arytenoid. Cartilages and muscle found in the **larynx**.

Astrocytomas. See **tumours of central nervous system**.

Ataxia. See **cerebral palsy**.

Athetosis. See **cerebral palsy**.

Atrophy. The wasting away of structures in any part of the body. It is often used referring to the wasting of part of the **brain**, which may produce such **communication disorders** (1) as **dysarthria** or **aphasia** (both 1). *See Gilroy et al. (1982).*

Auditory nerve. See **cranial nerves**.

Autonomic nervous system. Part of the nervous system which innervates **smooth muscle**. It is divided into two parts:
1. **sympathetic nervous system**;
2. **parasympathetic nervous system**.
It supplies the **heart**, sweat glands and digestive glands. *See Green (1978): 130.*

Autosomal dominant. See **chromosomes**.

Autosomal recessive. See **chromosomes**.

Autosomes. A human has 23 pairs of chromosomes, of which 22 are autosomes while the 23rd pair are sex chromosomes (see **chromosomes**). *See Hosking (1982): ch. 6.*

B

Babinski reflex. A reflex obtained as part of the **plantar response** during a neuro-

logical examination. The reflex takes the form of the hallux being extended with extension of the other toes which separate in the shape of a fan. *See Gilroy et al. (1982): 44.*

Basal ganglia. This structure is filled with grey matter at the base of the **brain**. The nuclei found in this structure include the caudate nucleus and lentiform nucleus. As the two nuclei have a stripe effect because of the way in which the grey and white matter are formed, both of these together are known as the corpus striatum. If this structure becomes diseased, **tremor** and **rigidity** (see **Parkinson's Disease**) may occur. *See Barr (1979): 164.*

Bell's palsy. A facial paralysis of the peripheral type produced by a disorder of the **facial nerve** (see **cranial nerves**). Its cause is unknown but it could be a result of a viral infection which involves the geniculate ganglion. Bell's palsy occurs often in the middle-aged and elderly. There is facial paralysis which progresses steadily to a severe weakness and even to total loss of function on one side of the face. The affected side presents a sagging face and an eye which can hardly close and, at times, it is impossible to close because of weakness in the **obicularis oculi** (see **muscles of facial expression**). The eye waters continuously but with the involvement of the **geniculate ganglion** can produce loss of tears resulting in dry eye. Initially, treatment is given by aspirin but later **corticosteroids** are often given. The eyes are treated with eye drops. There is a good prognosis and patients can recover within a two to three week period. About 15 per cent continue to have facial weakness and excessive lacrimation. However, old age provides a poor prognosis. *See Gilroy et al (1982): 311.*

Bifurcation. A division into two parts or branches such as the point at the bottom of the **trachea** where the two **bronchi** divide and lead into the **lungs**.

Bilateral. An occurrence which takes place on two sides of a structure. For example, **vocal nodules** (1) are said to be bilateral as there is one nodule on each of the **vocal cords** (3).

Bobath method. A particular treatment technique used in **physiotherapy**. This technique is aimed at producing symmetry of the body for those who suffer from **hemiplegia**. The therapist tries to get the patient to use their weak side, thus removing **anosognosia**. It is important that the patient learns to position the body correctly.

Bolus. See **swallowing**.

Bone. A type of **connective tissue** which can be of different strengths according to how it is made up. In other words, it can be very strong or decrease in strength until it becomes very brittle. Bone has a matrix, i.e., its formation, formed in a concentric tubular pattern. The outer surface has a layer of fibrous tissue known as periosteum. The bones which appear denser are compact bones while those which are more open on the inside are cancellous bone. Classification of the bone is according to shape. There are five types—long, short, flat, irregular and sesamoid bones. *See Tortora et al (1984): 124–134.*

Bradykinesia. See **Parkinson's disease**.

Brain. Comprises two **cerebral hemispheres**—the left and the right connected by the **corpus callosum**. The motor and sensory areas run in parallel lines on either side of the central fissure down to the lateral fissure. Below the cerebral **cortex** is the **thalamus** (acts as sensory relay station to cerebral cortex), **hypothalamus** (controls temperature, metabolism and endocrine balance), **reticular system** (arousal system which activates regions of cerebral cortex), **cerebellum** (controls muscles, balance and coordination of voluntary movement) and the **medulla oblongata** (controls breathing, swallowing, digestion and heart beat). *See Barr (1979): passim.*

Brain abscess. Acts like a **tumour of the central nervous system**. It distorts the brain structures by compressing its various parts. It is caused by bacteria from the **ear** (6), usually **suppurative otitis media** (see **otitis media**, 6), resulting in an abscess occurring in the **temporal lobe** (see **cerebral hemispheres**). The bacteria can also come from the blood. The symptoms produced are those of fever, **aphasia**, (1), **convulsions**, coma and headaches. Diagnosis is carried out by **CT scan**, X-rays of the **skull** and an examination of bacteria from the areas given above. Treatment is by surgical excision, anti-parasitic drugs and sulphadiazine and penicillin to reduce localized infection. *See Gilroy et al. (1982): 224–227.*

Brainstem. This structure within the **brain** comprises the **medulla oblongata**, the **pons** and the **midbrain**. Each of these three parts has structures particular to each as well as tracts and fibres which are common to all three. *See Barr (1979): chs 6 and 7.*

Bronchi. Two branchings to the left and right of the **trachea** which lead to the left and right **lungs** respectively. There are three differences between the two bronchi:

1. The right bronchus is shorter than the left.
2. The right bronchus is vertical while the left is almost horizontal.
3. The right bronchus is wide while the left is narrower. *See Joseph (1979): 125.*

Buccal nerve. See **mouth**.

Buccinator. See **muscles of facial expression**.

Bulbar palsy. A palsy caused by a disorder in the pathways the nuclei of which arrive in the **medulla oblongata**. This disease produces weakness in the affected muscles which can deteriorate over a period of time. The disease affects four muscle groups:

1. **muscles of mastication**;
2. **muscles for swallowing**;
3. muscles of the **tongue**;
4. muscles of the face.

It is a progressive disease which begins with difficulty of tongue movement, progressing to immobility of the tongue. The **obicularis oris** (see **muscles of facial expression**) muscles are affected in the early stages making it difficult to close the lips producing excessive drooling. The **soft palate** (see **mouth**) fails to close which allows food to be regurgitated down the **nose**. The final stage of the disease is a failure to swallow and close the jaw. In many cases, prognosis is poor and it can lead to death in one to two years of onset due to aspiration pneumonia. If the muscles are affected by an **upper neurone disease**, (see **neurone**) there is **spastic** (see **spasticity** and **cerebral palsy**) rather than **flaccid** (see **flaccidity**) weakness. This is also known as Pseudo-Bulbar Palsy. There is no cure, only ways to make life bearable, e.g., liquidized food for easy **swallowing**, or drugs for reducing muscle pain. *See Draper (1980): 167–168.*

C

Cafe-au-lait syndrome. See **neurofibromas** (**tumours of the central nervous system** (3)).

Canal. Any passage or tube-like structure within the body. For example, the **ear canal** (see **ear**, 6) situated in the **outer ear** (see **ear**, 6) is an air-filled tube closed at one end by the **eardrum** (see **ear**, 6).

Cancellous bone. See **bone**.

Cancer. A layman's term used to describe the existence of a **tumour**. There are various types of cancerous growths or **tumours**. They can occur in the brain (**tumours of the central nervous system**), the **larynx**, and commonly, in the female breast. The term 'cancer' usually describes tumours when they are **malignant**.

Carbamazepine. See **epilepsy**.

Carcinoma. A **malignant** growth which can appear in any part of the body, removal of which requires an operation. *See Pracy et al. (1974): passim.*

Carotid artery. One of the main arteries in the neck. As it rises it branches into the internal and external carotid arteries. The external carotid artery serves structures within the neck and head such as the **larynx, tongue, external ear** (see **ear**,

6), and **muscles of mastication**, etc. The internal carotid artery supplies parts of the **brain**. *See Joseph (1979): 98–100.*

Cartilage. A type of **connective tissue**. There are three types of cartilage—hyaline, fibrous and elastic. The hyaline type is found in the costal cartilages, the fibrous type is found in discs among the vertebrae, while the elastic type is found in the **pinna** (see **ear**: 6) and the **epiglottis**. *See Tortora et al. (1984): 12–13.*

Catarrh. A symptom of nasal irritation. The commonest products in the atmosphere to cause catarrh are dust, alcohol and tobacco. Commonly described as a 'stuffy nose'. *See Pracy et al. (1974): 61–65.*

Central nervous system. The system within the body which produces reflexes when one part of the body is particularly stimulated. Most of these responses come from the **brain** via the **spinal cord**. Its opposite is the **autonomic nervous system**. *See Taverner (1983): ch. 13.*

Centrencephalic epilepsy. See **congenital neuronal dysfunction**.

Cephalic. Usually a suffix to describe disorders in or of the head, for example,

microcephalic (an abnormally small head).

Cerebellar. A description of structures found around the **cerebellum** and of disorders which occur within the cerebellum, producing **dysarthric** characteristics (see **dysarthria**, 1) in the patient's speech.

Cerebellum. Comprises a cortex of grey matter, a central area in the middle of white matter and four pairs of central nuclei. The cerebellum is connected to the **medulla oblongata, pons** and the **midbrain** by the inferior, middle and cerebellar peduncles respectively. The cerebellum organizes the person's motor movements. The synchronous movements of muscles will be affected adversely if there is a lesion to this part of the **brain** affecting the person's speech, producing **cerebellar dysarthria** (1). *See Barr (1979): ch. 10.*

Cerebral. A description of structures or disorders which occur within the **brain**.

Cerebral abscess. See **brain abscess**.

Cerebral artery. The artery which runs through the **brain**. The major part of the artery is the middle cerebral artery which is situated in the lateral fissure between the **frontal** and **temporal lobes** (see **cerebral hemispheres**). During a **CVA**, this artery bursts and blood spreads over the brain which affects areas such as Broca's area (see **cerebral hemisphere**) as it supplies this area. Thus, a rupture of the artery can cause **aphasia** (1). *See Barr (1979): 294.*

Cerebral hemispheres. The **brain** has two hemispheres, right and left, connected by the **corpus callosum**. Both hemispheres have four lobes—frontal, temporal, parietal and occipital. The left hemisphere in the majority of people is known as the **dominant hemisphere** (see **dominance**) and it controls the right side of the brain. It contains the language centres of the brain. In particular, Broca's area can be found in the frontal lobe while Wernicke's area can be found in the parietal lobe. Both hemispheres have a motor and sensory strip from which signals are sent to the nerves innervating the muscles of movement, touch and smell, etc. The occipital lobe is concerned with vision. The right hemisphere has centres for rhythm, artistry, arithmetic and control of muscles used for speaking and eating. *See Barr (1979): ch. 13, 194–195.*

Cerebral infarction. See **cerebrovascular accident**.

Cerebral palsy. A group of disorders of movement and posture due to slow development and non-progressive disorders of the **brain**. There are several possible causes of cerebral palsy which can occur at various times around the child's birth.

1. During the **prenatal**, i.e., before birth, period, the possible causes are congenital infections, e.g., **TORCH**, congenital malformations within the brain, radiation or nutritional deficiency.

2. During the **perinatal**, i.e., process of delivery, period, the possible causes are periventricular haemorrhage, birth asphyxia, birth trauma, hyperbilirubinaemia or venous stasis/thrombosis.

3. During the **postnatal**, i.e., after birth, period, the possible causes are **meningitis, encephalitis, trauma** or metabolic disorder.

There are four types of cerebral palsy:

1. Spastic cerebral palsy. The commonest type of **CP** which accounts for about 70 per cent of children so affected. The damage to the brain, which produces **hemiplegia** and **bilateral** hemiplegia, is centred on the **corticospinal tracts** (see **pyramidal system**). Bilateral hemiplegia produces a **pseudobulbar palsy** (see **bulbar palsy**) which produces speech with **dysarthric** characteristics (see **dysarthria**, 1), impaired **swallowing** and a poor **gag reflex**.

2. Ataxic cerebral palsy. Damage to the brain in the **cerebellum** which produces **hypotonia**, a broad base gait, tremor and **dysmetria**. The patient's speech is **dysarthric** (see **dysarthria**, 1) although **intelligence** (4) is normal.

3. Dyskinetic cerebral palsy. Damage to the brain, causing involuntary movements and reduced voluntary movements, is found around the **basal ganglia**.

a) Athetosis. A subtype of dyskinetic **CP** producing slow, writhing movements and severely **dysarthric** speech (see **dysarthria**, 1) caused by damage to the **extrapyramidal system** in the brain, asphyxia at birth or anoxia to the **basal ganglia**.

b) Chorea. A subtype of dyskinetic **CP** producing fast, jerky movements in the upper extremities caused by a disease to the **basal ganglia**.

c) Dystonia. A subtype of dyskinetic **CP** producing increase in muscle tone, no contractures and persistence of primitive reflexes. Distorted postures are maintained for long periods of time and produce rotation, adduction of limbs and extension of the spine. It affects the

agonist and **antagonist** muscles.

4. Mixed cerebral palsy. A form of **CP** which has characteristics of (1)–(3).

Those who are involved with treatment will be the **physiotherapist, speech therapist** (1), **educational psychologist** (4) and, possibly an **ENT** surgeon. *See Gilroy (1982): 63–64; Hosking (1982): ch. 7; Illingworth (1983): ch. 16 (diagnosis of CP) and 258–259.*

Cerebrospinal fluid. Fluid which flows round the **brain** coming from **ventricles** (see **third ventricle** and **fourth ventricle**) in the **brain** and the central **canal** of the **spinal cord**. Most of the **CSF** consists of water, cells and little protein. It has also sugar and sodium chloride. The **CSF** is used to diagnose diseases of the **meninges** and **central nervous system**. *See Barr (1979): 309–312.*

Cerebrovascular accident. The medical term which encompasses the different ways in which a 'stroke' occurs. There are two disorders which affect the blood vessels supplying the **brain**— haemorrhage and cerebral infarction. A haemorrhage occurs when a vessel bursts either in the brain itself or in the **subarachoid space**. The commonest cause is berry anneurysms. The vessel wall is weakened and the dilating artery bursts through the defective part. Ninety per cent of berry anneurysms are found on the **circle of Willis**. The rupture of anneurysms can affect **cranial nerves III** and **Vi** and **Vii**. They form usually at the junction in the **cerebral artery**. The majority of patients suffer the following symptoms:

1. severe generalized headache with pain in the neck;
2. nausea and vomiting;
3. transient vertigo;
4. feelings of faintness and confusion.

Arterio Venous Malformations are a haphazard grouping of blood vessels which appear in the **parietal lobe** (see **cerebral hemispheres**) although it can occur elsewhere in the brain. The part of the brain which is affected is stained by numerous small haemorrhages. The symptoms are generalized or partial **seizures**, headaches on the side of the malformation, a 'bruit' is heard over the orbits in the **skull** and 50 per cent of malformations bleed into the **subarachnoid space**. Treatment is given for the seizures by anticonvulsant drugs while surgery can be used to remove the malformation.

There are two types of cerebral infarction—embolism and thrombosis.

1. An embolism begins as a thrombus on the wall of the left atrium (see **heart**) of a fibrillating heart. When it becomes detached it comes to rest in a branch of the left **middle cerebral artery** (see **cerebral artery**). **Hemiplegia**, unconsciousness or **aphasia** (1) occurs within a few seconds of onset. Fifty per cent of all **strokes** are caused by a blood vessel blockage.

2. A thrombosis causes a blockage to the **internal carotid** or vertebral arteries as well as the cerebral arteries and their branches. Mostly, cerebral infarction follows thrombosis of an atherosclerotic vessel. It occurs also as a complication from other diseases. In general, cerebral infarction will occur only when there is a critical reduction of blood flow to the brain. *See Gilroy et al. (1982): chs 8 and 9.*

Chorda tympani nerve. See **tongue**.

Chorea. See **cerebral palsy**.

Chromosomes. A baby receives 22 pairs of chromosomes plus a sex chromosome from each parent. In a male these chromosomes are an X and a Y, while in the female they are an X and an X. As this is an equal division of the chromosomes, the child has half the characteristics of each parent. If there is an abnormality in the chromosomes, certain syndromes can result, e.g., **Downs Syndrome**. Some syndromes and diseases are described in terms of the type of autosomal or sex chromosome abnormality. A dominant autosomal disorder is inherited by several members of the family, while a recessive autosomal disorder is inherited by fewer members of the family. Disorders can be produced by an abnormality of the X part of the sex chromosome. An X-linked recessive disorder appears in males as they have only one X chromosome and so will have the abnormal gene. However, females who have an abnormal gene in one X chromosome have a second X chromosome which cancels out the first. For an X-linked disorder to be present in females both X chromosomes have to be affected. *See Hosking (1982); 32, ch. 6.*

Chronic. A description of a disease or illness which has a slow onset or its symptoms are slow to appear. It is opposed to **acute**.

Circle of Willis. A circular artery in the **brain** which is the endpoint for various **cerebral arteries** and around which the blood flows. The arteries which end in the circle of Willis are the anterior communicating, anterior cerebral, internal carotid, posterior communicating and posterior cerebral arteries. If damage occurs in one of the major arteries. it is possible for blood to flow round the other arteries because of the circle of Willis. *See Barr (1979): 298.*

Circum vallate papillae. See **taste buds**.

Clavicular. A description of the use of the chest. For example, some patients suffering from **dysarthria** (1) will not produce normal **abdominal-dia-phragmatic respiration**, but, instead, breathe from their chest. This is known as clavicular respiration.

Clavicular respiration. See **clavicular**.

Cleft palate. In the normal development of the **mouth** the palatal shelves come together to form the **hard palate** (see **mouth**) as the **tongue** falls down into the cavity. A cleft palate is the embryological failure of the **hard palate** to fuse together while the child is in utero. A cleft lip is caused by failure of the tissue surrounding the lip to fuse together during the same period. A cleft lip and palate occurs when both the hard palate and lip have failed to form in utero. Clefts can occur unilaterally or bilaterally. Most child who have this condition at birth can be helped by surgery. A cleft lip will be repaired around 3 months of age while a cleft of the palate will be closed at 6 months of age. Carrying out an operation at such an early age allows the surgeons to make use of the continual growth in the tissues of the affected areas. Thus, healing is more natural and few scars are left. A submucous cleft palate has a divided **uvula**, a whitish line down the midline of the **soft palate** and a bony notch on the ridge between the soft and hard palates. The muscles of the soft palate do not function correctly and **velopharyngeal incompetence** (see **velopharyngeal**) may result. Occult submucous cleft palate exists when the situation just outlined occurs but the white line is obscured by muscle, the bony notch is not evident and there is no bifiduvula either. *See Edwards and Watson (1980): ch. 3, 100–103, ch. 12.*

Clonic. See **epilepsy**.

CNS, Central nervous system.

Compact bones. See **bone**.

Compound racemose gland. See **salivary glands**.

Computer axial tomography. Another name for **computer tomography**. *See Draper (1980): 107.*

Computer tomography. A non-invasive technique used to locate space occupied by lesions. It differs from ordinary X-ray techniques in that it uses a narrow, moving beam which scans the brain. The results are processed by computer which distinguishes the different densities of brain tissue. Thus, lesions can be picked out quickly, some having a greater or lesser density than the surrounding brain tissue. A **CT** scan can pick out haemorrhages, **tumours** (see **tumours of the central nervous system**), cysts as well as atrophy, oedema, necrosis and **multiple sclerosis**. *See Barr (1979): 208–209; Gilroy et al. (1982): passim.*

Congenital muscular dystrophy. A congenital myopathy. This is different from the muscular **dystrophy** from which children can suffer in later years. It is not so much progressive weakness of muscles as a collection of more than one symptom. The severe physical breakdown of the muscle is similar to other forms of dystrophy but those who are affected may get better gradually. The underdevelopment of the joints is present at birth. Treatment is given through **physiotherapy**. *See Gilroy et al. (1982): 343; Hosking (1982): 174.*

Congenital neuronal dysfunction. A condition which produces sudden, abnormal discharges of neurones in the **brain**, producing epileptic **convulsions**. This occurs in the **reticular system** in the centrencephalon. Thus, the type of **epilepsy** produced is known as centrencephalic epilepsy. *See Draper (1980): 85.*

Connective tissue. Made up of cells in a ground substance comprising fibres. There are two types determined by the type and quantity of fibres in the ground substance—packing **CT** and supporting **CT**. In the former there are two groups —reticular tissue and loose/dense **CT**, while in the latter there are **bone** and **cartilage**. *See Tortora et al (1984): 90–98.*

Contrecoup effect. See **head injury**.

Convulsion. The sudden onset of **seizure**-like, involuntary movements e.g., **grand-mal epilepsy** (see **epilepsy**), **ferbrile convulsions**.

Cordectomy. A description of the surgical removal of a **vocal cord** (3) caused by **laryngeal nerve palsies** (1) or **tumours** on the cord. When one cord is removed, the one which remains will usually compensate completely; if this does not happen, it might require a **teflon injection** (1) to enable it to do so.

Coronoid process. See **mandible**.

Corpus callosum. A part of the **brain** found in the **thalamus**. It links the two **cerebral hemispheres** and covers the **lateral ventricle** (see **third ventricle**).

Its main body is about 8cm long and it carries information from one hemisphere to the other. The fibres from each lobe run around it. *See Barr (1979): 201.*

Cortex. A covering of grey matter which covers the two **cerebral hemispheres**. It is a hard layer shaped into folds. Its total weight is about 40 per cent of the weight of the **brain**. It is full of neurons, other fibres and is 1–4mm thick. *See Barr (1979): ch. 14.*

Cortical. A term for describing structures or disorders found in or near to the **cortex**.

Corticosteroids. Used for treating some diseases by reducing inflammatory reaction in the nerve itself and preventing the adverse effects of prolonged pressure within a **canal**. *See Tortora et al (1984): 118.*

CP. Cerebral palsy.

Cranial nerves. Nerves which leave the **brain** to innervate different muscles throughout the body. Lesions to these nerves may produce **dysarthria** (1). There are 12 nerves:

I.   Olfactory—affects the sense of smell
II.   Optic—affects vision
III. Oculomotor—supplies· extraocular muscles
IV.   Trochlear—supplies superior oblique muscles
V.   Trigeminal—consists of three parts:
      i   ophthalmic
      ii maxillary (upper jaw)
      iii mandibular (lower jaw)
VI.   Abducens—supplies lateral rectus
VII. Facial—supplies **muscles of facial expression** (**motor** component) —supplies sensation of **taste**
VIII. Vestibulocochlear—supplies balance and hearing
IX.   Glossopharyngeal—supplies general sensation and **taste** —supplies sensory component of pharyngeal plexus
X.   Vagus—supplies **parasympathetic** component of cardiac oesophageal and pulmonary plexi —sensory component supplies the superior laryngeal nerves and recurrent laryngeal nerves
XI.   Accessory—supplies the spinal and cervical areas of the spine
XII. Hypoglossal—supplies all **intrinsic muscles** and all **extrinsic muscles** of the **tongue** except the palato glossus (see **mouth**).

These nerves cross over as they travel through the body. As they leave the **brain**, those from the left side cross to the right side of the body, while those from the right side of the brain cross to the left side of the body. Thus, if a person suffers a **CVA** in the left **cerebral hemisphere**, he will have a **hemiplegia** down the right side, as the nerves from the left hemisphere will be affected. *See Gilroy et al (1982): 10–36.*

Cricoarytenoid. See **larynx**.

Cricoid cartilage. See **larynx**.

Cri du chat syndrome. A **syndrome** found in children which produces **mental handicap** (1 and 4). The child produces a high pitched cat-like cry during infancy, more frequent in females, of low birth weight, with **microcephaly** and some facial abnormalities. It is a chromosomal disorder. *See Hosking (1982): 88.*

CSF. **Cerebrospinal fluid**.

CT. Connective tissue.

CT Scan. **Computer tomography scan**.

Cuneiform cartilages. Found in the **larynx**. There are two such cartilages. They look like small mounds and appear in the ary-epiglottic fold. *See Tortora et al (1984): 545.*

CVA. **Cerebrovascular accident**.

Cyanosis. A condition found in people who suffer from anoxia, either from anoxic anoxia or stagnant anoxia producing a lack of oxygen in the blood. *See Tortora et al (1984): 476, 515.*

Cytomegalovirus. One of the diseases which can produce disorders in the children if the mother suffers from it during the **prenatal stage** of the child's development. It can result in **mental handicap** (1 and 4), **cerebral palsy** and other handicaps in the child. It is part of the **TORCH** classification of conditions which can affect the foetus during the **prenatal** period. *See Hosking (1982): 199.*

D

Dandy-Walker malformation. A malformation in an abnormally large head. It occurs in the **fourth ventricle** while the child is growing. It is associated with **hydrocephalus** while the brain tissue around it fails to grow adequately. *See Hosking (1982): 71–72.*

Degeneration. The progressive wasting of part of the body or structures within the body caused by disease. Nerves in the peripheral nervous and **central nervous system** can degenerate by Wallerian degeneration. Its opposite is regeneration. *See Barr (1979): 39–41.*

Deglutition. Another word for **swallowing**.

Dejerine syndrome. The only **acquired dyslexia** (1) which has precise neurological lesion sites, described by Dejerine in 1892 and more fully explained in Geschwind (1965). It causes patients to read letter by letter. It is caused by the link between the **angular gyrus** in the left **cerebral hemisphere** and the visual input system in both hemispheres being broken. Since the angular gyrus is unaffected *per se*, writing is relatively unimpaired but because of the disconnection, the written input cannot reach the gyrus and so reading is severely affected. *See Patterson and Kay (1982): 411–441.*

Dementia. The progressive destruction of brain cells producing changes in a person's character especially in old age. This destruction may be caused by **trauma**, infections to **CNS**, **tumours**, metabolic disorders, infarctions or haemorrhages (see **cerebrovascular accident**). The principal dementias are **Alzheimer's Disease** or **senile dementia**, **multi-infarct dementia** (4), **Pick's disease** (4), normal pressure **hydrocephalus**, **Jacob-Creutzfeldt disease** and **Huntington's chorea** (4). *See Gilroy et al. (1982): 169.*

Dendrite. A type of **neurone** which is short, chubby and has branches emanating at one end while at the other there is a long axon. *See Tortora (1984): 271.*

Depressor anguli labii inferioris. See **muscles of facial expression**.

Diaphragm. See **abdominal-diaphragmatic respiration**.

Diastematomyelia. A rare condition in which a bony projection produces a cleft of the **spinal cord**. There is weakness in the muscles in legs and feet deformity.

Sensory impairment may also exist. Surgery can provide relief from some of the symptoms in some cases. *See Gilroy et al. (1982): 57.*

Diazepam. A possible drug treatment for **epilepsy**.

Diencephalon. A structure in the **brain**, also known as the **forebrain**, which appears immediately above the **midbrain**. It has two branches which become the **cerebral hemispheres**. As they grow forwards, they form the frontal lobes (see **cerebral hemispheres**), growing backwards, the **occipital lobes** (see **cerebral hemispheres**) and to the sides, the **temporal lobes** (see **cerebral hemispheres**). The hemispheres hide the other structures of the brain to such an extent that the only way they can be seen is from below. The structures of the **thalamus**, **hypothalamus** and **third ventricle** are also found in this area. *See Barr (1979): 141–163.*

Digastric muscles. See **muscles of mastication**.

Distocclusion. A type of **malocclusion** found in a person's teeth. See **orthodontics**.

Dominance. Most patients who are right-handed will have a left **cerebral hemisphere** dominance for controlling **language** (3) and other movements and a right cerebral dominance which controls **speech** (1) and rhythm. The same is true for the majority of left-handed people. For the other left-handed people (about 2 per cent), the language and speech centres are in the opposite hemispheres. Sperry (Nobel Prize Winner, 1981) carried out experiments where the two hemispheres were split so that he could find out accurately the specialization of each hemisphere. This is also known as cerebral dominance. *See Atkinson et al. (1983): 44–50.*

Down's syndrome. In the mid-1860s, Dr Langdon Down identified the characteristics of this **syndrome** to which he gave his name. It is also called by a nickname 'Mongolism' because sufferers of Down's Syndrome look like Mongolians. This syndrome is produced by Trisomy 21. In other words, an extra chromosome is produced, bringing the total of chromosomes in the person suffering from Down's Syndrome to 47 instead of 46. The physical features which characterize Down's Syndrome are:

1. Epicanthic folds, i.e., slanting eyes;
2. **Hypotonic** (see **hypotonia**) limbs, i.e., floppy;
3. square-shaped faces;
4. small noses and ears;
5. tongues which come forward more than in normal children;
6. teeth appear much later than normal children;
7. little fingers curve inwards;
8. a wider gap between big and second toes.

Neurological problems such as **epilepsy** are very rare, milestones are almost always delayed, **intelligence** (4) is low, they tend to have heart malformations and are prone to upper respiratory tract infection. People who suffer from this condition comprise 22 per cent of the whole **mental handicap** (1 and 4) population in Great Britain. There is an equal distribution throughout the world. One in every 666 live births results in Down's Syndrome. *See Cunningham (1982): passim.*

Duchenne muscular dystrophy. See **dystrophy**.

Dyskinetic cerebral palsy. See **cerebral palsy**.

Dysmetria. The loss of the ability to work out the distance between the person and the object. It is caused by a lesion in the **cerebellum**. *See Gilroy et al (1982): 36, 200.*

Dystonia. The abnormal movement or posture caused by a disorder affecting the **agonist** and **antagonist** muscles. Dystonia musculorum deformans is a movement disorder caused by a disorder in the axial and limb muscles. It can be inherited as an autosomal dominant or recessive trait. The condition progresses from a mild movement disorder to involvement of the lower limbs and in its final form to inability to walk. There is no particular drug therapy. However, there is often spontaneous remission. Acute dystonic reaction is caused by the sudden onset of dystonic movements in the facial muscles and a movement disorder in the eyes. Meige's Disease affects movements of face, mouth and jaw. This is also known as Breugel's Disease. *See Gilroy et al. (1982): 96, 107, 108.*

Dystrophy. Usually describes the weakness and **degeneration** of muscles fibres caused by genetically controlled myopathies. There are several dystrophies which all have different characteristics. The main type is Duchenne muscular dystrophy which is a sex-linked recessive disease. As with all dystrophies the disease is progressive. It occurs predominantly in males in the ratio 20 : 100,000. Babies are normal at birth and reach their early milestones at a normal rate although there may be some delay in standing and walking. The patient develops a clumsy, waddling gait and has difficulty in climbing stairs. **Gower's sign** appears at this stage. By about 10 years, the patient is confined to a wheelchair. Prognosis is not good, death is likely in the teens or early twenties. Facioscapulohumeral dystrophy is an autosomal dominant disease. It begins between 10 and 20 years. The patient suffers minimal disability. Scapuloperoneal dystrophy is an autosomal dominant or sex-linked recessive disease and occurs in early childhood. No treatment is required and there is a full-life expectancy. Limb girdle dystrophy is an autosomal recessive disease, occurring between the ages of 10–20. The patient may be confined to a wheelchair after 40 years of age. Distal dystrophy is autosomal dominant, occurring in adults. There is full-life expectancy. Oculopharyngeal dystrophy is autosomal dominant and occurs in the middle years and it is slowly progressive. *See Gilroy et al. (1982): 337–340.*

E

EEG. **Electroencephalography**.

Electroencephalography. A technique for studying the electrical activity within the **brain**. These emanate from the cerebral **cortex**. The patient either lies on a bed or sits upright and electrodes are put over the **skull**. The waves are plotted on an electroencephalogram by a machine known as an electroencephalograph. There are four types of wave which can appear on the printout:

(1) Alpha waves appear at a frequency

of 10–12 cycles per second and appear in most people while awake.

(2) Beta waves appear between frequencies of 15–60 cycles per second and occur while the nervous system is functioning.

(3) Theta waves appear at frequencies of 5–8 cycles per second and occur when the person is under emotional **stress** (4).

(4) Delta waves appear at frequencies of 1–5 cycles per second and occur while the person is asleep. If they occur and the adult is awake, this could indicate brain damage. It is used in the diagnosis of **epilepsy, tumours of the central nervous system**, and infectious diseases such as **meningitis** and **trauma**. *See Tortora et al (1984); 329, 357, 358.*

Embryo. The intrauterine organism which after about two months develops into the fetus. *See Haines and Mohiuddin (1972): passim.*

Embryonic. A description of an **embryo**.

Encephalitis. The result of a viral infection which invades the **central nervous system**. It occurs mainly in the frontal and temporal lobes (see **cerebral hemispheres**) of the **brain**. The virus produces a fever, **focal sites**, **convulsions** and coma. Treatment takes the form of antiviral agents, steroids and anticonvulsants. **EEGs** are used as means of **diagnosis** (1) of encephalitis. *See Gilroy et al. (1982): 246–251.*

Encephalitis lethargica. A cause of postencephalitic Parkinsonism, found during the worldwide epidemic in 1917–1928. *See Gilroy et al. (1982): 103.*

Endocrine system. This system comprises glands which do not have ducts and secrete directly into the bloodstream. It is the opposite of the exocrine glands. The endocrine glands include the pituitary and thyroid glands, four parathyroids, two adrenal glands, two gonad glands and the pancreas which can function in both the endocrine and exocrine systems. The fluid secreted by these glands is known as a hormone. *See Green (1978): 114–120.*

ENT. Ear, Nose and Throat. *See Pracy et al. (1974): passim.*

Epiglottis. A structure at the top of the **larynx** and behind the hyoid bone. *See Tortora et al. (1984): 545.*

Epilepsy. Epilepsy is not a disease in itself but a symptom of a disease. While the symptom lasts, there is an abnormal amount of electrical activity reaching the cerebral **cortex** from a **focal site** in the **brain**. It occurs in the following diseases

—**congenital neuronal dysfunction, systemic metabolic disorder** and **structural brain disease**. The symptom shows itself in different ways:

1. Grand-mal epilepsy takes the form of a generalized seizure. It begins with feelings of agitation and the 'attack' is sudden. The patient finds himself in a dreamy state, collapses and will probably turn a shade of 'blue' because of stenosis. During the **tonic** phase, he lets out screams, grits teeth and the body is rigid. This stage lasts about 30 seconds. The clonic phase begins with the patient waving his limbs wildly without control and he may become incontinent. Eventually, the patient falls into a deep sleep and within a few hours wakens normally. He will be unable to remember any of these events.

2. Petit-mal epilepsy is found mainly among children. They have a momentary loss of consciousness, i.e., one to two seconds, during which they either blink or stare into space. It looks often as if they have poor or limited attention span. At worst, it can occur hundreds of times a day, at best, when controlled by drugs, only rarely. There is no collapse and recovery follows immediately with no other side-effects. It is always due to **congenital neuronal dysfunction**. There can be remittance in adolescence. It is much commoner than grand-mal epilepsy.

3. Status epilepticus consists of a series of **fits** between which the patient does not recover consciousness. It can last for hours with the minimum duration being about one hour and requires immediate treatment with drugs. The cause is usually split 50/50 between those patients who have been removed suddenly from a drug regime or have removed themselves and those who suffer from **structural brain disease**. Generalized seizures take place in the form of grand-mal, petit-mal attacks, or tonic/clonic seizures or myoclonus.

4. Myoclonus consists of non-repetitive shock-like contractions of muscles or muscle groups. It is caused by electrical discharges from many levels of the **central nervous system**. It can also occur in metabolic encephalopathy, including hypoxia, hepatic and uremic encephalopathy and in many infections and **degenerative** (see **degeneration**) diseases of the **brain**, **brainstem** and **spinal cord**.

The popular drug treatment for adults suffering from epilepsy is phenytoin but it can produce facial hair, acne rash, thickness of facial features and may cause problems to the **mouth**. Carbamazepine is given if phenytoin causes problems from its side-effects. However, carbamazepine causes atrophy of the **cerebellum** and the gums may become thickened. It can also interfere with the liver and with vitamin D. Sodium-valproate can reduce grand-mal and petit-mal seizures but it may cause an increase in weight and gastro-intestine problems. Ethosuximide is used for **petit-mal epilepsy** sufferers. Its side-effects include drowsiness, headache, photophobia, dizziness, hiccoughs, bone marrow suppression and vomiting. Diazepam is given intravenously for those who suffer from status epilepticus. *See Gilroy et al. (1982): ch. 4.*

Epithelium. Epithelial cells form themselves into membranes which can be of one layer or several layers. The former is simple epithelium while the latter is stratified epithelium. The three types of epithelial cells which form themselves into these membranes are squamous cells (flat and thick at the nucleus), cuboidal cells (similar in height and width and are many-sided) and columnar cells (polygonal in shape, height is greater than width). The three types differ in their appearance depending on whether they form simple or stratified epithelial membranes. *See Leeson and Leeson (1970): ch. 5.*

Ethmoid plate. See **nose**.
Ethosuximide. See **epilepsy**.
External carotid artery. See **carotid artery**.
Extrapyramidal system. A system of fibres which operates the whole motor system within the **central nervous system**, excluding the **pyramidal system**. *See Barr (1979): 271–275.*
Extrinsic muscles of the tongue. There are three extrinsic muscles of the **tongue**.

1. The genioglossus muscle runs from the superior genial tubercle of the **mandible** and inserts itself under the tongue. It is supplied by the lingual artery, lingual vein and **cranial nerve IX**. This nerve supplies the surface of the back one-third of the tongue, the **circum vallate papillae** (see **taste buds**).

2. The styloglossus muscle runs from the **styloid process** to the **tongue**. It pulls the tongue back and upwards. It is supplied by the **lingual nerve** and **cranial nerve Viii**.

3. The hyoglossus muscle runs from the hyoid bone (see **muscles for swallowing**) to the tongue and pulls it backwards and downwards. It is supplied by the hypoglossal nerve. *See Tortora et al (1984): 587.*

F

Facial nerve. See **cranial nerves**.
Facioscapulohumeral muscular dystrophy. See **dystrophy**.
Falx cerebri. A sickle-shaped structure within the **brain** attached at the top along the midline of the skull and crossing over the **corpus callosum**. At one end it is attached to the tentorium cerebelli. *See Barr (1979): 305.*
Fascia. There are two types of fascia—superficial and deep fascia. The former is a loose **connective tissue** while the latter is a dense **connective tissue** made up in sheets. *See Tortora et al (1984): 204.*
Fasciculus. A bundle or a group of nerve or muscle fibres (e.g., **arcuate fasciculus**). *See Tortora et al (1984): 225–27.*
Fauces. See **mouth**.
Febrile convulsions. A condition which occurs during a fever associated with an acute systemic infection disease. They are not caused by infection to the **central nervous system**. Most children with this condition have a history of neurological or developmental abnormality. The movements during these convulsions are of the **tonic** and **clonic** (see **epilepsy**) type. A poor prognosis exists if the child has associated neurological problems. However, if the child suffers from febrile convulsions per se, there is a better prognosis. When convulsions last for longer than 30 minutes, the brain is deprived of oxygen and scarring in the temporal lobe can produce a permanent focus for **epilepsy** in adulthood. Drug treatment is provided. Phenobarbitone is given if the convulsion lasts for longer than five to ten minutes. **Sodium-valproate** (see **epilepsy**) can also be used. If this condition is suspected before birth, the mother is given **diazepam** (see **epilepsy**) rectally or intravenously as it has a very fast absorption rate. Children should

always be kept cool during a convulsion. It occurs in 3 per cent of all children, the highest incidence being between 10 months and two years of age. About 30 per cent have a family history. *See Gilroy et al. (1982): 71.*

Festinant gait. See **Parkinson's disease**.

Fetal alcohol syndrome. A condition from which the child suffers if the mother has been an alcoholic during pregnancy. It can produce **mental handicap** (1 and 4) and give the child a particular facial appearance—a small nose, slit eyes and a convex top lip. The child is often irritable, is **hypertonic** (see **hypertonia**) and suffers from tremor and **tonic** seizures. The irritability can be treated by **chlorpromazine** (4). *See Gilroy et al. (1982): 277.*

Fibreoptic laryngoscope. A machine which at one end has a length of tubing which contains glass fibres with illumination. It has an eye piece. The patient's nose is anaesthetized so that the tube can be passed along the floor of the **nose**, down the back of the **nasopharynx**, **oropharynx** and **laryngopharynx** (all see **pharynx**) to the **velopharyngeal area** (see **velopharyngeal**) where any muscle weakness or growths anywhere in the **larynx** can be observed. *See Edels (1984): 10.*

Fibrous meningiomas. A type of **meningioma** (see **tumours of the central nervous system**) which results from **connective tissue** elements and consists of strands of intertwining spindle cells with long fibrils. *See Gilroy et al. (1982): 206.*

Filliform. See **taste buds**.

Fistula. A hole or opening which remains after surgery to various parts of the neck and face, e.g., after surgery to close a **cleft palate**. *See Edwards and Watson (1980): 20, 22, passim.*

Fit. A layman's term for a **seizure**.

Flaccidity. A description of a child or adult whose muscles are hypotonic, making it difficult for the child to stand or sit upright. It may also produce **dysarthric** (see **dysarthria**, 1) characteristics of speech. *See Tortora et al. (1984): 214.*

Flexion. A description of the forward movement of joints, e.g., head moving forward on neck, etc. *See Tortora et al (1984): 183.*

Focal sites. A specific part of the **brain** from where symptoms of diseases and disorders can occur. In **aphasia**, the focal sites could be Broca's area, Wernicke's area (see **cerebral hemispheres**), etc., or the electrical discharges in **epilepsy** have a focal site from where they discharge. *See Gilroy et al. (1982): 68.*

Foramen. A description of an opening or passage within the body. There are several and are called foramina. *See Tortora (1984): 139.*

Foramen caecum. See **tongue**.

Forebrain. See **diencephalon**.

Fourth ventricle. A structure within the brain which acts as a **canal** in the **hindbrain**. It has a diamond-shaped floor while its roof is tent-like and covered by the **cerebellum**. The floor is covered with symmetrical elevations caused by the grey matter of the **cranial nerves**. Compression of this ventricle by fluid produces **hydrocephalus**. *See Barr (1979): 74–76.*

Fragile X syndrome. A sex-linked **chromosome** disorder. It produces varying degrees of **mental handicap** (1 and 4) and the facial appearance of large forehead, large **mouth** and ill-formed **ears** (6). Carriers can be affected. The child's **expressive language** (1) is superior to **comprehension** (1) while **perseveration** (1) may also be found.

Friedreich's ataxia. A degenerative disease affecting the tracts of the **spinal cord**. It occurs during adolescence and early adulthood. The condition is inherited as an **autosomal recessive trait** (see **chromosomes**). It produces **dysarthric** (see **dysarthria**, 1) characteristics of speech, spastic gait and intention tremor. The **CSF** is normal. It is progressive, patients cannot walk five years after the symptoms have appeared, with death occurring 10 to 20 years after **respiration** problems have set in. *See Gilroy et al. (1982): 175–176.*

Frenulum. See **tongue**.

Frontal lobe. See **cerebral hemispheres**.

Fungiform. See **taste buds**.

G

Gag reflex. The description of the act of **swallowing** caused by the stimulation of the walls of the **oropharynx** (see **pharynx**). *See Joseph (1979): 140.*

Geniculate ganglion. Found in **cranial nerve VII**, it houses the cells which pick up the sense of taste. It attaches to the lingual branch of the **mandibular nerve** the fibres of which go to the **taste buds** on the front two-thirds of the **tongue**. *See Barr (1979): 109.*

Genioglossus muscle. See **extrinsic muscles of tongue**.

Gilles de la Tourette syndrome. An inheritable, metabolic disorder which produces tics. These tics begin in the face and, in time, they increase and begin to affect the shoulders and upper limbs. As breathing becomes poor, the patient's speech is affected. There are only minor neurologic signs. The disease does not interfere with the patient's life-expectancy. Prognosis is good for those who are treated with haloperidol. It is also known as tic convulsif (see also 4). *See Gilroy et al. (1982): 99.*

Glioma. The commonest type of **tumour**. *See Gilroy et al. (1982): 196.*

Glossal. A description of structures and disorders with tongue involvement.

Glossopharyngeal nerve. See **cranial nerves**. (Also known as **cranial nerve IX**.)

Glottis. The space which appears when the **vocal cords** (3) open. *See Tortora et al. (1984): 545.*

Gower's sign. A symptom found in Duchenne muscular **dystrophy**. During this disease, the patient can have difficulty in standing from either a sitting or lying position. Gower's sign is the means used by the patient to establish a standing position. The patient rolls over and pulls himself onto his hands and knees, pushes up till he has a firm base on his hands and feet. The last stage is to make his feet walk up towards his hands until he can stand upright. *See Gilroy et al. (1982): 338.*

Grand-mal epilepsy. See **epilepsy**.

Granulation tissue. A granular formation which can occur, for example, in the **arytenoid** region, sometimes occurring as other growths, e.g., **contact ulcers** (1) try to heal and ulceration is produced. *See Tortora et al. (1984): 101.*

Greater horn of hyoid. See **pharynx**.

Greater wing of sphenoid. See **muscles of mastication**.

Griffiths' test. A test for developmental milestones devised by Ruth Griffiths. It involves four elements of the child's development which have to be closely observed:

1. Does the child kick vigorously?
2. Does the child enjoy the bath?
3. Does the child push the feet against the teacher's hand?
4. Does the child have strong arm movements?

All children from 1 to 3 months of age may be put through this test. *See Illingworth (1983): 2, 5, 9.*

Guillain-Barre syndrome. A condition producing lymphocytic attacks on the peripheral nerves at the point where demyelination occurs. It results in motor weakness with associated pains in the shoulders and back. Breathing can be affected and a **tracheostomy** should be undertaken. In very severe cases, there can be **dysarthria**, **dysphasia** (both 1) and diplopia. The paralysis ascends through the body. *See Gilroy et al. (1982): 332–333.*

Guthrie test. A test is given to newly born babies to check for such conditions as **phenylketonuria**. The heel is given a prick to remove some blood for examination. *See Hosking (1982): 121.*

Gyrus, Gyri. The **cerebral hemispheres** are covered in grooves and smooth areas. The smooth areas, between the grooves, are the gyri. There are several gyri each with a specific name, e.g., **angular gyrus**. *See Barr (1979): ch. 13.*

H

Hallux. See **plantar response**.

Hamulus. See **pharynx**.

Hard palate. See **mouth**.

Hare lip. The layman's term for cleft lip (see **cleft palate**).

Head injury. A **trauma** to the **brain** which can have widespread effects on the person's daily life. A closed head injury is caused by the brain being knocked against the back of the skull. This is known as the contrecoup effect. In essence, the brain is a mass of tissue surrounded by fluid, so any harsh blow to the head, e.g., punch, hitting it on the ground from a fall, will result in it moving rapidly to the back of the skull.

Such sudden movement can cause the blood vessels to snap. It is the deceleration caused by the back of the skull which causes the resulting disorders. The consequences are concussion and bruising which causes haemorrhages and clots. **Focal** (see **focal sites**) deficits produce **hemiplegia**, **aphasia** (1), and problems with the **cranial nerves**. Global deficits produce loss of consciousness, disinhibition and memory deficits. Later complications can include post-concussion syndrome, **hydrocephalus**, **dementia** and **fits**. Medical treatment takes the form of steroids. The patient whose symptoms are minor has a good prognosis but those severely impaired need a structured therapeutic programme, preferably in a rehabilitation centre for the best recovery results. *See Gilroy et al. (1982): 292–294.*

Heart. The heart is divided into four areas—the right and left atria and the right and left ventricles. These make up the four quarters of the heart. The heart pumps blood around the body. Blood enters the heart by the inferior and superior vena cavi into the right atrium which contracts and pushes the blood through the tricuspid valve to the right ventricle. The ventricle pushes the blood through the pulmonary valve into the pulmonary artery from where it goes to the **lungs** where it picks up oxygen and it turns bright red and returns to the heart by four pulmonary veins and enters the left atrium. When it contracts, the blood is pushed through the mitral valve into the left ventricle which in turn pushes the blood through the aortic valve into the aorta. As it goes along this artery, it passes into other arteries of the body, arterioles (smaller arteries) and the capillaries where it loses oxygen and becomes dark blue. From these different areas of the body, the blood flows back to the heart and begins the cardiac cycle again. When the heart is active, it is a period of systole, when it is at rest, it is known as a period of diastole. *See Tortora et al (1984): ch. 20.*

Hemiplegia. The result of a **CVA**, **head injury** or other disease which produces a **focal** (see **focal sites**) lesion in the **brain**. Two limbs are affected, usually the arm and leg on one of the sides of the body. If the lesion occurs in the left **cerebral hemisphere**, the hemiplegia will affect the patient's right side. In such circumstances **anasognosia** can occur (1). Hemiplegia is treated by **physiotherapy**.

Hemisphere of the brain. See **cerebral hemisphere**.

Herpes simplex. An **encephalitis** which can be fatal and occurs in the **temporal lobe** (see **cerebral hemispheres**) of the **brain**. It produces cold sores. Both children and adults are affected with an equal sex ratio. The patient presents symptoms similar to those of flu, e.g., headache, fever, followed by irritation to the meninges and becomes disorientated in space. Later, **psychosis** (4) and **memory** (4) problems can occur as well as **aphasia** (1) and monoparesis (one limb is affected by weakness). The final stage is a coma. If a mother suffers from this infection during pregnancy, it can cross the placenta and cause disorders to the fetus. It is part of the **TORCH** classification of infections which can affect a fetus. *See Gilroy et al. (1982): 250–251.*

Hindbrain. Part of the **brain** which comprises the **pons, medulla oblongata** and the **cerebellum**. It is found below the **midbrain**. *See Barr (1979): ch. 7.*

Homeostasis. The body has to keep in balance its intake and output of substances. Intake refers to what a person consumes while output refers to the working of the excretory pathways via the kidneys. *See Green (1978): 92.*

Hormones. See **endocrine system**.

Hydrocephalus. A condition occurring in the **brain** caused by a **tumour** in close proximity to the **fourth ventricle** with evidence of **intracranial pressure**. It can be treated by ventricular drainage. The Arnold-Chiari malformation may also produce hydrocephalus. This malformation is produced by a disorder to the **medulla oblongata** and **cerebellum** causing an obstruction to the **CSF**. There are three types which differ mainly by severity. *See Gilroy et al. (1982): 58–595, 203.*

Hyoid bone. See **muscles for swallowing**.

Hypernasality. A condition caused by the failure of the **soft palate** (see **mouth**) to close when producing speech. This produces sounds which are both **nasal** (see **articulation**, 3) and **oral** (3). This can be caused by enlarged **adenoids**.

Hyperplasia. The excessive coming together of cells. *See Tortora et al. (1984): 429.*

Hypertonia. A description of an abnormal amount of power in a person's limbs.

Hypoglossal nerve. See **intrinsic muscles of tongue**.

Hypoglossus muscle. See **extrinsic muscles of tongue**.

Hypoplasia. A description of an

anatomical structure which has not developed fully as it should. *See Tortora et al. (1984): 429.*

Hypothalamus. A structure in the brain found below the middle of the **thalamus**. It is important to regulate sleep, thirst, hunger and temperature within the body. It affects the **autonomic nervous system**. *See Barr (1979): 155–162.*

Hypotonia. A description of **flaccidity** found in a person's muscles. *See Draper (1980): 18–19.*

I

ICP. Intracranial pressure.

Idiopathic. A disease which has no known cause. *See Tortora et al. (1984): 338.*

Impairment. A disease or injury which causes people certain difficulties in functioning. For example, if a lesion in the **brain** affects the motor coordination of the speech mechanism producing **dysarthria** (1), the patient is said to have an impairment in that area of the brain.

Inferior constrictor muscle. See **pharynx**.

Infra-. A description of the area below the structure to which the suffix is attached.

Infraglottic. A description of the whole area including the structures below the **glottis**.

Inspiration. The process of taking in a breath. A more precise term for this process is **abdominal-diaphragmatic respiration**. *See Tortora et al. (1984): 556–558.*

Intension tremor. A disorder caused by a disorder of the **cerebellum**. The patient's limb produces an observable tremor when specific movements are made. *See Gilroy et al. (1982): 36.*

Internal carotid artery. See **carotid artery**.

Intracranial pressure. Pressure within the cranium produced by the amount of **CSF**, blood and size of **brain**. If the pressure varies slightly in one area, another area can compensate but large lesions to a particular area may be so significant that no compensation can take place and the pressure is increased. This is raised intracranial pressure. *See Hosking (1982): 155–158.*

Intraoral. A description of structures or disorders which appear in the mouth itself.

Intraoral pressure. The build up of pressure in the mouth to allow a person to produce the sounds for speech. For those who suffer from **cleft palate**, this pressure is usually lacking.

Intrinsic muscles of the tongue. The **tongue** has three intrinsic muscles which, with the three **extrinsic muscles**, control its movement. The intrinsic muscles are named longitudinal, transverse and vertical. They are supplied by the **hypoglossal nerve** (see **cranial nerve XII**). The vertical muscle fibres pull the sides of the tongue down while the transverse muscle fibres help lengthen the tongue. *See Tortora et al. (1984): 587.*

Ipsilateral. A description of structures and nerves, etc. which are on the same side of the body. It is opposed to contra-lateral.

J

Jacksonian seizure. A **clonic**-type seizure (see **epilepsy**) which gradually spreads throughout the body, involving **ipsilateral** structures. The focal lesion is in the precentral **gyrus** of the **brain**. *See Gilroy et al. (1982): 68, 200.*

Jakob-Creutzfeldt disease. A spongioform encephalopathy affecting the **central nervous system**. It progresses quickly throughout the **CNS** and produces **dementia**. (see also 4). *See Gilroy et al. (1982): 254–255.*

Jaw. See **mandible**.

Jugular vein. There are two parts of this vein—the **internal** and **external carotid artery** (see **carotid artery**). The latter receives some of the branches of the external carotid artery while the former receives blood from arteries inside the skull. *See Tortora et al. (1984): 504.*

K

Kleinfelter syndrome. One of the most common **sex chromosome** (see **chromosomes**) abnormalities. Although not severe, it is associated with **mental handicap** (1 and 4). It is caused by the presence of two X **chromosomes** along with the Y chromosome. Males who are affected do not develop secondary sexual characteristics at puberty and the characteristic appearance is of a person who is tall and thin with long legs and arms. *See Salmon (1978): 371–372.*

L

L-dopa. Levodopa.
Lacrimal duct. See **nose**.
Laryngopharynx. See **pharynx**.
Laryngoscope. The different devices used by **ENT** consultants to carry out **laryngoscopy**.
Laryngoscopy. There are three types of laryngoscopy which can be administered:
1. Direct laryngoscopy. After anaesthesis, a rigid laryngoscope is placed along the floor of the mouth and down the back of the patient's throat. A light system shows up the **subglottic** and **supraglottic** areas of the **larynx**. If any tumours are found, tissue can be taken for further analysis by using long-handled forceps.
2. Indirect laryngoscopy. This is the first examination using a mirror to view the relevant parts of the **larynx**. If there appears to be a growth, a direct laryngoscopy will be undertaken.
3. Microlaryngoscopy. The process of removing small growths from the **vocal cords** (3) without damaging the cords. It is carried out by looking through an operating microscope. *See Edels (1984): chs 1 and 2.*
Larynx. The organ of the **voice** (3). It extends from the back of the **tongue** to the **trachea**. It is 4.5cm long, 4cm in transverse section and 3.5cm from front to back. It is smaller in the female than in the male after puberty. It comprises **cartilage** held together by **membrane** and ligament. The **hyoid bone** (see **muscles for swallowing**) is at the top, the thyroid cartilage in the middle and the cricoid cartilage at the bottom. The thyroid cartilage is made up of two quadrilateral structures joined in the midline at the laryngeal prominence to which the vocal ligament is attached. The cricoid cartilage is like a ring. The arytenoid cartilage is attached to the lamina of the cricoid and has an apex and three roughly triangular surfaces. The larynx is controlled by the following muscles:
1. Cricothyroid muscle has two parts—vertical and oblique. The muscle tilts the cricoid up or thyroid down and tightens the **vocal folds** (3).
2. Arytenoid muscle—the transverse and oblique arytenoid muscles control the arytenoid cartilages and go up either side of the aryepiglottic folds.
3. Posterior crico-arytenoid muscle runs up to attach to the muscular process of the arytenoid. When it contracts, it abducts the **vocal cords** (3) by rotating the arytenoid cartilage; when it pulls the arytenoid cartilages backwards, the vocal cord tenses.
4. Lateral crico-thyroid muscle is attached to the superior border of the cricoid cartilage passing upwards and backwards and attached to the muscular process of arytenoids. When it contracts it adducts the vocal fold by rotating the arytenoid cartilage inwards.
5. Thyro-arytenoid muscle is attached to the front of the inner surface of the laryngeal prominence. It passes backwards and upwards and becomes attached to the antero-lateral surface of the arytenoid cartilage and its muscular process.
6. Vocalis—part of it is attached to the lateral aspect of the vocal ligament and some of its fibres run up to the aryepiglottic fold. When it contracts, the arytenoid cartilages rotate medially to adduct the vocal cords, while in pulling the arytenoid cartilage forward, the vocal cords relax.
7. Thyrohyoid muscle leaves the thyroid cartilage and attaches to the greater cornu of the hyoid bone. It raises the

thyroid cartilage and pushes down the hyoid bone.

The larynx houses the vocal cords which produce **voice** (3). *See Tortora et al. (1984): 237, 545.*

Lateral pterygoid. See **muscles of mastication** (4).

Lesser horn of hyoid. See **pharynx.**

Levator anguli labii superioris. See **muscles of facial expression.**

Levodopa. A drug which provides dopamine to those patients who have an insufficiency of dopamine in the **brain.** It can be used with those who suffer from **Parkinson's disease** as it has a significant effect on **bradykinesia** (see **Parkinson's disease**). However, it can cause nausea, **depression** (4), and **dyskinesia** (see **cerebral palsy** 3). *See Gilroy et al. (1982): 104.*

Light for dates. A light birth weight is a third of normal birth weight. The child is born at or near to full term. This condition is caused by placental insufficiency produced by toxaemia, multiple pregnancy or smoking, intrauterine infections, e.g., **TORCH**, and **chromosomal abnormalities** (see **chromosomes**). The babies are very alert, thin, wasted and with wrinkled skin; they have a poor stress response. There is fetal distress in labour and passes meconium after the first day of delivery. If the child inhales meconium in the juices around it and starts poor breathing, producing meconium aspiration syndrome, this causes brain damage and can lead to death. *See Illingworth (1983): 87.*

Lingual frenulum. See **tongue.**

Lingual nerve. See **mouth.**

Lingual tonsil. A structure formed by some lymphoid tissue at the back of the **tongue.** *See Tortora (1984): 523, 544.*

Longitudinal muscle. See **intrinsic muscles of tongue.**

Lumbar puncture. A technique for diagnosing such infections as **meningitis.** A certain quantity, usually about 1ml, of **cerebrospinal fluid** is drawn off the **meninges** to check for infection. With patients suffering from meningitis, the fluid is clouded by the presence of organisms. Normal CSF fluid is clear. *See Gilroy et al. (1982); 217, 219.*

Lungs. There are two lungs in the thoracic cavity covered by a pleura lining. Air reaches the lungs by the **trachea** and the **bronchi** which branch into the right and left lung. The right lung is divided into three lobes by an oblique fissure and transverse fissure. The left lung is divided into two lobes by an oblique fissure. Each lobe contains part of the bronchus, an artery and a vein. They are necessary for respiration. The microscopic structure of the lungs is seen as a series of passageways. The **bronchi** become bronchioles, which turn into respiratory bronchioles. These bronchioles divide into alveolar ducts, subdividing into alveolar saccules which produce alveoli at their end. *See Tortora et al (1984): 552–556.*

M

Macrocephaly. An abnormally large head caused by an increased amount of brain tissue. It is opposed to **microcephaly.**

Macroglossia. An abnormally large tongue. The condition may be **congenital** (1). It has been proposed that children suffering from **Down's Syndrome** have such a condition as their tongue seems to protrude more than with normal children who do not suffer from this syndrome. However, the tongue may just seem very large because the child has a particularly small upper or lower jaw. Surgery can be used to reduce its size. **Articulation disorders** (1) can occur. *See Travis (1971).*

Malignant. A **tumour** which can grow inside the body destroying any neighbouring tissue. It is opposed to benign. *See Tortora et al. (1984): 74.*

Malocclusion. See **orthodontics.**

Mandible. The lower jaw. It is used in the act of chewing or mastication. It has four muscles attached to various parts of its body—**temporalis muscle, lateral pterygoid, medial pterygoid** and **masseter** (see **muscles of mastication**). At the top of the ramus of the mandible, there is the **coronoid process** and the head, between which is the **zygomatic arch.** The Stylomandibular ligament stretches from the **styloid process** down to the **angle of the mandible.** The **salp-**

ingopharyngeus muscle runs from the auditory tube (6) to the mandible. The symphysis menti shows the midline where the two halves of the jaw have joined together. *See Tortora et al. (1984): 150.*

Mandibular nerve. The mandibular nerve is part of the **trigeminal nerve** which is **cranial nerve V**. To distinguish this nerve from the other two which form the Trigeminal nerve, the mandibular nerve is denoted as **Viii**. The sensory part of the nerve supplies the back two-thirds of the **tongue**, part of the face and scalp, the **mandible** and lower teeth and the mucous membrane of the floor of the mouth. *See Tortora et al. (1984): 333.*

Masseter muscle. See **muscles of mastication**.

Maxilla. The upper jaw. It is formed by the fusion of the palatal shelves during intrauterine growth. The maxilla comprises the **hard palate** (see **mouth**), the floor and sides of the nasal cavities, the floor of the orbits and the part of the nasolacrimal canal. The teeth in the top dentition are rooted in the maxilla. *See Tortora et al. (1984): 146, 147.*

Maxillary nerve. A sensory nerve which supplies some of the skin of the scalp, part of the face, the lower eyelid, part of the inside of the cheek, the mucous membrane of the nasal cavity, palate and maxillary sinus and the upper teeth and gum. It is part of the **trigeminal nerve** which is **cranial nerve V**. To distinguish the maxillary nerve from the other two parts of the nerve, the maxillary nerve is denoted as **Vii**. *See Tortora (1984): 333.*

Meatus. See **nose**.

Meconium. See **light for dates**.

Meconium aspiration syndrome. See **light for dates**.

Medial pterygoid muscle. See **muscles of mastication**.

Medulla oblongata. Part of the **brainstem**. It is about 3cm long. The **spinal cord** ends in the medulla with two lumps which contain grey matter. There are several tracts which it has in common with the **pons** and **midbrain**. *See Barr (1979): 70–72.*

Megalencephaly. A condition found in children who have an oversized head and overweight **brain** without neurological disorders. When these children are born, they have an abnormally large head and big bodies. Anatomic megalecephaly is inheritable as an autosomal dominant trait and can be familial. In a study in 1972, out of 18 children the incidence

was 4 : 1 in favour of males and half of the children were familial cases. *See De Meyer (1972): 634–643.*

Membrane. A layer or sheet of tissue which can surround cells, structures, line **canals** and separate structures. *See Tortora (1984): 98; Leeson and Leeson (1970): passim.*

Meninges. A membranous covering of the **brain** and **spinal cord**. If it becomes infected, **meningitis** occurs. *See Barr (1979): 304–308.*

Meningiomas. See **tumours of the central nervous system**.

Meningitis. An infection of the **central nervous system**. It is also known as a droplet infection as it occurs when youngsters get together and an organism sticks and increases in the **nasopharynx** (see **pharynx**). Viruses are the commonest cause. The symptoms are headaches, neck stiffness, fever and vomiting. Diagnosis has to be made from the **cerebrospinal fluid** which looks milky. The **CSF** is extracted by the **lumbar puncture** technique. Treatment is by antibiotics with Benzylpenicillin being the first choice. *See Gilroy et al. (1982): 219–227.*

Meningocoele. A mild form of **spina bifida**. It is caused by the partial or incomplete closure of the neural tube. The **meninges** are abnormal as are the vertebrae. *See Hosking (1982): 63–66.*

Meningothelial meningioma. A type of **meningioma** (see **tumour of the central nervous system**) coming from arachnoid cap cells, consisting of sheets of cells which contain large, vascular nuclei. *See Gilroy et al. (1982): 214.*

Metastasis. A **tumour** which begins in the **lung**. It produces neurological symptoms and occurs between 40 and 70 years of age. Most of these tumours travel through the arteries to the **CNS**. They develop in the **cerebral hemispheres** and can push out the contents of the hemispheres across the midline. This is shown up on **computer tomography**. The symptoms are headache and partial or generalized **fits**. Treatment is by **corticosteroids** with a possibility of **radiotherapy** for multiple tumours. *See Gilroy et al. (1982): 212–213.*

Microcephaly. In this condition, the child has an abnormally small head accompanied by a small brain. They have depressed levels of **intelligence** (4). It can be divided into primary microcephaly and secondary microcephaly. The former is inherited as an autosomal recessive trait. It can occur in other conditions associated with chromosomal and non-chromosomal deficiencies. The latter is produced by infection or other problems which may arise in the **perinatal** period. *See Hosking (1982): 72.*

Microglossia. An abnormally small **tongue**. The condition is relatively rare. It is caused by the failure of the anterior two-thirds of the tongue to grow normally. It occurs in the **prenatal** period. The patient's speech can sound muffled and treatment is by **speech therapy** (1). *See Travis (1971).*

Micrognathia. The failure of the **mandible** to develop normally.

Midbrain. Part of the **brain** which is found above the **pons**. It is the smallest of the three main parts of the brain—**hindbrain, forebrain** and midbrain. It is about 1.5cm long, 2.5cm wide and 2cm thick. There are ascending and descending tracts of **cranial nerves III** and **IV.** The floor of the **third ventricle** is formed at the front between the cerebral peduncles. The substantia nigra which, when it loses its blackness, causes **Parkinson's disease** is situated in the midbrain. *See Barr (1979): 90–97.*

Middle constrictor muscle. See **pharynx.**

Mixed cerebral palsy. See **cerebral palsy.**

Mobius syndrome. A congenital disorder which produces weakness of the facial muscles and the failure of the eyes to **abduct** (see **abduction**). It is an **idiopathic** condition which can run in families. *See Gilroy et al. (1982): 59.*

Molar teeth. See **teeth.**

Motor area. See **brain.**

Motor neurone disease. A progressive disease which causes failure in the motor neurones in the **spinal cord**, loss of motor neurones in the **brainstem**, a loss of Betz cells in the cerebral **cortex**. Only motor cells are affected. The cause is uncertain. There is complete loss of motor control which produces **dysarthria** (1), loss of hand function and mobility. There is no sensory loss and no **dementia**. Treatment is aimed at making the patient's life as comfortable as possible since the disease progresses steadily until death. There can be remission but this may be just for a few weeks or months. *See Gilroy et al. (1982): 177–179.*

Mouth. Often called the oral cavity. The mouth has a roof which is formed by the hard palate and soft palate at the back of the mouth. This part of the mouth is supplied by the greater palatine and nasopalatine nerves, the fibres of which travel in the **maxillary nerve**. The floor of the mouth is formed by the **tongue** and supplied by the **lingual nerve** (see **tongue**) while the walls of the mouth, i.e., the cheeks, are supplied by the buccal nerve, both of these are branches of the **mandibular nerve**. In the back wall of the mouth is the isthmus of fauces (fauces are arches) which is also known as the oro-pharyngeal passage. Between the arches, the **uvula** (3) hangs. Behind the uvula is the palatine tonsil or true tonsil. The **palatopharyngeus muscle** (see **muscles for swallowing,** 2) runs to the palate from behind this tonsil. The front wall is formed by the **teeth** which are set in the upper and lower dentitions or dental arches. The alveolar ridge is behind the upper teeth. *See Tortora et al. (1984): 585–594.*

Mouth breathing. A symptom of **adenoidal** problems. The child's **mouth** is affected as he will have a high arched maxilla. He will also have narrow nostrils, **flattening of affect** (4), and the pharyngeal **tonsil** will be enlarged. This will produce the typical 'look', i.e., adenoidal facies, of a child who suffers from adenoidal problems. The sense of smell will be affected and he will lose taste, thus providing a possible reduction in the child's appetite. There could also be a **conductive hearing loss** (6). *See Travis (1971): 751–752.*

Mucous membrane. A sheet of **epithelium** which is wet by mucous supported by basal lamina and, finally, by **connective tissue.** *See Leeson and Leeson (1970): 292.*

Multiple sclerosis. A disease of the **spinal cord**. It is caused by an influx of lymphocytes (inflammatory protein) which produces demyelination in the **CNS**. It affects all the areas of the **brain** around the **ventricles** (see **third ventricle** and **fourth ventricle**), **spinal cord** and **brainstem.** The symptoms are optic neuritis, double vision, **dysarthria** (1), **ataxia, spastic** gait (see **cerebral palsy**), **hemiplegia** and, occasionally, **dementia**. The diagnosis is made following tests such as visual evoked responses and an examination of the **CSF** which should show evidence of the lymphocytes. It can follow a remission-relapse course. There is also the 'five-year rule' which means the disability may last for five years at a time. Treatment takes the form of **corticosteroids, physiotherapy** and **speech therapy** (1). *See Gilroy et al. (1982): ch. 7.*

Muscles of facial expression. These

muscles are supplied by **cranial nerve VII**. There are two types of muscle—sphincters which close off openings and dilators which will cause structures to open. They modify the expression of the face and can add extra force and/or meaning to what is being said. The obicularis oculi surrounds each eye and can be used to screw up the eyes. The obicularis oris muscle allows the person to pout his lips. This muscle is supplied by the buccal and mandibular branches of the **facial nerve**. The buccinator allows a person to smile while the levator anguli labii superioris and depressor anguli labii inferioris allow the person to elevate and lower the lips respectively. All these facial muscles are derived from the second pharyngeal arch. *See Tortora et al (1984): 229.*

Muscles of mastication. There are four muscles which control the function of chewing (i.e., mastication):

1. Temporalis muscle is the shape of a fan whose fibres reach a tendon which goes to the **zygomatic arch**. They are inserted on the **coronoid process**. The anterior and superior fibres raise the **mandible** while the posterior fibres retract it. The muscle is supplied by the deep temporal nerves which are branches of the anterior division of **mandibular nerve**.

2. **Masseter muscle** begins at the bottom and the middle part of the **zygomatic arch**. The fibres go downwards and backwards and are attached to the lateral aspects of the **ramus of the mandible** (see **mandible**). It is supplied by the **mandibular nerve**. Its function is to lift the mandible, covering teeth during the process of chewing.

3. Medial pterygoid muscle has a deep head starting at the middle of the lateral pterygoid plate. Its fibres go downwards, backwards and laterally and end in the middle part of the angle of the mandible (see **mandible**). It is supplied by the **mandibular nerve** and it helps in raising the mandible.

4. Lateral pterygoid muscle has an upper and lower head. The former begins at the infratemporal surface of the greater wing of sphenoid while the lower head begins on the surface of the lateral pterygoid plate. Both heads meet and insert themselves in the front of the **mandible** neck and articular disc of the **temperomandibular joint**. It is supplied by the anterior division of the **mandibular nerve**. Its function is to pull forward the neck of the mandible by the articular disc as the mouth opens. It causes also the rotating which produces the action of chewing. Knowledge of such muscles is important for those patients who have a disorder of chewing. *See Tortora et al (1984): 232.*

Muscles for swallowing. Two main muscles are used in the process of **swallowing**:

1. Mylohyoid muscle stretches along the mylohyoid line of the **mandible**. The fibres go downward and forward. The posterior fibres end in the hyoid bone while the anterior fibres end in the body of the hyoid bone. It is supplied by the mylohyoid branch of the inferior alveolar nerve. Both mylohyoid muscles raise the floor of the mouth and the hyoid bone during the first stage of swallowing. The hyoid bone can also function to lower the jaw to open the mouth.

2. Digastric muscle has three parts:

a) Posterior belly is supplied by the **facial nerve** (see **cranial nerves**) and begins in the middle of the **mastoid process** (see **ear**, 6) of the temporal bone and ends in the intermediate tendon, having crossed the carotid sheath, i.e., tissue which surrounds the **carotid arteries**.

b) Intermediate tendon crosses the stylohyoid muscle and is kept in place by a loop of deep **fascia** which holds to the junction of the body and greater cornu of the hyoid bone.

c) Anterior belly is supplied by the mylohyoid branch of the **mandibular nerve**. It goes forward and is attached to the lower edge of the **mandible**. It lowers the jaw and raises the hyoid bone. There are also two other muscles used in swallowing:

1. Stylopharyngeus muscle which begins at the side of the **styloid process** and inserts itself in the side of the **pharynx** near to the **thyroid cartilage** (see **trachea**). This muscle raises the **larynx** and expands the pharynx to allow an easy passage for the bolus of food.

2. Palatopharyngeus muscle has its origin at the soft palate (see **mouth**) and inserts itself into the **thyroid cartilage** and the side and back walls of the pharynx. It raises both the larynx and pharynx and closes the **nasopharynx** (see **pharynx**) during the process of **swallowing**.

Knowledge of such muscles is important for speech therapists who are concerned with patients with disorders of swallowing. *See Joseph (1979): 59–60.*

Myelomeningocoele. A form of **spina bifida**. The legs are **flaccid** and there is paralysis of the bladder and bowel. There is an abnormality to the skin, **spinal cord**, vertebrae and **meninges**. It is often associated with **hydrocephalus**. *See Hosking (1982): 62–66*.

Mylohyoid muscle. See **muscles for swallowing**.

Myoclonus. A movement disorder characterized by sudden jerks. It can occur in the normal population while asleep but it

becomes a disorder when associated with **epilepsy** producing 'tea cup epilepsy' (cf. the dropping of a tea cup when nudged) and is a symptom of acquired brainstem diseases, e.g., **Jakob-Creutzfelt disease** which causes **degeneration** of the **basal ganglia**, hypoxic brain damage or drug dependency. *See Gilroy et al. (1982): 97–98*.

N

Nasal. A description of any structure or disorder related to the **nose**.

Nasopalatine nerve. See **mouth**.

Nasopharynx. See **pharynx**.

Neurilemoma. A **benign tumour** (see **malignant**) which affects **cranial nerve VIII**, the acoustic nerve (see **vestibulocochlear nerve**; **cranial nerves**). It produces **tinnitus**, **progressive hearing loss** (both 6) and episodic vertigo. As it increases in size, it involves the other **cranial nerves** and structures of the **brain** such as the **cerebellum**. Such interference can produce cerebellar **ataxia** (see **cerebral palsy**). Treatment is by surgery. *See Gilroy et al (1982): 206–208*.

Neurofibroma. See **tumours of the central nervous system** (3).

Neurone. The cell which is responsible for passing nerve impulses to muscles. Some neurones are called **dendrites** because of their particular structure. Motor neurones receive information which makes movement possible. When there is a lesion affecting both upper and lower motor neurones, there is physical handicap as well as **dysarthric** (see **dysarthria**, 1) characteristics of the person's speech. *See Tortora et al. (1984): ch. 12*.

Nose. The front part of the nose has two U-shaped cartilages forming the nostrils. At the posterior of the nose, there is an opening to the **nasopharynx** (see **pharynx**). The **nasal** cavity is formed by a roof, floor and wall. The floor is the top surface of the **hard palate** and the roof is

divided into three parts—the front or anterior part is the slope or bridge of the nose, the middle part is the ethmoid or cribiform plate, while the posterior part is formed by the anterior and inferior surfaces of the cribiform plate. Both cavities are divided by the nasal septum. The lateral walls are formed by the superior, middle and inferior conchae or folds. Between these folds are the superior, middle and inferior meati. Around the middle meatus, there are the four openings of the frontal sinus, the anterior ethmoid sinus, the maxillary sinus and the middle ethmoid sinus. At the lower edge of the cavity, just above the floor is the naso-lacrimal duct. This structure draws tears from the eyes down the nose through a flap in the nose. When the nose is blown, it stops material being blown upwards. If the flap does not shut and the nose is blown, bubbles may appear at the side of the eyes. Blood is carried to the nose by the ophthalmic, maxillary and facial artery while the nerve supply comes from nerves of a similar name. *See Tortora et al (1984): 542, 543*.

Nystagmus. A rhythmical movement of the eyes which can occur at rest or when they move. It can happen to both eyes or just to one and is caused by a disorder to structures of the **brain** or some of the **cranial nerves**. The involuntary movements of the eyes can be horizontal, vertical, oblique, or circular. They can also be swinging or jerky in appearance. *See Gilroy et al. (1982): 23–24*.

O

Obicularis oculi. See **muscles of facial expression**.

Obicularis oris. See **muscles of facial expression**.

Occupational therapy. An occupational therapist works with patients who have difficulty in coping at home on their own. They are shown how to carry out everyday activities and are given an opportunity to demonstrate their handiwork in the making of tea-trays, mats, stools, etc, to help develop muscles in their hands and arms which may have been affected by a **CVA, head injury**, etc.

Oesophagus. A structure which is 25cm long and starts at the level of the sixth cervical vertebrae and ends about the level of the eleventh cervical vertebra where it enters the stomach. It narrows at the **pharynx**, where it passes into the **diaphragm** (see **abdominal-diaphragmatic respiration**) and at the bottom of the thorax. It has an inner circular layer of muscles and an outer longitudinal layer of muscles. The top part of the oesophagus is covered with **striated muscle** while the bottom of it is covered with **smooth muscle**. It is possible to use the upper part for producing **oesophageal speech** (1) as it has striated muscle. Smooth muscle cannot operate in this fashion. The blood supply is from the inferior thyroid artery. It runs behind the **trachea**. *See Tortora et al (1984): 594, 595.*

Olfaction. A description of the way in which people use their sense of smell.

Olfactory. See **cranial nerves**.

Oligodendrogliomas. See **tumours of the central nervous system**.

Optic nerve. See **cranial nerves**.

Oral cavity. See **mouth**.

Oropharynx. See **pharynx**.

Orthodontics. The study of teeth formation and other structures in the mouth which require treatment from the placement of various prostheses to realign the dental arches if they are deformed. There are three descriptions of teeth formation: Class I refers to teeth which are well-related to each other as are the two dental arches, i.e., top teeth at front cover one-third or half the bottom teeth when clenched; Class II (division 1) refers to an increase in overjet, i.e., top teeth are protruding away from the bottom teeth by more than 2–4mm; Class II (division 2) refers to an increase in overbite where the lower incisors are completely covered; Class III refers to a condition where the lower teeth completely cover the top teeth when clenched. Classes II–III are known as malocclusions. Orthodontists can also be involved with the treatment of children suffering from **cleft palate** as the teeth may be formed in a haphazard formation. *See Edwards and Watson (1980): ch. 13 (orthodontics and cleft palate).*

P

Palatal lift. See **prosthesis**.

Palatal shelves. See **Pierre–Robin syndrome**.

Palatine tonsil. See **mouth**.

Palatopharyngeus muscle. See **muscles for swallowing**.

Papillae. See **tongue**.

Papilloma. Benign growths appearing in any part of the **larynx** which can cause dyspnoea, i.e., difficulty with breathing. They are little bunches of pinkish wart-like growths which are found in the dark, moist caverns of the airways. If it is adversely affected, a **tracheostomy** is required. Papillomata tend to disappear at puberty but when they appear initially, surgery may be required. If surgery is required, it takes the form of conventional excision surgery, laser beam, ultrasonic and radiation therapy. The person may require **speech therapy** (1) after surgery. *See Fawcus (1986).*

Parasympathetic nervous system. Part of the **autonomic nervous system** which produces the opposite effect of the **sympathetic nervous system**. It operates at its maximum potential during sleep, it slows down the heart. It is used to enervate the muscles, controlling the digestive system as well as defecation and micturition. Its activity is restricted to the trunk and skull as there are no fibres in the arms and legs. *See Green (1978): 133–134.*

Parkinson's disease. Caused by disorders to the **basal ganglia**. The main areas of the **brain** affected are the caudate nucleus and the **substantia nigra** (see **midbrain**). The disorder is concentrated mainly in the substantia nigra which loses its blackness. The disease itself can be caused by viruses, e.g., encephalitis lethargica, drugs given for other disorders, e.g., **chlorpromazine**: (4), and poisons, e.g., manganese producing a neural loss in Basal ganglia, **cerebellum** and substantia nigra. There are three main symptoms:

1. Tremor which is the least disabling but, perhaps, most embarrassing as it can produce **pin rolling**. It may disappear but during **anxiety** (4) can become worse.

2. Rigidity occurs when the basal ganglia can no longer produce automatic movements including facial expression.

3. Bradykinesia which produces a slowness in carrying out what the person wants to do. The typical posture of the patient is a hunched forward appearance with head down against the chest, shoulders pushed forward with the arms hanging loosely at the side. Forward movement produces a festinant gait, i.e., a faster and faster progression. This symptom can also produce disorders for which **speech therapy** (1) is required. The preferred drug treatment is **levodopa (l-dopa)**. *See Gilroy et al. (1982): 100–106.*

Parotid duct/glands. See **salivary glands**.

Perinatal period. The time when the delivery of the baby takes place. At this time, there are several factors which can produce a delay in the child's future development. Among these are birth asphyxia (the umbilical cord ties itself around the baby's neck), birth trauma (the method of delivery may have caused problems), preterm babies and those who are **light-for-dates**. *See Illingworth (1983): 17, 199.*

Peristalsis. See **swallowing**.

Petit-mal epilepsy. See **epilepsy**.

Pharyngeal tonsil. See **tonsil**.

Pharyngeal tubercle. See **pharynx**.

Pharyngo basilar fascia. See **pharynx**.

Pharynx. A structure which begins at the base of the skull and stretches downwards to the sixth cervical vertebra where it becomes continuous with the **oesophagus**. The pharynx is divided into three parts:

1. Nasopharynx which starts at the posterior openings of the **nose** and ends above the **mouth**.

2. Oropharynx which continues from the end of the nasopharynx, passes the posterior opening of the oral cavity and ends close to the **larynx**;

3. Laryngopharynx continues from the end of the oropharynx and continues to the top of the oesophagus.

The **adenoids** are found in the nasopharynx while the **tonsils** can be found in the oropharynx. The pharynx consists of three muscles:

1. The superior constrictor muscle fibres leave the hamulus, pterygomandibular ligament and from the **mandible**, the upper fibres end at the pharyngeal tubercle while the lower fibres mingle with the middle constrictor muscle and attach themselves to the posterior wall of the pharynx;

2. The middle constrictor muscle fibres leave the stylohyoid ligament, the lesser and greater horns of hyoid and attach themselves to the posterior wall of the pharynx;

3. The inferior constrictor muscle fibres leave the oblique line, the side of the **cricoid cartilage** (see **larynx**) and insert themselves to the posterior wall of the pharynx. **Cranial nerve IX** provides the sensory nerve input to the pharynx while **cranial nerve X** provides motor nerve input. The pharynx-basilar fascia is a **membrane** which runs down in front of the vertebrae. As the person swallows all these muscles lift up together. The salpingopharyngeus muscle leaves the **auditory tube** (6) and inserts itself into some of the fibres of the **palatopharyngeus muscle** (see **muscles for swallowing**). This muscle raises the top part of the side wall of the pharynx and opens the auditory tube. *See Tortora et al (1984): 543–555.*

Phenylketonuria. An **autosomal recessive** (see **chromosomes**) condition. It is an inborn error in metabolism as the gene lacks a certain chemical. An entirely preventable condition if found by the **Guthrie test**. The child is on a special diet for the rest of his life. If it is untreated, **mental handicap** (1 and 4), **microcephaly** and **seizures** can result. *See Hosking (1982): 121–122.*

Phenytoin. A drug treatment for **epilepsy**.

Physiology. The study of how the body functions. While an anatomist studies structures of the body, a physiologist studies how these structures function. Thus, some of the subjects which interest a physiologist are the workings of the heart, the breathing system, the **autonomic** and **central nervous systems** and the way food is digested. *See Green (1978): passim.*

Physiotherapy. The   physiotherapist

works with physically handicapped patients. This handicap may be **congenital** (1), e.g., **cerebral palsy**, or **acquired** (1) such as a **hemiplegia** due to a **CVA** or **head injury**, etc.

Pierre–Robin syndrome. A syndrome caused by the failure of the tongue to fall into place during the seventh week of in utero growth. The neck does not grow normally and so the lower jaw is pushed against the chest and there is no room for the tongue to fall down into the **mouth** and the palatal shelves fail to close to form the **hard palate** (see **mouth**). The four characteristics of this syndrome are:

1. **Cleft palate** but not cleft lip;
2. Respiration problems;
3. A small **mandible**;
4. Glossoptosis (drooping of the tongue backwards).

See Edwards and Watson (1980): 123–128.

Pin rolling. The manifestation of the **tremor** (see **Parkinson's disease**) suffered by those who have **Parkinson's disease**. It appears at the fingers which with the thumb produce a rolling motion as if there were a pin between them.

Placenta. A sack-like structure within which the fetus develops during pregnancy. *See Tortora et al (1984): 510, 511.*

Plantar response. A response obtained by stimulating the sole of the foot with a blunt object. If the response exists, the hallux will flex. If there is extension, this is an abnormal response and is recorded as an extensor plantar response. *See Gilroy et al. (1982): 44.*

Pons. A structure within the **brain**. It is part of the **hindbrain**, measures about 3.5cm wide and 3cm long, and is situated above the **medulla oblongata**. It comprises fibres which make up the middle cerebellar peduncles, while further into its centre, it is essentially a continuation of the medulla oblongata. It is associated with **cranial nerves V, VI, VII** and **VIII**. The **cerebellum** is found above the pons. *See Barr (1979): 73–74.*

Posterior pharyngeal wall. The area at the back of the **pharynx** to which the **superior, middle** and **inferior constrictor muscles** (see **pharynx**) insert themselves.

Postnatal. The period in the baby's life following delivery. At this time, the child is at risk of infection from **meningitis, encephalitis, trauma** and metabolic disorders.

Prader-Willi syndrome. A child suffering from this syndrome will be obese and floppy. There will be varying degrees of **mental handicap** (1 and 4), an enormous appetite and breathing problems which could result in death. Their eyes will be almond-shaped. Parents should be advised of a suitable diet. It is not passed on to other children. The child has difficulty with **short-term memory** but **long-term memory** (see **memory**: 4) is unaffected. *See Hosking (1982): 176.*

Prenatal. A stage occurring during pregnancy. At this time, the fetus can be affected by infections from the mother (e.g., **TORCH**), radiation or nutritional deficiency. *See Illingworth (1983): ch. 2.*

Preterm. The description of a baby who is born before the normal end of the pregnancy, usually before 37–38 weeks into the pregnancy. A preterm baby can be caused by a trauma, e.g., car accident, a multiple pregnancy, or cervical incompetence. As the lungs are immature, breathing problems occur. The child is kept prone in an incubator. Liver problems occur producing a high level of bilirubin in the **brain** producing kernicturus (a condition involving **cerebral palsy** and **hearing loss**: 6) and the child also has immature bone marrow producing anaemia and lack of protection from infections such as **meningitis**. *See Illingworth (1983): 25–27.*

Prime mover. See **agonist, antagonist**.

Prolabium. The middle part of the top lip which tends to protrude down further than the rest of the lip.

Proprioception. The ability to orientate one's limbs or joints in space, e.g., to touch one's nose with the eyes closed. Such skills are used in a person's daily life, e.g., eating, walking, speaking, etc. If speech is dysarthric (**dysarthria**, 1), it may be caused by loss of proprioception, e.g., difficulty in moving the mouth to make the correct sounds, so neuromuscular facilitation is given in **speech therapy** (1).

Prosthesis. The technical name for a 'brace' used to correct the positioning of teeth in the dental arches. For those suffering from **cleft palate**, there are devices to put in the mouth to help the baby to feed, and for older children the palatal lift which raises the **soft palate** (see **mouth**) to reduce the **nasalization** (3) in the child's speech.

Psammomatous meningiomas. A type of **meningioma** (see **tumours of the central nervous system**). They take the form of curly, spindle-like cells. The central part of the tumour degenerates, calcifies and forms a psammoma body. *See Gilroy et al. (1982).*

Pseudobulbar palsy. See **bulbar palsy**.

Pterygoid plate. See **muscles of mastication**.

Pyramidal system/tract. The fibres of the **upper neurone** (see **neurone**) make up this system. As they go into the brain by the **spinal cord**, they become known as the corticospinal tracts. They are responsible for voluntary movements. *See Barr (1979): 268–271.*

Q

Quadriparesis. See **quadriplegia**.

Quadriplegia. A physical handicap which affects all four limbs. Often found in types of **cerebral palsy**. Also known as quadriparesis. *See Hosking (1982): 26, 93.*

R

Radiogram. See **radiology**.

Radiologist. See **radiology**.

Radiograph. See **radiography**.

Radiography. The process of observing structures within the body on film. The commonest technique for obtaining such images is using X-ray. The plates of film on which the images are printed are known as radiographs. *See Tortora et al. (1984): 21.*

Radiology. A diagnostic technique which uses barium to show up lesions within various structures such as the **oesophagus** and **larynx**. The images found using this technique are called radiograms. The operators are known as radiologists. *See Pracy et al. (1974): 97.*

Radiotherapy. A therapeutic technique used to remove **tumours** without the patient undergoing surgery. Radiotherapy sometimes follows surgery and it is this combination which is most effective for removing a tumour completely. *See Pracy et al. (1974): 89, 108, 118, 134.*

Raised intracranial pressure. See **intracranial pressure**.

Ramsay-Hunt syndrome. A complication which can set in during the Herpes Zoster, i.e., the chickenpox virus, disease. It involves the **geniculate ganglion** and causes a rash on the **pinna**, **external auditory meatus** and **eardrum** (6). There is also an **ipsilateral** paralysis of the face. *See Gilroy et al. (1982): 312: 331.*

Ramus of mandible. See **Zygomatic arch**.

Recessive condition. See **chromosomes**.

Recurrent laryngeal nerve. See **trachea**.

Reserve air. See **reserve volume**.

Reserve volume. In breathing, the full capacity of the **lungs** is not used all the time. Most people keep within the level of the **tidal volume**. The rest of the air which could be used is the reserve volume of which there are two types:

1. The inspiratory reserve volume—the volume of air which can be used during varying degrees of deep inspiration;
2. The expiratory reserve volume—the volume of air which can be used for varying degrees of breath expiration. *See Green (1978): 56.*

Residual air. The air remaining in the **lungs** as **residual volume**.

Residual volume. An amount of air which is always left in the **lungs** after total expiration. *See Green (1978): 56.*

Respiration. The process of breathing using the **lungs** and the diaphragm. There are two elements to respiration: inspiration (breathing in), and expiration (breathing out). The normal type of breathing is **abdominal-diaphragmatic respiration** while **clavicular respiration** (see **clavicular**) is often thought to be less normal. *See Green (1978): ch. 8.*

Respiratory capacity. Another name for **vital capacity**.

Reticular system. This system in the **brain** receives almost all sensory input from the whole **central nervous system**. It has a role in such functions of the brain as sleep-arousal cycle. Its neurones are connected to the motor areas of the brain and **spinal cord**. *See Barr (1979): ch. 9.*

Rhinitis. A disorder found in the **nose**, affecting its **mucous membrane**. *See Pracy et al. (1974): 46, 47.*

Rigidity. See **Parkinson's disease**.

Rubella. Also known as German measles. It forms part of the **torch** classification of infectious diseases which can adversely affect a fetus. If the fetus becomes infected, it will die or produce spontaneous miscarriage. When it occurs at less than eight weeks into the pregnancy, the fetus' life is threatened but it is not so life threatening if it occurs after eight weeks. If the child survives birth, there could be congenital heart disease, the **brain** is underdeveloped producing **cerebral palsy**, **autism** (4) and **mental handicap** (1 and 4). The eyes will suffer from cataracts and there will be a **hearing loss** (6). The disease can be prevented by the mother undergoing immunization during child bearing years. The latest research shows immunization of 10 year old or older girls is successful. *See Hosking (1982): 199.*

S

Salivary glands. There are three pairs of large salivary glands. The ducts from these glands open into the **mouth**. The glands are:

1. Parotid gland—a wedge shaped structure lying behind the **mandible** and below the **ear** (6) and in front of the **mastoid process** (6). It grows at the same rate as the person. The sternomastoid muscle runs behind the gland. The **cranial nerve VII** ends in this gland. The duct runs over the **buccinator muscle** (see **muscles of facial expression**) and exits at the second molar (see **teeth**). This is a wholly **serous** producing cell producing water-like fluid.

2. Sub-mandibular gland—opens through a duct in the floor of the **mouth** and runs back far under the mandible. The gland measures 2–3cm deep, wide and high. The duct opening is at the side of the **lingual frenulum** (see **mouth**). It is a mixed serous/**mucous** producing cell.

3. **Sublingual salivary gland**—situated under the **membrane** of the **mouth** and is both the shape and size of an almond. It opens into the mouth by several ducts. It is a mixed serous/**mucous** producing cell.

The glands are operated by secretory motor nerves. The parotid gland is supplied by the parasympathetic fibres from the **glossopharyngeal nerve** (see **cranial nerves**) while the other two salivary glands are supplied by the **facial nerve** (see **cranial nerves**). The salivary glands are compound racemose glands because they branch into several parts: lobes—lobules —branching ducts—dilated alveoli. The three glands together produce 1–1½ litres of saliva per day. *See Tortora et al (1984): 590, 591.*

Salpingopharyngeus muscle. See **pharynx**.

Sarcoma. A **tumour** which arises from hard tissue. Thus, a fibro-sarcoma arises from fibrous tissue, an osteo-sarcoma arises from **bone** while a chondro-sarcoma arises from **cartilage**. *See Tortora et al. (1984): 75.*

Schwann cell. A cell which covers the myelin sheath covering the nerve's axon. It is divided into the sections of the nerve between the nodes of Ranvier. The myelin is formed by the membrane of the Schwann cell. When Wallerian degeneration takes place, it is the Schwann cells which are affected. *See Barr (1979): 34–36.*

Secretory motor nerves. See **salivary glands**.

Seizure. A way of describing **fits** or **convulsions** (cf. **epilepsy**).

Senile dementia. See **Alzheimer's Disease**.

Serous cells. These produce a water-like substance. See **salivary glands**.

Sex chromosomes. See **chromosomes**.

Shunt. A device fitted into the brain to drain the fluid causing pressure against the **fourth ventricle** where the patient suffers from **hydrocephalus**. There are two types of shunt treatment—the Spitz-Holter shunt and the Pudenz shunt. *See Hosking (1982): 69–71.*

Sinus. See **nose**.

Skull. A structure formed by the main **bones** of the head and **mandible**. The bones all fit together strongly except for the mandible which swings quite freely so that the **mouth** can open and close.

The largest area of the skull is occupied by the **brain**. Other areas of the skull are the orbits which are filled by the eyes and their respective nerves and muscles, the nasal cavities (see **nose**) and the **mouth**. *See Tortora et al (1984): 138–151.*

Smooth muscle. Produces slow contraction over long distances. It is supplied by the **autonomic nervous system**. Its fibres are spindle-like and have thin ends while the central part is thicker containing the nucleus of the muscle. It is found in the gut, respiratory passages, urinogenital system, iris of eye and blood vessel walls. *See Leeson and Leeson (1970): 155–160.*

Sodium valproate. A drug treatment for **epilepsy**.

Soft neurological signs. A possible diagnosis for children who have a few problems but are not so severe as to produce **mental handicap** (1 and 4). These may arise from a forceps delivery, when part of the brain has been damaged causing a mild **hemiplegia** or **language delay** (1).

Soft palate. See **mouth**.

Somatic nervous system. See **striated muscle**.

Spastic cerebral palsy. See **cerebral palsy**.

Spasticity. A condition produced by a lesion to the upper motor **neurones** causing a tightening of the muscles which continues for the duration of the lesion. The patient's speech is characterized by a **spastic dysarthria** (1). *See Tortora et al. (1984): 355.*

Spina bifida. A **congenital** (1) abnormality of the **central nervous system**. The commonest form of this condition is spina bifida occulta. It occurs between the lumbar vertebra 5 and the saccral vertebra 1. There is a failure in the fusion of the vertebral arch and an abnormality in the overlying skin. Twenty per cent of children with a closed lesion have normal **intelligence** (4) and no physical handicaps. *See Hosking (1982): 62.*

Spinal cord. A cylinder-like structure which is situated in the canal of the vertebral column. It is about 45cm long and about 1cm wide. It extends up through the magnum foramen to the **medulla oblongata**. At the end of the spinal cord is the cauda equina (a collection of lumbosacral roots), in the middle of these roots is the filum terminale which attaches to the coccyx. There are two enlargements which enervate the limbs—cervical enlargement supplies the upper limbs and the lumbosacral enlarge-ment supplies the lower limbs. It is composed of grey and white matter. *See Barr (1979): ch. 5.*

Status epilepticus. See **epilepsy**.

Sternocleidomastoid muscle. A muscle in the neck which runs from behind the **ear** (6) to the top of the chest. The right part of the muscle turns the head to the left and raises up the chin. *See Tortora et al. (1984): 231.*

Sternohyoid muscle. See **larynx**.

Stoma. A hole left in the neck after **laryngectomy** (1) or **tracheostomy**. It is used for breathing. *See Edels (1984): 40, 194–196.*

Striated muscle. This type of muscle is also known as skeletal muscle. It is enervated by the somatic nervous system. *See Leeson and Leeson (1970): 161–169.*

Sturge-Weber syndrome. Its main characteristics are **mental handicap** (about 30 per cent) (1 and 4), **Hemiplegia** (1) (about 30–40 per cent), a port-wine stain on the side of the face and **epilepsy** (about 90 per cent). The developing blood vessels in the **parietal** or **temporal lobes** (see **cerebral hemispheres**) will be abnormal. *See Salmon (1978): 94–96.*

Stroke. The layman's term for a **cerebrovascular accident**.

Structural brain disease. A possible cause of **epilepsy**. Almost any disease of the **brain** which produces a focus for discharging neurones which causes epileptic convulsions. The disease could be due to a **tumour of the central nervous system**, a **brain abscess** or degenerative disorders causing **degeneration** of **neurones**, etc. *See Draper (1980): 86.*

Styloglossus muscle. See **extrinsic muscles of the tongue**.

Styloid process. A projection found in the **skull** which extends down and forward from the temporal bone and measures 2cm long and 3mm wide. It is the starting point for muscles and ligaments which are marked by using stylo-as a prefix to their complete name. *See Tortora et al. (1984): 145.*

Stylohyoid muscle. See **muscles for swallowing**.

Stylopharyngeus muscle. See **muscles for swallowing**.

Subarachnoid space. Part of the **brain** which forms from the pia mater. It contains fluid. Berry anneurysms (see **cerebrovascular accident**) cause bleeding around the subarachnoid space as well as into the brain itself producing a **CVA**. *See Barr (1979): 308.*

Subglottic. A description of the position

of all structures or lesions found below the **glottis**.

Sublingual salivary gland. See **salivary gland**.

Submandibular salivary gland. See **salivary gland**.

Submucous cleft palate. See **cleft palate**.

Sulcus. In the **brain**, a sulcus appears as a groove surrounded by flat areas called **gyri**. *See Barr (1979): ch. 13.*

Sulcus terminalis. See **tongue**.

Superior constrictor muscle. See **pharynx**.

Supraglottic. A description of the position of structures or lesions found above the **glottis**. It is opposed to **subglottic**.

Swallowing. The transfer of the food bolus from the mouth to the stomach avoiding the airway, i.e., **trachea**. Also known as the process of deglutition. The bolus goes through stages before it reaches the stomach after it is prepared by saliva from the **salivary glands**.

1. The bolus is moved to the back of the **mouth** by the tip of the **tongue** being raised (see **mouth**). As the tongue contracts, the bolus is moved nearer to the **pharynx**. This is a wholly voluntary process.

2. The bolus moves into the oropharynx (see **pharynx**), the muscles of which are stimulated from the **medulla oblongata** via the **glossopharyngeal nerve** (see **cranial nerves**). The bolus could leave this area by four exits—the mouth, nasopharynx (see **pharynx**), **larynx/trachea** or **oesophagus** but vari-

ous muscle contractions occur to shut off three of the exits except the one to the oesophagus.

3. As the oesophagus is a flat tube with no opening the bolus has to wait for the muscle at the top to relax and produce an opening and a contraction to push the food into it. The bolus is propelled down the oesophagus by a series of peristaltic waves. When the bolus reaches the end, there is a sphincter into the stomach which the last peristaltic contraction opens to allow the bolus to enter the stomach. *See Tortora et al (1984): 594.*

Sympathetic nervous system. Becomes highly active when the patient becomes very excited. Thus, it is often known as the 'fight, fright, flight' system. The chemical transmitted to the muscle is noradrenaline. As part of **ANS**, it enervates **smooth muscle**. *See Green (1978): 130–133.*

Symphysis menti. See **mandible**.

Synapse. A junction between two nerves where there is a transfer of nerve impulses by the emission of chemicals from one to the other. *See Green (1978): 130.*

Syndrome. A grouping of several characteristic clinical features common to a particular disease or condition.

Systemic metabolic disorder. A disorder which is associated often with **epilepsy**. It is produced by toxic substances in the body resulting in hypoxia, hypoglycaemia, pyridoxine deficiencies. When the patient produces a **fit**, it takes the form of centrencephalic discharges. *See Draper (1980): 86.*

T

Tactile. A description of the action of touching an object. *See Tortora et al. (1984): 347, 348.*

Taste. The **tongue** is the organ of the body which is responsible for the sense of taste. For this purpose, it is divided into the following parts:

1. The front of the **tongue** which detects a bitter taste;

2. The back of the tongue which detects a salt/sweet taste;

3. The sides of the tongue which detect a sour taste.

The anterior two-thirds of the tongue (except **taste buds**) are supplied by the chorda tympani nerve, a branch of cra-

nial nerve VII. If this nerve becomes damaged, the chorda tympani can also suffer. *See Green (1978): 47, 163.*

Taste buds. These produce the sensation of **taste** and are found in the papillae which cover the two-thirds of the front of the **tongue**. There are three types of papillae:

1. Circum vallate papillae—mushroom-shaped and surrounded by a ditch or moat in which are found rows of taste buds (8–12 in a row) in front of the sulcus terminalis;

2. Fungiform—little puff-like balls with a moat around them in which are found more taste buds;

3. Filliform—small, conical-shaped lumps which contain no taste buds.

The taste buds are supplied by **cranial nerve IX**. *See Tortora et al. (1984): 375.*

Teeth. Set into the gums formed by layers of **mucous membranes** which cover the alveolar processes of the upper and lower jaws. Each person has two incisor teeth, one canine, two premolars and three molars. The wisdom teeth appear last. *See Tortora et al. (1984): 591–593.*

Teeth malocclusions. See **ortho-dontics**.

Temporalis muscle. See **muscles of mastication**.

Temporal lobe. See **cerebral hemis-phere**.

Temporomandibular joint. A joint which is at the same level as the **ear** (6). It allows the jaw to open and close.

Temporomandibular joint syndrome. The failure of the joint to allow the jaw to open and close which leads to difficulty in chewing (see **muscles of mastication**). There may be other characteristics to the syndrome affecting the patient's hearing as well as causing discomfort in the muscles and a clicking of the joint.

Tensor veli palatini muscle. The muscle which operates the **soft palate** (see **mouth**) and is shaped like a triangle as it starts from the skull and runs along the **eustachian tube** (see **ear**, 6). It has its apex at the pterygoid hamulus. Its nerve supply comes from **cranial nerve Viii**. Its functions are to open the **auditory tube** (6) and, on contraction, to tense the soft palate. *See Edwards and Watson (1980): 58.*

Thalamus. A large part of the **dien-cephalon** which measures about 3cm. It comprises two oval shaped pieces of grey matter and it forms the side of the **third ventricle**. Each piece can be found deep in the **cerebral hemispheres** above the **midbrain**. Various nuclei can be found within it (e.g., those for hearing, vision and general sensations plus taste). Some of the other nuclei act as synapses con-trolling voluntary motor actions and arousal. It acts also on information from the senses such as temperature, touch and pressure. *See Barr (1979).*

Third ventricle. It is divided by the **thal-amus** and between the lateral ventricles, which are linked to the third ventricle by the interventricular foramen. The **cerebro-spinal fluid** flows into the third ventricle from its initial starting point in the lateral ventricles and before it enters the **fourth ventricle** from where it passes around the rest of the **brain**. *See Barr (1979).*

Thyrohyoid muscle. See **larynx**.

Thyroid cartilage. See **larynx**.

Thyroid gland. See **trachea**.

Tidal volume. The amount of air used when breathing normally. See **reserve volume**. *See Green (1978): 54.*

Tongue. The floor of the **mouth** is formed by the tongue, which when lifted is held down to the **mucous membrane** by the lingual frenulum. On either side of the frenulum are two papillae or bumps on top of which are the openings of the sub-mandibular **salivary glands**, while below the tongue, there are two swel-lings which are called sub-lingual **saliv-ary glands**. The tongue can be divided into two parts and the line where the division occurs is the sulcus terminalis, i.e., the inverted 'v' shape. The foramen caecum is at the apex of the 'v' or small depression. The surface is covered by stratified squamous epithelium partly keretinized. The front two-thirds are covered by papillae while the underside is smooth **mucous membrane** similar to the rest of the surface. In these papillae, the **taste buds** can be found. The back one-third is covered by the lingual tonsil. Immediately behind the tonsil are two depressions or valleys called valecula while behind this ridge is the **epiglottis**. The tongue is moved by six muscles —three **intrinsic muscles** and three **extrinsic muscles**. The tongue is an **active articulator** (see **articulation**, 3) used in speech and is also used in the processes of **swallowing** and chewing. *See Tortora et al (1984): 587, 589.*

Tongue thrust. The involuntary forward movement of the **tongue**, often found in children suffering from **cerebral palsy**. It can produce **articulation delay** or **articulation disorder** (both 1), and affect the eating process as the food can be pushed out by the tongue. Treatment for both problems can be given in **speech therapy** (1).

Tongue-tie. The layman's term for **ankyloglossus**.

Tonic. A stage which occurs during a fit in **grand-mal epilepsy**. It can also be a minor fit producing muscle contractions keeping the muscles tight. *See Gilroy et al. (1982): ch. 4.*

Tonsil. There are three tonsils at the back of the **mouth**—the pharyngeal, palatine, and **lingual tonsil**. *See Tortora et al (1984): 523, 544.*

Tonsillectomy. The operation which removes infected and enlarged **tonsils**.

The palatine tonsil or true tonsil is removed. It may produce **hypernasality** which can be treated by **speech therapy** (1). *See Pracy et al. (1974): 101.*

TORCH. An acronym for the four conditions which can affect a fetus which are:

1. **toxoplasmosis;**
2. **rubella;**
3. **cytomegalovirus;**
4. **herpes simplex.**

Toxoplasmosis. An infection which is not serious to adults but can cause brain damage if transferred in utero through the placenta to the fetus. It is caused by ingestion of food which has come into contact with organisms found in cat feces. It forms part of·the **torch** classification of infections which can affect a fetus. *See Gilroy et al. (1982): 244.*

Trachea. The trachea is commonly referred to as the windpipe. It is about 10cm long and 2cm wide, extending from the sixth cervical vertebrae down to the fifth thoracic vertebrae. At this point, it divides into the left and right **bronchi**. In outline, it is more or less circular but it is actually flattened at the back since running down its whole length is the **oesophagus**. It is surrounded by three large vessels of the neck—**carotid artery**, **jugular vein**, **vagus nerve** (see **cranial nerves**). The nerve behind the trachea is the recurrent laryngeal nerve which supplies nearly all the muscles of the **larynx**. It can be easily picked out on X-ray as it has 20 tracheal rings made of hyaline cartilage while the rest of the wall comprises **connective tissue** and **smooth muscle**. It is lined by ciliated columnar **epithelium** with **mucous** cells. At the front, opposite the third tracheal ring is the thyroid gland. On inspiration, the trachea lengthens and changes shape as its walls are elastic. Its main function is to provide air during inspiration. *See Tortora et al. (1984): 547, 548, 550.*

Tracheal rings. See **trachea**.

Tracheostomy. An operation to remove the **trachea** when the patient suffers from severe problems in breathing. Tubes are inserted into a hole in the neck to aid **breathing** (1). *See Pracy et al. (1974): 142–152.*

Tracheotomy. See **tracheostomy**.

Transverse muscle. See **intrinsic muscles of the tongue**.

Trauma. Any injury which occurs to parts of or structures in the body or severe feelings of **stress** (4) caused by the external environment.

Treacher Collins syndrome. Forty per cent of patients suffering from this syndrome have a **cleft palate**. There is a characteristic facial appearance with downward slanting eyes with an underdeveloped **mandible** and **maxilla**. There are also abnormalities in the **ear** such as a lack of a **pinna** causing **hearing loss** (6). This hearing loss may cause learning difficulties but the syndrome is not associated with **mental handicap** (1 and 4). *See Edwards and Watson (1980): 84, 101, 257.*

Tremor. See **Parkinson's disease**.

Trigeminal nerve. See **cranial nerve V**.

Triplegia. A physical handicap which affects three limbs—usually both legs and one arm—and is often found in those patients who suffer from **cerebral palsy**.

Trisomy-21. See **Down's syndrome**.

True tonsil. See **mouth**.

Tuberous sclerosis. A condition which has three principal features—**epilepsy**, **mental·handicap** (1 and 4) and skin disorders called adenoma sebaceum. The child has small tumours which grow throughout the body. However, not every child suffers from these three features but 40 per cent have a skin disorder, 60 per cent suffer from mental handicap and almost all suffer from epilepsy. Prognosis depends on the site and size of the tumours and whether they are **malignant**. *See Hosking (1982): 200–201.*

Tumour. The medical term for a **cancerous** growth found in tissues in the body.

Tumours of central nervous system. These are some of the commonest cancerous growths which form in the glia of the brain:

1. Oligodendrogliomas. These tumours which may become **malignant** produce a greyish-red area in the **brain** producing a honeycomb effect. It is most often found in the **frontal lobe** of the **cerebral hemispheres**. As they grow slowly, they produce a gradual headache and a generalized **seizure**. They appear in patients between the ages of 30 and 40 years. They comprise five per cent of all gliomas. Treatment takes the form of removal followed by **radiotherapy** with the post-operative life span likely to be about five to seven years.

2. Meningiomas. These comprise 10 per cent of all intracranial tumours and are of four types:

a) **meningothelial meningiomas;**
b) **fibrous meningiomas;**
c) **psommomatous meningiomas;**
d) **angiomatous meningiomas.**

These types appear in the later years of

life and are commoner in women. Treatment takes the form of surgical removal. The prognosis is good as long as complete removal has taken place. Otherwise the **tumour** may reappear and necessitate a second operation a few years later.

3. Neurofibromas. This type of tumour can be inherited as an **autosomal dominant trait** (see **chromosomes**). It appears on the **cranial** or peripheral nerves of the **brain** and **spinal cord** and is quite common on **cranial nerve VIII**. It can produce raised pressure in the head, **aphasic** symptoms (see **aphasia, 1**), **hemiplegia**, problems in the visual fields as well as **seizures**. Headaches are not a common symptom. The condition is often called the cafe-au-lait syndrome because of the coffee coloured marks which appear on the face. The tumours are usually multiple.

4. Astrocytomas. These tumours are represented by a grey mass which has unclear boundaries. They appear most commonly in the **frontal lobes**, next the temporal lobes, parietal lobes (see **cerebral hemispheres**), **basal ganglia** and occipital lobes (see **cerebral hemispheres**) in decreasing order of frequency. Headaches are often felt on one side of the **brain** which become more general-ized and **raised intracranial pressure** (see **intracranial pressure**) develops. Treatment takes the form of surgical removal followed by **radiotherapy**.

5. Medulloblastomas. These grow very quickly and are very invasive from metastatic seeding. These tumours account for 21 per cent of all intracranial tumours in childhood. They are common in children below the age of 10 years and rarer in older children. The posterior fossa is the site for these tumours. As they grow near to the **fourth ventricle**, hydrocephalus can often develop. Treatment takes the form of surgical removal followed by **radiotherapy** while the hydrocephalus can be treated with ventricular **shunts**. The prognosis depends on how much of the tumour has been removed and the efficacy of the **radiotherapy**. *See Gilroy et al. (1982): ch. 15.*

Turner's syndrome. A **sex-chromosome disorder** (see **chromosomes**) where 45 **chromosomes** are present with one X but no Y chromosome. It is not particularly associated with **mental handicap** (1 and 4). However, there are disorders of the neck, kidneys, ovaries and heart. The child is likely to have learning difficulties such as reading problems. *See Salmon (1978): ch. 15.*

U

Ultrasonography. A non-invasive technique to assess the growth of the fetus. It can show how the fetus is placed in the placenta, the amount of fetal growth which has taken place and can identify any disorder of the spine, thus showing any possibility of the child suffering from **spina bifida**. It may also show if there are to be multiple births. *See Tortora et al (1984): 745.*

Unilateral. A lesion or disease which affects one side of the body or structure in the body. It is opposed to **bilateral**.

Upper neurone disease. See **neurone**.

Uvula. A piece of tissue hanging down from the back of the **soft palate** and between the isthmus of the fauces (see **mouth**). The uvular muscle runs along the middle of the **soft palate** (see **mouth**) and moves the uvula. Although this may not have been thought to be of much use, research now suggests that the muscle contracts and leads to a **velopharyngeal closure**. *See Edwards and Watson (1980): 59, 94.*

Uvular muscle. See **uvula**.

V

Vagus nerve. See **cranial nerves**.
Valecula. See **tongue**.
Vascular. A description of structures or

problems in the blood supply to the body.
Velopharyngeal. A description of struc-

tures or disorders between the **soft palate** (see **mouth**) and the back wall of the **nasopharynx** (see **pharynx**). When the structures in this area close, it is known as velopharyngeal closure. This closure takes place during speech and swallowing so that the **oropharynx** (see **pharynx**) is separated from the nasopharynx by the raising of the **soft palate** and the moving inward of the walls of the **pharynx**. A failure of this closure is known as velopharyngeal incompetence. If the soft palate or velum fails to reach the back wall of the **pharynx** because of damage or because it is too short to reach the wall, it is called velopharyngeal insufficiency. *See Edwards and Watson (1980): 59–62, 91–95.*

Velopharyngeal closure. See **velopharyngeal**.

Velopharyngeal incompetence. See **velopharyngeal**.

Velopharyngeal insufficiency. See **velopharyngeal**.

Ventricles. See **third ventricle; fourth ventricle**.

Vertical muscle. See **intrinsic muscles of the tongue**.

Vestibulocochlear nerve. Also known as **acoustic nerve** (6). See **cranial nerves**.

Vital capacity. The greatest **tidal volume**, i.e., the biggest breath a person can take in and let out, a person can produce. *See Green (1978): 57.*

Vocalis muscle. See **larynx**.

Z

Zygomatic arch. The crescent moon shape at the top of the ramus of the mandible. The bones which form the arch and the protruding part of the cheek are the zygomatic bones. *See Tortora et al. (1984): 145, 149, 150.*

Zygomatic bones. See **zygomatic arch**.

REFERENCES

Atkinson, R. L., Atkinson, R. C. and Hilgard, E. R. (1983). *An Introduction to Psychology*. Harcourt, Brace, Jovanovich.

Barr, M. L. (1979). *The Human Nervous System: An Anatomical Viewpoint*. Harper and Row.

Cunningham, C. (1982). *Down's Syndrome: An Introduction for Parents*. Souvenir Press.

De Meyer, W. (1972). 'Megalencephaly in Children'. In *Neurology*, 22, pp. 634–643.

Draper, I. T. (1980). *Lecture Notes on Neurology*. Blackwell.

Edels, Y. (1984). *Laryngectomy: Diagnosis and Rehabilitation*. Croom Helm.

Edwards, M. and Watson, A. C. H. (1980). *Advances in the Management of Cleft Palate*. Churchill Livingstone.

Fawcus, M. (Ed.) (1986). *Voice Disorders and their Management*. Croom Helm.

Gilroy, J. and Holliday, P. L. (1982). *Basic Neurology*. Macmillan.

Green, J. H. (1978). *Basic Clinical Physiology*. Oxford.

Haines, R. W. and Mohiuddin, A. (1972). *Handbook of Human Embryology*. Churchill Livingstone.

Hosking, G. (1982). *An Introduction to Paediatric Neurology*. Faber & Faber.

Illingworth, R. S. (1983). *The Development of the Infant and Young Child: Normal and Abnormal*. Churchill Livingstone.

Joseph, J. (1979). *Essential Anatomy*. MTP Press.

Leeson, T. S. and Leeson, C. R. (1970). *Histology*. W. B. Saunders.

Patterson, K. and Kay, J. (1982) 'Letter-by-letter Reading: Psychological Descriptions of a Neurological Syndrome'. In *Quarterly Journal of Experimental Psychology*, 34A, 411–441.

Pracy, R., Siegler, J. and Stell, P. M. (1974). *A Short Textbook of Ear, Nose and Throat*. Hodder and Stoughton.

Salmon, M. A. (1978). *Developmental Defects and Syndromes*. HM + M Publishers.

Taverner, D. (1983). *Taverner's Physiology*. Hodder & Stoughton.

Tortora, G. J. and Anagostakos, N. P. (1984). *Principles of Anatomy and Physiology*. Harper & Row.

Travis, L. E. (1971). *Handbook of Speech Pathology and Audiology*. Prentice-Hall.

Section 6

Hearing

A

ABLB. Alternate binaural loudness balance test.

AC. Air conduction.

Acoupedics. See **oral approach**.

Acoustic. The ability to hear sounds by the hearing mechanism in every human. *See Fry (1979): 3.*

Acoustic impedance. See **impedance**.

Acoustic impedance audiometry. See **impedance audiometry**.

Acoustic method. See **multisensory approach**.

Acoustic nerve tumours. Growths which are found in the hearing system causing a very mild **hearing loss** with a significant degree of problems in **speech discrimination**. They are **malignant** (5) but can be removed by surgery.

Acquired hearing loss. The onset of a **hearing loss** occurring after the **acquisition** (1) of speech and language. Such causes are produced by disease, tumours, natural ageing, excessive noise, ototoxic drugs and trauma.

Acuity. The sounds which the **ear** can pick up. These can vary depending on how near the sound source the person is. *See Denes and Pinson (1973): 100–105.*

Air-bone gap. See **pure tone audiometry**.

Air conduction. See **pure-tone audiometry**.

Air conduction hearing aid. See **hearing aids**.

Alternate binaural loudness balance test. A test for **recruitment** used with those who have a unilateral **hearing loss**. It attempts to match the loudness level of two tones. It requires a two-channel audiometer to send a signal to each **ear**. The tester presents a tone of 20dB SL to the better ear and the same tone to the poorer ear. The tone is increased until it is heard at the same loudness level in each ear.

Audiogram. See **audiometry**.

Audiologist. See **audiology**.

Audiology. A science concerned with the hearing mechanism used by humans. An audiologist uses various tests for finding out the degree of **hearing loss** from which a person suffers and the type of hearing loss. A decision is then made as to the type of **hearing aid** suitable for a particular patient. If a child is found to have a hearing loss, the effects on that child's education will have to be evaluated.

Audiometer. See **pure tone audiometry**.

Audiometric tests. Tests which are carried out by an audiologist (see **audiology**) to find out if a person is suffering from a **hearing loss**. The commonest test is **pure tone audiometry**. If the patients are found to have particular problems in the hearing mechanism other tests are used specifically for the problem. When younger children are presented to have their hearing tested, the audiologist may use **distraction tests** or **free field audiometry**.

Audiometric zero. A sound which is produced by the **audiometer** (see **pure tone audiometry**) but is just audible at 0dB. It is also known as clinical zero.

Audiometry. The process used by **audiologists** to test a person's hearing. The commonest test is **pure tone audiometry**.

Auditory canal. See **ear**.

Auditory discrimination. The ability to distinguish sounds from other sounds dependent on different frequencies and intensities of that sound.

Auditory method. See **multi-sensory approach**.

Auditory speech perception. A learnt skill for accepting auditory information. The various parts of this skill which has to be learnt by the child are:

1. Awareness of the presence of the sound;

2. Localization of the sound, so that the child knows from where it comes and so can pick up on linguistic cues as well as see the person producing the sound;

3. Cut out background noise and focus his attention solely on the sound he perceives;

4. Extract linguistic information from the **acoustic phonetic** (3) characteristics of the **phonemes** (see **phonology**, 3) produced;

5. Use of **memory** (4), particularly the short-term **memory** (4), to retain and process the **utterances** (2) produced by the speaker. However, if the child

suffers from a **hearing loss** during this period, these skills are more difficult to acquire:

1. Those who have a **conductive loss**, have a problem of receiving information (4 above) and so will require a **hearing aid** or the speaker to speak louder for him to receive such information;

2. Those who have a **sensory hearing loss**, have a problem in receiving information and also in discrimination (3 and 4 above);

3. **Neural/central hearing loss** have a

problem in obtaining meaning from the information they receive.

4. **Mixed hearing loss** will have elements of the difficulties found in (1)–(3).

See Sanders (1977): passim.

Auditory training. See **multisensory approach**.

Aural rehabilitation. See **education of hearing-impaired children**.

Auricle. See **ear**.

Average evoked response audiometry. See **evoked response audiometry**.

B

Basilar membrane. See **ear**.

BC. **Bone conduction**.

Bekesy audiometry. A procedure used in **pure tone audiometry**. Earphones are placed over the listener's ears and he is given a button to control the **intensity** (3) of the tones. The button must be pressed in order to make the tone audible and released when it is audible (causing the intensity to decrease again). The whole range of frequencies should be tested from low to high frequencies. The **audiometer** (see **pure tone audiometry**) does the sweep automatically and different tracings indicate different pathologies. Two frequency sweeps are carried out—one with a continuous tone and another with a pulsed tone. The person's threshold is traced by a stylus linked to the audiometer.

Binaural. A description of using both ears in hearing or an action being taken on the two ears such as testing both ears.

Bone conduction. See **pure tone audiometry**.

Bone conduction hearing aid. See **hearing aid**.

Brainstem evoked response audiometry. An **audiometric test** to check the early responses from the **brainstem** (5). It is the first of four classes of auditory evoked responses which consists of seven peaks. There are three electrodes of which the active electrode is placed on the **cortex** (5), the reference lobe is placed on the ear lobe, and the earth is placed on the other ear or neck. It is a non-invasive technique, does not affect the state of the patient and is regarded as a good objective idea of the patient's threshold. However, it is not frequency specific and the better ear might have to be **masked**.

BSER. **Brainstem evoked response audiometry**.

C

Calibrate. See **pure tone audiometer**.

Carhart's notch. A special feature found on a **pure tone audiogram**. It is represented on the audiogram by a dip in **bone conduction** at 2000Hz and is associated with **otosclerosis**.

Central hearing loss. This type of **hearing loss** is produced by a pathological condition occurring along the path of the **auditory nerve** from the **brainstem** to

the cerebral **cortex** (all 5). It produces a problem in **auditory speech perception** rather than just hearing. It is not usually reversible.

CERA. **Cortical evoked response audiometry**.

Clinical audiology. The description of **audiology** when it is used to evaluate the effects of a **hearing loss** on the person's daily life and giving him the means to cope with **communication** (1).

Cochlea. See **ear**.

Cochlear nerve. See **ear**.

Cochlear reflex. See **ECochG**.

Cochlear window. See **ear**.

Compliance. A description of the way in which the **tympanic membrane** and the **middle ear** function. If there is compliance, the easier it will be for the two to function and for sounds to be transmitted through this part of the hearing mechanism. It is opposed to **impedance**.

Conditioning tests. Tests used with some young children (from about 2½ years of age) who are too young to be tested by **pure tone audiometry**. It is based on **operant conditioning** (4). The child is told to do a specific action, e.g., put brick in box, peg in peg board, when it hears a specific sound. The sounds are **pure tones** (see **pure tone audiometry**). When the child responds accurately and consistently then the **intensity** (3) is reduced until the child's hearing threshold is reduced. The child should receive a **reinforcement** (4) after a correct response.

Conduction. The movement of sounds through the **outer** and **middle ears** into the **inner ear** (see **ear**).

Conductive hearing loss. A **hearing loss** caused by a pathology affecting the conduction of sound through the **outer ear**, **middle ear** and the fluids of the **inner ear** (see **ear**). The structures of the former two parts of the ear are affected while those of the inner ear are normal. It can affect **auditory speech perception**.

Congenital hearing loss. A **hearing loss** which occurs before the period of language development occurs. It can be caused by the **TORCH** (5) diseases affecting mothers during pregnancy.

Cortical evoked response audiometry. An **audiometric test** to check the late responses of the **brainstem** (5). The results are displayed as stage III on the graph of auditory evoked responses. The electrodes have a similar placement as for **BSER**. The patient is given a series of tone bursts with slow rise and fall on each **frequency** (3). It is non-invasive, frequency-specific and gives an objective measure of the patient's response. However, it is a very slow test and does not get very close to the hearing threshold.

Cross hearing. A phenomenon in which the sounds heard in one ear could have come from the other ear via bone conduction or the air around the head. This is a problem when testing hearing as it may be the sound heard in the tested ear has come from the non-tested ear by the routes already described.

D

Dactylology. See **fingerspelling**.

Damping. A description of how vibrations reduce in amplitude in a vibrating object. For example, a tuning fork begins to vibrate when it is struck against an object or hit and **resonates** (3) at a particular frequency. If the tuning fork is touched when it is vibrating, the **amplitude** (3) of the vibrations is reduced and dies away.

Deaf. A description of a person whose hearing is not used as the primary modality of **auditory speech perception** and language acquisition though it may be used as a supplement to vision or touch.

Diagnostic audiometry. The testing of a person's hearing to find out the severity of a **hearing loss** and the type of hearing loss, e.g., **conductive hearing loss**, **sensory-neural loss**, etc.

Difference limen. The smallest change in frequency needed to recognize a change in the **pitch** and **loudness** (both 3) of a sound. For example, if a sound of 200Hz is produced and a difference in pitch is heard at 203Hz but not at 202Hz, then the difference limen is 3Hz.

Distraction tests. Tests used with very young children (from 6 months to 18 months) who are not able to cope with **pure tone audiometry**. The child sits either by himself or on his mother's knee. A person sits in front of the child and produces toys to distract him while the **audiologist** (see **audiology**) stands behind him and produces tones either by a **warble** device, rattle, etc. The tester has to observe the child's reaction by turning his head. The only problem is the child could respond to other stimuli in his immediate environment.

E

Ear.   The ear comprises three parts:

1. The outer ear consists of the auricle or pinna. The external auditory canal is used to gather the sound and send it to the tympanic membrane or eardrum.

2. The middle ear is responsible for changing the sound waves from the medium of air to the medium of fluid. It comprises four walls which lead to the inner ear, mastoid, eustachian tube and tympanic membrane. It contains three ossicles which prevent loud sounds damaging the inner ear. These ossicles are the maleus (hammer), incus (anvil) and the stapes (stirrup) which has its end (or footplate) in the oval window. The vibrations of the eardrum are transferred by the hammer to the anvil to the stirrup. The oval window acts as the entrance to the inner ear. The round window or cochlear window allows fluid to return to the middle ear. The eustachian tube links the middle ear to the air in the **mouth** (5). It is used to equalize the pressure within the skull with the air outside, and so in an aircraft a person's ears are likely to crack as the pressure is equalized when it takes off and lands.

3. The inner ear contains the bony, coiled snail's shell known as the cochlea. The vibrations from the middle ear are changed into nerve impulses. The canals of fluid lead to the **acoustic nerve** (5) and the **brainstem** (5). *See Denes and Pinson (1973): 86–99.*

Eardrum.   See **ear**.

Earmold.   See **hearing aid**.

ECochG.   **Electrocochleography**.

Education of hearing-impaired children.   There are two main educational approaches to help the child suffering from a **hearing loss**:

1. The oral approach which depends mainly on spoken communication but may include **fingerspelling** or **lipreading**. Two approaches within the oral approach are: (i) acoupedic approach in which emphasis is placed totally on hearing for teaching speech and language. Its aim is to integrate the hearing-impaired into the hearing world. It was devised by Pollack. (ii) multisensory approach in which both hearing and visual stimulation are used. The child is encouraged to use lipreading but no **sign languages** or **systems** (1) are allowed. When language is being taught it should be in a mean-

ingful context. However, lipreading can be confusing as some sounds are very difficult to see although others are quite easy to see. Its efficacy depends on the speaker making the sounds as clear as possible and the conversation must take place in good light. As it is not a language system, it is not a particularly good way for a child to develop language. The main aim is to prevent the child from becoming a 'deaf ghetto' (Van Uden, 1970).

2. The manual approach which uses **sign languages** such as **British Sign Language** (1) and **sign systems** such as the **Paget-Gorman sign system** (1). Van Uden's comment already quoted is perhaps the best argument against this approach. However, it can expand the child's communication capabilities as sign languages do have their own language systems. Many deaf parents ask for their children to be taught **BSL** and it is less ambiguous than lipreading.

3. Total Communication is used to allow the child to use as many approaches as possible to communicate and develop speech and language. Thus, no one approach is emphasized more than another.

4. Rochester Method is an oral approach used with **fingerspelling**.

5. **Cued speech** (1).

See Northern and Downs (1984): 263–271.

Educational audiology.   A part of **audiology** which is designed to give advice on the educational needs of the child suffering from a **hearing loss**.

Electrocochleography.   An objective hearing test to find out very early responses. There are three electrodes of which the active electrode is placed on the promontory in the **inner ear** (see **ear**) which has the **oval window** (see **ear**) at the top and the **round window** at the bottom, while another electrode is placed on the ear lobe and the earth is placed on the forehead. It picks up the potential generated in the **cochlea** (see **ear**) and **auditory nerve** (5). It is a good objective test of a hearing threshold, it is rapid, each ear can be tested individually and the state of the patient is not affected. However, children may need to be anaesthetized. An ENT surgeon is required to place the electrode in the ear and it cannot test individual frequencies.

Eustachian tube.   See **ear**.

F

Fingerspelling. A form of communication used with patients suffering from **hearing loss**. Words are spelled out on the fingers, each finger formation forming one letter. It can be used in conjunction with **BSL** where only one finger spelling is given to represent the initial letter of a word for which there may not be a sign. The Rochester Method uses fingerspelling. It is sometimes called 'visible speech'.

Footplate. See **ear**.

Free-field audiometry. An **audiometric test** for very young children who cannot use earphones. It usually takes place in two rooms. The patient sits in one, equidistant from two loudspeakers. Live or prerecorded voices are presented. However, the child's ears cannot be tested individually. It is used in **speech audiometry**.

G

Glue ear. See **serous otitis media**.

Gradual fall. See **pure tone audiometry**.

H

Hard of hearing. A description of a person whose hearing, though impaired, is used as the primary modality for **auditory speech perception** and language acquisition.

Hearing aid. A device given to those who suffer from a **hearing loss**. It works by taking in the sound vibrations from the **ear** and converts them into electrical signals. These signals are amplified and converted back to sound waves which are sent via the earmold to the ear. To allow this procedure to happen, the hearing aid consists of a microphone (for picking up the sound and converting it to electrical signals), amplifier (makes the signal stronger), receiver (receives the signal and converts back to a sound signal, sending it through the tubing to the earmold in the auditory canal), battery (to power the aid) and the earmold (to make sure aid works well). If the earmold does not fit in the canal correctly, sound leaks out causing feedback (a whistling sound). There are also buttons and dials used to control volume, switch it on/off (O = off, M = microphone (on), T = telephone (to be used where there is a loop system)).

There are different types of aid such as:

1. Body aids where the receiver is far from the microphone and amplifier. The sound signals are taken by a **Y-cord** to the earmolds in both ears.

2. Ear Level Aids have the microphone at the bottom or top of the body of the aid facing forward. These are relatively inconspicuous but feedback is commoner than with body aids.

3. In-the-Ear Aids are only suitable for low losses: (i) Contralateral routing of signals; (ii) Bilateral contralateral routing of signals. The contralateral routing of signals occurs where the microphone is placed on one side of the head and the amplifier and receiver are placed on the other.

4. Loop system involves a magnetic loop wired into a room. The hearing aid is set to T position and picks up a signal transmitted by the magnetic loop. *See Miller (1972): passim.*

Hearing level. The level at which a sound is heard above 0dB. It is used in **pure tone audiometry**.

Hearing loss. The type of deafness from which a patient suffers after an **audiometric test** has been carried out. There are several types of hearing loss such as a **conductive hearing loss, sensory-neural loss, mixed hearing loss, central hearing loss, congenital hearing loss** and an **acquired hearing loss**.

Hearing threshold level. The smallest sound with a given frequency which the patient can hear 50 per cent of the time.

High frequency hearing loss. The person suffering from this type of hearing loss is unable to perceive sounds of a high frequency such as some of the **fricatives** (see **articulation**, 3).

HL.   **Hearing level**.

HTL.   **Hearing threshold level**.

I

Impedance. The opposition offered by an object to the transmission of sound or some acoustic energy. The greater the impedance, the less sound will be transmitted. It is opposed to **compliance**.

Impedance audiometer. See **impedance audiometry**.

Impedance audiometry. There are three types of **impedance** measures:

1. Static impedance which is measured by when the pressure in the external auditory canal equals the atmospheric pressure and the muscles of the **middle ear** (see **ear**) are at rest;

2. Dynamic impedance is measured when the **tympanic membrane** (see **ear**) is moved suddenly from its position at rest by the contraction of the **stapedius** (see **ear**) muscle, i.e., shows the amount of reflected energy as a function of change in the position and stiffness of the tympanic membrane;

3. Tympanometry measures changes in impedance with variations of pressure in the **external auditory canal** (see **ear**). The impedance bridge or impedance audiometer comprises three small rubber tubes which are attached to a small metal probe. One is a miniature microphone which picks up the sound in the canal, another is a loudspeaker which puts a **pure tone** (see **pure tone audiometry**) of 220Hz into the ear, and the third is an air pump which creates either a positive or a negative pressure in the canal. An airtight seal is created when the probe is placed in the canal. The results from static compliance are not particularly useful for making a diagnosis while the results from dynamic impedance are important. If there is a stapedius reflex, it indicates that hearing is normal, the middle ear is functioning normally (if obtained at normal HL) or there is a **sensory hearing loss** (if obtained at a low SL). If there is no stapedius reflex, this indicates a **facial nerve** (see **cranial nerves**, 5) lesion is present on the side of the tested ear, there is a problem with the **ossicles** (see **ear**), a **conductive loss** on side of earphone (i.e., sound is not loud enough in ear to elicit reflex), or a severe to profound **sensory-neural hearing loss** in the earphone ear. The results from tympanometry are in the form of diagrams. Jerger found five types:

1. Type A indicates normal middle ear function;

2. Type As (shallow) indicates normal middle ear pressure and a partially immobilized stapes (possible **otosclerosis**);

3. Type AD (deep) indicates malfunctioning of the ossicles producing high compliance;

4. Type B indicates the middle ear is filled with fluid, which makes it impossible to find a point of maximum compliance;

5. Type C indicates negative pressure in the middle ear produced by a blockage in the **eustachian tube** (see **ear**) causing **serous otitis media**.

Impedance bridge. See **impedance audiometry**.

Impedance tests. See **impedance audiometry**.

Incus. See **ear**.

Industrial hearing loss. See **noise-induced hearing loss**.

Inner ear. See **ear**.

K

Kendal toy test. A hearing test used with children from 2½ years of age. Objects are placed on the table in front of the child. The tester checks that all the toys are known, then stands behind the child and names an object. The child must point to it. The test requires no verbal response from the child. The tester looks at the pattern of errors. For example, a confusion between 'duck' and 'bus' indicates a **high frequency hearing loss**, as the high frequency sounds are missed. The test consists of three sets of 15 toys. *See test manual.*

L

Laddergram. The graphic form of results obtained from tests of loudness balance such as the **alternate binaural loudness balance test**.

Lipreading. A form of communication used with people who suffer from **hearing loss**. The person concentrates on lip movement alone to try and understand what is being said. However, only about one-third of sounds produced can be clearly seen, e.g., **bilabials**, **labiodentals**, **interdentals**, some **alveolars** (see **articulation**: 3) and **vowels** (see **cardinal vowel systems**, 3). Another difficulty is that many of these sounds can look the same such as /p,b,m/. **Speech-reading** is now preferred where the person takes into account not only lip movement but also facial expression and gesture, etc.

M

Malleus. See **ear**.

Manual approach. See **education for hearing-impaired children**.

Masking. During **audiometric tests** such as **pure tone audiometry**, there is a possibility that the results will be contaminated by **cross hearing**. On such occasions, masking is necessary. It does not matter if masking is used too much but it does matter if it is not used enough. Masking should be used when **air conduction** (see **pure tone audiometry**) thresholds in the test ear measure 40dB or are poorer than **bone conduction** (see **pure tone audiometry**) in the non-test ear because sound is then loud enough to set the skull in vibration and stimulate the **cochlea** (see **ear**) of the non-test ear. In bone conduction testing, if the thresholds are better than the air conduction thresholds, masking should be used.

Mastoid. See **ear**.

Middle ear. See **ear**.

Multisensory approaches. See **education for hearing-impaired children**.

N

Noise-induced hearing loss. When exposed to a loud noise for any length of time, a person will eventually suffer a noise-induced hearing loss which is sensory-neural in character. The degree of loss depends on how long the person was exposed to the sound and its **intensity** (3). If a depressed threshold goes back to normal after a few hours, it is called temporary threshold shift (TTS) but if the exposure is for a longer time, it can become a permanent threshold shift (PTS). This form of hearing loss is also known as industrial hearing loss. **PTS** can also occur if there is a sudden burst of noise. This is acoustic trauma and is found on an **audiogram** (see **pure tone audiometry**) by a dip at 4000Hz and a recovery at 8000Hz. The loss is **sensory-neural**.

O

Oral-manual controversy. See **education for hearing-impaired children**.
Oral approach. See **education for hearing-impaired children**.
Organ of corti. See **ear**.
Ossicles. See **ear**.
Otitis media. An infection which causes problems in the **middle ear** for children. There are two types:

1. Suppurative Otitis Media. An infection of the lining of the middle ear causing swelling and an accumulation of pus in the middle ear space. The infection can occur either from the **eustachian tube** (see **ear**) or from a ruptured **tympanic membrane** (see **ear**). The symptoms of the condition are fever, pain in the ear, and a red tympanic membrane. These symptoms can be slow or sudden to appear. The **hearing loss** which it produces is **conductive** and **flat** (see **pure tone audiometry**) across all **frequencies** (3). Treatment takes the form of antibiotics for the infection or else a surgical incision can be made in the tympanic membrane to suction out the pus. If the membrane is ruptured, there may have to be a vein graft (i.e., myringoplasty). It is an easy condition to detect as the child will complain of a sore ear and have a temperature.

2. Serous Otitis Media. If the eustachian tube fails to equalize the pressure in the **middle ear** (see **ear**), the air in the middle ear will be absorbed by mucous lining, producing a negative pressure in the cavity and the tympanic membrane is pulled inwards. This lining secretes fluids but they cannot move down the tube as it cannot open, so are sucked into the middle ear cavity until it is filled and the tympanic membrane is being pushed out. A **conductive hearing loss** results. If the fluid stays in the cavity, it will solidify and produce the condition of glue ear and exacerbate the hearing loss. As serous otitis media is not an infection, there are no symptoms and so any hearing loss is thought to be poor attention, naughtiness, etc., rather than that the child did not hear what was said to him. Gromets are inserted into the tympanic membrane to allow the fluid to drain and aerate the middle ear. After a few months, the gromets will fall out and the membrane will close by itself. *See Pracy et al. (1974): chs 4 and 5*.

Otorhinolaryngology. A name used in some countries to refer to the study of the **ear**, **nose** and **throat** (5).
Otosclerosis. A disease which begins in the bony labyrinth of the **inner ear** (see **ear**) and produces 'spongy' (sclerotic) bone. When it reaches the **middle ear** the **footplate** of the **stapes** (for all terms, see **ear**) becomes stuck to the **oval window** (see **ear**) producing a **conductive hearing loss**. The disease is progressive and can affect both ears. It happens in a person's 20s with an incidence of about 2:1 in favour of women. It may also produce **tinnitus**. The **audiogram** (see **pure tone audiometry**) will show a low frequency conductive loss with an **air-bone gap** (see **pure tone audiometry**) during the early stages, followed by **Carhart's notch**, and in the later stages a flat loss. The hearing loss may become **sensory-neural** when the structures in the bony labyrinth are affected. Treatment takes the form of removing the stapes and replacing it with a piston-type structure which acts in its place. *See Pracy et al. (1974): 38*.

Outer ear. See **ear**.
Oval window. See **ear**.

P

Paediatric audiology. A part of **audiology** in which hearing tests are carried out on children to find out the severity and type of **hearing loss** from which the children suffer. The **audiologist** (see **audiology**) has to counsel the child's parents as to the effects of a hearing loss both in the short term and long term.

Pinna. See **ear**.

Play audiometry. See **conditioning tests**.

Postlingual hearing loss. See **acquired hearing loss**.

Prelingual hearing loss. See **congenital hearing loss**.

Presbycusis. A **hearing loss** which results from the normal **ageing** (4) process. The symptoms are a **sloping sensory-neural hearing loss** which may have also a **conductive** component due to changes in the **middle ear**. The patient loses **speech discrimination** although patients can have a good understanding of speech if the speaker speaks slower rather than louder. There may also be general slowing down of processing ability.

PTA. **Pure tone average**.

Pure tone. See **pure tone audiometry**.

Pure tone audiometry. Pure tone testing involves the presentation of seven **frequencies** (3) (125, 250, 500, 1000, 2000, 4000 and 8000Hz) at decreasing or increasing **intensities** (3) in the range of −10–120dBHL until the patient identifies the tone as being present 50 per cent of the time or two-thirds of the time. The tones are given using two pathways of hearing:

1. Air conduction where the sound waves enter the **external auditory canal** and are transmitted via the **tympanic membrane** to the **ossicles** in the **middle ear** to the **oval window** from where they join the fluids of the **inner ear**. This action stimulates the hair cells on the **basilar membrane** (see **ear** for all terms). **AC** involves the whole hearing system, so any damage to any part of it will result in depressed thresholds for air conduction.

2. Bone conduction where sound waves hitting the head will set the skull vibrating if their **intensity** (3) is high enough, e.g., 40–50dB above **AC** thresholds. These vibrations of the skull set the **cochlea** of the **inner ear** in motion. Thus, **BC** does not affect the **outer ear** or **middle ear** (see **ear** for last four terms) but transmits sounds straight to the inner ear. Depressed thresholds will only occur in **BC** if there is a lesion or damage to the inner ear. A **conductive hearing loss** will have depressed **AC** thresholds but normal **BC** thresholds while a **sensory-neural hearing loss** shows depressed thresholds in both pathways.

The machine which is used to carry out these tests is an audiometer. It produces the frequencies by means of an electronic oscillator. Pure tones are not used in everyday speech but their use in testing gives a good idea of how the person will cope with complex speech signals as they are made of pure tones. When testing for **AC** thresholds all seven frequencies are used while in **BC** only five are used (125Hz and 8000Hz are not used as the former requires such an intensity that it produces a sensation, so the patient may react to sensation and not to tone. Present audiometers cannot produce an intensity for making 8000Hz audible). In **AC** testing earphones are placed over both ears while **BC** requires a bone conduction vibrator placed on the **mastoid** in the **ear**. The results of pure tone audiometry are graphically displayed on an audiogram. This gives frequencies along the horizontal axis and intensities up the vertical axis. The audiologist uses symbols to show which pathway has been tested and in which ear (see below).

When analyzing the results on the audiogram, the tester should look for the presence of an air-bone gap i.e., the difference between the **AC** and **BC** curves. This will reveal if the hearing loss is conductive, sensory-neural or mixed. The degree of hearing loss is determined by the pure tone average. The **AC** thresholds for 500, 1000, 2000Hz are

				AC	BC	Unmasked:	AC	BC
Right ear	—	red	R	O	[		△	<
Left ear	—	blue	L	X	]		△	>

added and divided by 3. This gives only a reasonable prediction of the degree of hearing. The slope of the curves is also an important feature:

Low Frequency Loss—usually conductive hearing loss;

Flat Loss across all frequencies —conductive or sensory neural;

Ski Slope/High Frequency/Sloping Loss—**sensory-neural** usually.

Audiograms can also show particular features of a person's hearing such as **Carhart's notch**, acoustic trauma, **noise-induced hearing loss** and **presbycusis**. There are a few classifications to show the degree of hearing loss such as Green (1978).

Pure tone average. See **pure tone audiometry**.

R

Recruitment. An accompanying problem to **sensory-neural loss**. It occurs when the **intensity** (3) level of the sound is given a small increase but to the patient it becomes almost unbearable. For example, an increase of 20dB may sound like an increase of 60dB. Tests used to detect recruitment include direct tests for recruitment such as **ABLB**, the **Stapedius reflex threshold** and indirect tests for recruitment such as finding out the **difference limen**, the **short increment sensitivity index** and **Bekesy audiometry**.

Retrocochlear hearing loss. A **hearing loss** which is caused by damage or a lesion behind the **cochlea** (see **ear**), just below the **brainstem** (5). It produces a **sensory neural hearing loss**.

Rochester method. See **education for hearing-impaired children**.

Round window. See **ear**.

S

Screening audiometry. **Audiometric tests** which are carried out quickly with groups of patients (usually children in schools or in a pre-school clinic). The frequencies are tested at a constant **intensity** (3) level. This is also known as sweep testing.

Sensation level. A measure of the loudness of a sound above the patient's hearing threshold. It is measured in dB. For example, if the hearing threshold is 60dBHL and a sound is presented at 90dBHL, the sensation level will be 30dBSL.

Sensory-neural hearing loss. This is caused by a lesion or damage to the **inner ear** (see **ear**) or in the **auditory nerve** (5) to below the **brainstem** (5). It can only improve with a **hearing aid**. Patients often talk too loudly because they cannot hear their own voice and sometimes they suffer from vertigo and often suffer from **tinnitus**. They have a difficulty picking up speech especially if they are in a noisy environment or having a conversation in a group. There is no **air-bone gap** (see **pure tone audiometry**) while the loss varies from a mild to severe loss.

Serous otitis media. See **otitis media**.

Ski slope. See **pure tone audiometry**.

SL. **Sensation level**.

Sloping hearing loss. See **pure tone audiometry**.

Sound pressure level. The pressure of a sound decreases the further it gets from its source. **SPL** is a measurement of the pressure at a particular point in its travel from its source. It is measured in dynes/cm^2 or Pascals (Pa). *See Denes and Pinson (1973): 41–42*.

Speech audiometry. An **audiometric test** to give the **audiologist** (see **audiology**) a better measurement of the person's hearing as real speech is used instead of **pure tones** (see **pure tone audiometry**) which are not used in every day speech. Those suffering from a **retrocochlear hearing loss** and a **cen-**

tral **hearing loss** may do reasonably well with pure tones but still have poor **speech discrimination**. This type of audiometry also allows the tester to assess the person's social disability, find a lesion in the auditory pathway, predict the outcome of surgery, assess the value of lipreading or auditory training, etc., and assess the efficiency of **hearing aids**. Any speech from monosyllabic **words** to **sentences** and **discourse** (all 2) is used. However, monosyllabic and bisyllabic words are used most often. Whatever linguistic material is used, it must be within the capabilities of the patient to understand it. The stimuli are usually presented by the tester in one room while the patient sits in the other room and hears the stimuli in earphones or loudspeakers. There is variability between testers but stimuli can be presented at a suitable speed for each patient. A prerecorded tape could also be used. A **free-field presentation** is used with children. Two types of assessment are carried out —**speech reception threshold** and **speech discrimination test**. *See Hood (1981).*

Speech discrimination test. A test used in **speech audiometry** for assessing the person's ability to understand speech at levels above his/her threshold of hearing. Lists of 25 or 50 monosyllabic words are used. The words have been phonetically balanced. One list is presented at + / − 30dB above **SRT**. Correct repetitions are scored as a percentage. The next list is presented as 10dB higher followed by another list at a further 10dB higher. The curve of discrimination scores is shown on a graph. *See Hood (1981).*

Speech reception threshold. The level measure in dB, at which 50 per cent of bisyllabic words are repeated accurately. Three words are presented at a level of + / − 25dB above **PTA**. The person repeats the words and then descends in 5dB steps until the patient fails to repeat one or more words. This is followed by six words at each level. The **SRT** is the level at which three to four words out of six are repeated correctly. *See Hood (1981).*

SRT. **Speech reception threshold**.

Stapedectomy. The removal of the **stapes** (see **ear**) by a surgical procedure. *See Pracy et al. (1974): 38.*

Stapedius reflex. See **impedance battery**.

Stapes. See **ear**.

Static impedance. See **impedance battery**.

Stirrup. See **ear**.

Stycar hearing test. An assessment devised by Mary Sheridan to be used with children between the ages of 6 months and 7 years. It uses very simple and familiar objects, words and pictures. Its aim is to test the child's ability to hear meaningful speech with different **frequency** and **intensity** (both 3) components. The test contains several different subtests for different age groups. These subtests take the form of toy tests, cube tests, doll vocabulary, picture vocabulary, word lists and sentences. Thus, the tester can identify sounds which are producing difficulties for the child. *See test manual.*

Suppurative otitis media. See **otitis media**.

Sweep testing. See **screening audiometry**.

T

Tinnitus. A condition which is found in **conductive** and **sensory-neural hearing losses**. The patient will often complain of rushing, roaring, ringing noises in their **ear**. It is a very annoying condition and there is no real treatment for it although it is possible to help the patient with a tinnitus masker which can be placed behind the ear to control the amount of tinnitus experienced by the patient. In many cases, the sound can only be heard by the person, but in more severe cases, other people can hear it.

Tinnitus masker. See **tinnitus**.

Tone decay. This can be measured by **impedance tests** for the **stapedius reflex** (see **impedance battery**). It is produced by a **retrocochlear hearing loss**. The **ear** adapts to the tone from the earphones very quickly and hears it as softer since the **amplitude** (3) decreases as the ear adapts to the tone. If the amplitude of the tone decreases by more than 50 per cent in 10 seconds, tone decay is present. The tone is presented 10dB above the reflex threshold. Those with normal hearing have some decay at 2000 and 4000Hz but not at 500 and 1000Hz.

Total communication. See **education of hearing-impaired children**.

Tympanic membrane. See **ear**.

Tympanogram. See **impedance battery**.

Tympanogram classification. See **impedance battery**.

Tympanometry. See **impedance battery**.

V

Vestibular. See **vestibular canal**.

Vestibular canal. A part of the **ear**. However, it is not used as part of the hearing mechanism but is used for balance. There are three semicircular canals which contain fluid. When this fluid is level in the canals, the person can keep his balance, however if it becomes unlevel, the person will fall over more to one side than another. It is found in the **inner ear** (see **ear**).

Vestibular membrane. The fluid which flows in the **vestibular canal**.

Visible speech. See **fingerspelling**.

W

Warble tone. A machine used with very young children during **distraction tests**. It produces a warble tone at varying **intensities** (3) and is held to each side of the child. If the child hears the tone, he will turn his head to the side where the tone has been presented. If he cannot hear the tone, he will continue to look at the person in front of him who is distracting him with toys.

Windows. See **ear**.

Y

Y-cord hearing aid. See **hearing aid**.

Z

Zero hearing level. A measurement of **SPL** which makes a **frequency** (3) just audible to a person with normal hearing.

REFERENCES

Denes, P. B. and Pinson, E. N. (1973). *The Speech Chain: The Physics and Biology of Spoken Language*. Anchor.

Fry, D. B. (1979). *The Physics of Speech*. Cambridge University Press.

Green, D. S. (1978). 'Pure Tone Air Conduction Testing'. In Katz, J. (Ed) (1985) *Handbook of Clinical Audiology*. Williams and Wilkins.

Hood, J. D. (1981). 'Speech Audiometry'. In Beagley, H. A. *Audiology and Audiological Medicine*. vol. 1, ch. 7.

Kiernan, C., Reid, B. and Jones, L. (1982). *Signs and Symbols*. Heinemann Educational Books.

Meadow, K. (1980). *Deafness and Child Development*. Edward Arnold.

Miller, M. H. (1972). *Hearing Aids*. Bobbs-Merrill.

Northern, J. and Downs, M. (1984). *Hearing in Children*. Williams and Wilkins.

Pracy, R., Siegler, J. and Stell, P. M. (1974). *A Short Textbook of Ear Nose and Throat*. Hodder and Stoughton.

Sanders, D. A. (1977). *Auditory Perception of Speech*. Prentice-Hall.

Note: As most of the terms in this section can be found in one text, it has not been detailed after each explanation. The text is: Martin, F. N. (1981). *Introduction to Audiology*. Prentice-Hall.

Section 7

Electronic Devices

B

Bodyspek 2000. Provides an objective assessment of an infant's hearing. It will identify a significant **hearing loss** (6) before the child begins to develop language. Electrodes are placed in front of the ear, behind the same ear and at the back of the child's neck. The test starts by pushing the switch to 60dB sound level, all other adjustments are automatic. The Bodyspek 2000 produces 2000 clicks until the post auricular myogenic response (PAM) is elicited and the test stops automatically. If the child fails at this sound level the child is retested at 80dB. The test usually lasts about ten minutes.

C

C-speech. Produces an analysis of speech on a television screen following the patient speaking into a microphone. Two bands appear on the screen. The top band can be used by the therapist to show the patient how a sound or word should be said and the lower band is for the patient's attempts. There is a variable timebase which means that sounds, words or complete phrases can be used with this system. Speech is analyzed into three displays:

1. chequed pattern for high frequency sounds, i.e., **fricatives** and **aspirated consonants** (3);
2. white band for low frequency sounds plus all **vowels** and the consonants /l,m,n,ng,r,v,w,y/;
3. black band represents silence.

Although developed for children with a **hearing loss** (6), the unit could be used with any **articulation** or **phonological disorders** (1) a child may have. Other patients who might benefit from C-speech include **dysarthric**, **dyspraxic**, **dysphonic** (all 1) and **cerebral palsied** patients (5).

Canon communicator. A mini-electronic typewriter which can be used with patients who have difficulty being understood because they have inadequate **expressive language** (1) or none at all. The keyboard has the 26 letters of the alphabet arranged in frequency order, i.e., the most used letters at the top of the keyboard. The vowels and consonants have different coloured keys, i.e., consonants are on light grey keys while vowels are on dark grey keys. Thermal tape is used for printing. There are also alternative keyboard covers for patients who might have a **tremor** (5) and press the wrong key. The communicator works off a battery pack which can be recharged. Patients suffering from a **hearing loss** (6), **aphasia**, **dyspraxia** and **dysarthria** (1) can benefit from using it. The machine measures $131 \times 85 \times 30$mm and it weighs 280g. It is produced by Canon Business Machines UK Ltd.

Chatterbox. A speech synthesizer which produces the words typed into it. It has a **QWERTY keyboard** (8) and a built-in amplifier unit with rechargeable batteries. There is a 12-character display screen which allows typing errors to be corrected before pressing the 'speech key'. The memory holds 74 sentences and phrases which the patient may need to be accessed quickly. These expressions are for emergencies, feeding, shopping and everyday conversation. It can be used with non-vocal patients who still have good motor coordination.

Communication board. See **possum**.

Convaid. A portable device which operates electronically. It has a built-in speech synthesizer which can use the voice of a male, female or child speaker. There is a touch-keyboard of 64 squares. When one of these squares is pressed, the synthesizer produces the word. There is also an alarm square.

Converse with Claudius. A machine which can be fitted to the patient's telephone and produces speech artificially. 'Claudius' (the Roman Emperor who suffered from a speech defect) stands for Calling Line Announcement Using Digitally Integrated Voice Synthesis. It consists of a keypad with 16 buttons which when pressed can produce 64 phrases including emergency messages for ambulance, fire or police. Both female and male voices can be produced. It can be used in a face-to-face conversation. It has been developed by British Telecom and manufactured by A. P. Besson.

D

Delayed auditory feedback. An electronic device which is used to make stuttering patients communicate more fluently. While it can make a stuttering patient more fluent, it has the opposite effect on non-stuttering patients. In general terms, DAF works on the principle of placing a delay between saying a word, phrase or sentence and hearing it through the normal feedback mechanism. So, if the speaker is reading a list of items, as he says one item there will be an electronic delay before he hears it, which may disorientate the fluent speaking patient and may make him become **dysfluent** (1).

E

Eyetyper model 200. A communication system operated by direct eye contact between the patient and the machine. The keyboard has a lens, a light and eight eye-gaze sensors plus a large display panel. The sensors can be used in two, four or eight combinations. A glance can produce a word, phrase or symbol which will appear on the display panel and be produced by the built-in speech synthesizer. Different overlays can be used. It can be interfaced to a **computer**, a **modem**, a **printer** (all 8) or other environmental control devices. It is portable and is produced by Ariel Enterprises.

F

Fo-indicator. An indicator to help improve three different aspects of speech production:
1. **pitch** of the voice (3);
2. **intonation** (3);
3. **phonation** (3).
Fo represents **fundamental frequency** (3). A contact microphone is held against the throat and the fundamental frequency, indicated by the movement of the vocal cords, is measured by the pointer. The frequency range is 50–550Hz (3). The upper and lower limits of the frequency range are indicated by the use of red and green lamps and set by red and green controls respectively. It can be used with children suffering from a **hearing loss** (6) whose sounds are not always used with an acceptable pitch level. It measures 190 × 190 × 100mm, weighs 1.3kg without batteries and is produced by SCI Instruments.

H

Hector speech aid. An aid to help patients who **stammer** (1) to become more **fluent** (1) speakers. It consists of a throat microphone placed against the **larynx** (5), a small amplifier and a control box which can be attached to a waist belt or put in a pocket. The microphone can be hidden under a high collar of a blouse, shirt or jumper. Its aim is to decrease the **rate** (3) of the patient's speech and hence allows the speaker to produce a type of **prolonged speech** (1). If the speaker has a very fast rate of speech, it is picked up by the microphone and a tone is produced through the amplifier. The volume of the tone can be turned up or down so that it can blend into the background noise. It can be used for practice at home and during speech therapy sessions.

Helpmate. A lightweight machine, requiring a mains power supply with a display which can hold 40 characters and a normal **QWERTY keyboard** (8). Each key has an associated word or phrase, so by touching the 'phrase key' followed by a letter, the preset word or phrase will come out of the memory. The memory can store a whole message of up to 250 characters in length. It has a rechargeable battery. Helpmate measures 350 × 199 × 100mm and weighs 2.7kg without the battery and 3.6kg with the battery. A clip-on finger guard is provided for those with motor difficulties. It is produced by Weyfringe.

L

Language master. A machine which can be used in a similar fashion to a tape recorder. It uses different sizes of cards with a two-track magnetic tape running along the length at the bottom of the cards. The cards can have sounds, words, phrases or pictures on them with the auditory stimulus on one of the two tracks spoken by the therapist for the patient to imitate on the second track of the tape. The patient can find out by listening carefully the difference between the way he says the stimuli as compared to the correct version by the therapist. It is produced by Bell and Howell. *See Code and Muller (1983): 175–176.*

Lightwriter. A twin-screen machine with a **QWERTY keyboard** (8) for patients who have difficulty using **expressive language** (1). The message is typed up on a screen facing the patient and another facing those to whom he is wanting to communicate. Each can hold up to 20 characters both upper and lower case. The memories hold fixed messages of 500 characters, entire messages for later use and the operating instructions. It has a rechargeable battery which, when fully charged, lasts for a continuous six hours' operation. It is especially useful for patients to use in a conversation involving groups of people since they can see the message straightaway. There is an optional printer which can be used.

M

Memowriter. A combined typewriter and calculator with the appropriate facilities for such a keyboard. There is a wide print roll which holds 20 characters as does the larger display screen. The screen can hold 120 characters before printing begins. The memories can hold 800 characters including emergency messages and personal information which can be accessed by using only three keys. The memowriter measures 225 × 142mm and is portable. It is produced by QED Ltd.

Microscribe. A small, portable word-processor. It has a **QWERTY keyboard**

(8) and an 80 character display in which the patient can write, edit, send, receive or delete text. The memory has a capacity of 8000 characters which can be put onto nine documents plus a ten-message memory capable of holding 80 characters. It can be used as a **word processor** (8), a voice synthesizer or it can be linked up to a microcomputer. It is battery operated with rechargeable batteries.

Microwriter. A machine with six keys, i.e., no **QWERTY keyboard** (8), which, when pressed in different combinations, produces a letter. The patient has to learn these combinations. It is said the patient can learn these in one hour and become proficient in their use after a few weeks. Its memory holds five pages of text which is still held in memory when the machine is switched off. It is portable and can be linked up to a speech synthesizer, printer or television.

Minivib 3. A tactile stimulator which can be used with patients who are hard of hearing or who have a severe **hearing loss** (6). The machine takes in sounds from around the person and changes them into vibrations. It works better for sounds which change rather than those sounds which remain constant. The vibrator unit is usually placed on the wrist. It can also act as a monitor for the patient's own voice. It weighs 55g while the vibrator weighs only about 2g. It is worked by a rechargeable battery.

Model 1600 voice analyzer. The voice analyzer can be used in the clinic, home, hospital or school. It is designed to pick up **fundamental frequency** (Fo) and **intensity** level (both 3) at the same time on a monitor. There are two lines which can be compared, the top one with the therapist's model and the lower one for the patient's attempts. Both can be superimposed on the other for an easy comparison. The machine can be linked up to a printer so that the therapist can keep accurate records of assessments and progress during therapy. It is produced by Millgrant Wells Ltd.

Motor assessment. By carrying out this assessment, the speech therapist has to find out which limb the patient can control best. The different parts of the body which must be considered are:

1. the head (including mouth for sucking and blowing and eye movement);
2. the hands (including the freedom of movement of the fingers, how far apart they can be spread and how mobile the hand is at the wrist);
3. the legs (including the amount of foot movement and the range of foot movement).

Having assessed all these limb movements, the speech therapist can gain an idea of the best switch for the patient's communication device.

N

N-indicator. An indicator to help those children who may suffer from speech problems due to **hyper/hypo-nasalization** (5). It operates by finding out how much vibration exists at the end of the **nose** (5) by having the patient place a contact microphone on this part of the nose and the amount of vibration is shown by the deflection of the pointer on the display unit. A green and red lamp shows if the pointer is less or greater than 50 per cent deflection. The indicator should be adjusted for each child. It may also be possible to show the degree of **phonation** (3). It measures $190 \times 190 \times 100$mm, weighs 1.3kg without batteries and is produced by SCI Instruments Ltd.

O

Orovox. A speech synthesizer with an unlimited vocabulary. The patient can program it to accept his/her own speech and 250 phrases can be pre-programmed. There is fast access to these phrases which can be obtained by depressing a single key. All programs are retained even when the computer is switched off. It can be used by itself or connected to a computer by using RS232 input and output to which a printer could be attached. It is produced by Speech Systems Ltd.

P

Personal aid for communication. An electronic box divided into squares with a light above each. Overlays are placed into the box and by pressing a switch, the patient can switch on the light above the appropriate picture, word or phrase. The patient can make a positive choice of eight symbols per card. This is the standard PAC. The PAC 6 is similar but the patient will have only six stimuli from which to choose. The PAC measures 215 × 130mm and weighs 450g. Both models are produced by Geoffrey King Enterprises.

Personal speech amplifier. An amplifier which can be used with those patients who have weak voices from **dysphonia** (1). It has a microphone which is attached over the ear and an amplifier which can be attached to a pocket or waist belt. There is an on/off switch, volume control plus a battery which is rechargeable. The patient can have free hands and complete freedom of movement. It is produced by Datamed.

Phonic ear vois 130. A portable machine with 45 **phonemes** (3), 352 words and 19 phrases plus four programmable levels. There is also an overlay for users of **blissymbolics** (1). By depressing the button, sounds, words or phrases can be produced by a speech synthesizer.

Phonic ear vois 135. This machine has a personal programmable memory which allows up to 5000 entries. The pre-programmed memory holds 46 words, 45 **phonemes** (see **phonology**, 3), 12 **morphemes** (see **morphology**, 2) and 10 commonly used phrases. There is a light touch sensitive display area with nine selectable functions. Speech can be edited by the use of the 'review' command and by combining the use of words, phonemes, morphemes and letters. The available vocabulary is unlimited. It is portable and a key guard is also available so that it can be used early by those patients with poor hand control.

Poligon. A smaller version of **Claudius**

converse. It has only two buttons. When depressed, one of them plays a tune (the 'signature of the communication handicapped') while the second produces the message, 'Hello, I have a speech handicap, please be patient with me.' At the time of writing, this is only a prototype produced by British Telecom for Speak Week 1987.

Porta-amp portable public address system. A system to be used with those patients suffering from **dysphonia** (1). It is good for patients who speak to groups (e.g., teachers). It increases the amplification of their voices. The loudspeaker can be positioned anywhere or carried around on the shoulder strap provided. It has rechargeable batteries. The system measures 231 × 175 × 94mm and weighs 1.95kg. It is produced by Raymed.

Possum. There are several devices produced by Possum to help patients suffering from **communication disorders** (1):

1. Porta-Scan Communicator. There is a built-in plate switch. Six pictures can be placed on the communicator and the required picture indicated by illuminating a small light at the top left-hand corner. It can be placed on a wheelchair easily.

2. Communicator Boards. All these boards are back-lit. The number following each name refers to the number of squares which can be lit up and hence the number of stimuli which can be placed on them. The Communicators 4, 16 and 32 all have pictures or words which can be lit individually square by square. However, the Communicator 100 has a 10 × 10 matrix, i.e., 100 cells/squares. The patient indicates which cell is required by illuminating a light in the top left-hand corner. The light can be used horizontally, vertically or diagonally. There are four overlays provided with the board although therapists can make up their own. The memory can hold a message using 40 cells. It has an alarm cell to obtain attention when in difficulty. Any type of Possum input can be used. It

measures 483 × 356 × 108mm and can be connected to a printer or speech synthesizer.

3. Typewriter systems.

a) Overdeck typewriter conversion. This can be placed on the patient's own typewriter.

b) Combination system. This system is supplied with a GCTW12 (an illuminating scanning board with letters and punctuation marks), PEK (Possum Expanded Keyboard) for use with those patients who have gross uncontrollable movements and a mini-keyboard for those patients with small controlled movements.

4. Text Processor Workstation. The most advanced communication aid developed by Possum. It comprises:

a) a tape library filing system;

b) an easy-read facility on TV screen (improves fluency and speed of reading and retrains visual scanning movements);

c) TV screen to precompose text before printing it or to store it in memory of the microprocessor for future use;

d) a vocabulary of 800 words and phrases provided to increase the speed of composition;

e) Tellink where two text processors can be connected to produce a telephone network.

S

S-indicator. An indicator to help the patient in producing a correct /s/ sound. An indicator panel with a needle plus a light give visual feedback as to the quality of the /s/. It can be used with the poorest of speakers. It can also be used for training other voiceless fricatives. Tests in Sweden have shown that it can be used effectively with children of 6 years of age. It measures 190 × 190 × 100mm, weighs 1.3kg without batteries and is made by SCI Instruments Ltd.

Splink. A system comprising a small electronic word board which has 950 basic words, letters, numerals, common phrases and various prefixes/suffixes plus instructions. It can fit on the patient's knee and transmits a signal by infra-red to a microprocessor box which is plugged into the aerial socket of an ordinary TV set. Thus, the words and so on appear on the screen. There are no wires but the patient must keep within 12–15 feet of the TV set. Two or more word boards can be used with a single microprocessor so that Splink can be used with groups. Splink stands for 'Speech Link'. *See Code and Muller (1983): 187–192.*

Switches. Each of the electronic devices described in this section can be operated by different switches depending on the patient's handicaps, e.g., hemiplegia, quadraplegia, etc. **Possum** have designed several types of switches to be used with their own electronic aids:

1. Flexitube on a microphone stand for the patient who can only operate the device by puffing or blowing;

2. Manual input by paddle switches which require the lightest touch downwards to operate the machine;

3. Plate switch which just requires a touch to operate the machine. There is a single and a double plate switch. In the latter, each half of the switch acts as a single switch;

4. Pressure pad which the patient can press either with his hand or foot;

5. Joy stick for the patient with good coordination who can push the lever backwards, forwards and sideways;

6. Wobblesticks for the patient with gross uncontrollable movements. They will operate the machine by just being knocked by hand or foot;

7. Danavox switch which can be operated by use of hand or foot but requires harder pressure to function;

8. Neck halter on which are placed two microswitches which can be operated by the chin;

9. Bifurcated flexitude with microswitches on a microphone stand which are operated by a side-to-side head movement;

10. Heavy duty foot switches mounted on an angled bracket which is operated by gross foot movement;

11. Footskate which requires fine foot control as it operates eight microswitches as it is moved up and down.

Quest Educational Designs have designed switches for their own electronic devices:

1. LA/1 Lever switch which only requires the lightest touch to operate the

communication device;

2. LA/2 Platform switch which has a microswitch at each corner and is used with patients who have gross motor movements;

3. LA/3 Sound-operated switch which starts a machine by the use of the patient's voice;

4. LA/4 Lever switch with twin flex —similar to LA/1;

5. LA/5 Graphics switchboard which is a control box with five switches ideal for use with a computer for drawing graphics;

6. LA/6 Heavy duty lever switch requiring a very light touch to make a device function;

7. LA/7 Sub-miniature lever switch which can be used as a 'head' switch;

8. LA/8 Puff switch interiors which are fitted into devices by the patient or relatives. There are three microswitches which function in turn as the puff pressure increases.

It is important that the therapist carries out a good **motor assessment**, so that the appropriate switch can be chosen to help the patient's ability to communicate.

T

Talking brooch. A machine comprising a display, a keyboard and a control box. The display is usually worn at the top of the patient's clothing like a 'brooch'. The message is typed out on the keyboard and appears on the display. The message runs from right to left across the display.

Toucan communicator. A portable device which can be used by those with a **communication disorder** (1) and who are physically handicapped. It is operated by two switches which can be used by hand, foot or chin. The display comprises two circles of coloured LED (i.e., Light Emitting Diode) lamps. The outer circle is the main circle as it contains the alphabet, numbers, common punctuation and control characters. The inner circle is used less. There are two displays, one facing the patient and one facing the person to whom he wishes to commu-

nicate. Each display can hold 80 characters. The memory can be accessed to provide urgently required phrases or to plan future conversations. All messages can be prepared in advance and retained in the communicator's memory. The speed at which the characters are chosen can be varied. There is an alarm button which can be used to call immediate attention. It can be connected to many types of microcomputer, printer and the Toucan Portable Speech Synthesizer. Patients who benefit most from the communicator would be those suffering from **cerebral palsy** (5), **CVA** (5) and **head injury** (5). It measures 265 × 205 × 125mm, weighs 2.5kg (approximately) and has rechargeable batteries. It is produced by Toucan (Communication Aids) Ltd.

V

Vocaid. A speech synthesizer. It is supplied with a set of printed overlay cards with 32 squares providing 35 utterances and an 'off' square. Each card covers specific subjects (e.g., bedside, leisure, etc.). Each card has a special code that chooses its program. As one of the squares is pressed, the word or phrase is produced. The back of each overlay card has blank squares so that it can be adapted for a system of symbols (e.g., photos, **blissymbolics** (1) or **rebus** sym-

bols (1). It measures 360 × 270mm and is easily portable. It is produced by Texas Instruments.

Voicette. An amplifier to be used with those patients who have a weak voice due to **dysphonia** (1). The amplifier can be held over the shoulder. The microphone is hand-held and attaches to the amplifier directly. It is suitable for patients who may need to talk to groups (e.g., teachers).

REFERENCES

Code, C. and Muller, D. J. (1983). *Aphasia Therapy*. Edward Arnold.
Fishman, I. (1987). *Electronic Communication Aids: Selection and Use*. Little, Brown and Company.

NOTE: As far as the author knows, there is no book which details these machines but further information can be obtained from the local Communication Aids Centre.

Section 8

Microcomputers

A

Access. A description of how to obtain data or other information from a disc in a **disc drive** or instructions from **memory** so that they can be carried out (e.g., from a program in the computer's memory).

Acorn computers. Acorn produce the BBC series of microcomputer. They began by producing the BBC B and BBC B+, but recently they introduced the Master series of BBC computers and the BBC Master compact. The Master 128 has 128K of memory and has built-in **software** including view **word processor**, viewsheet, spreadsheet, edit program and text editor, and **BBC BASIC**. Extra **rom** software can be easily added by inserting the eprom cartridge in one of the two plug-in slots. There are interface facilities for a disc drive and both serial and parallel interface for printers and other ports which include User port, 1 MHz bus, Tube, Analogue port, Monitor/TV ports and cassette interface. It uses also the Advanced Disc Filing System (ADFS). The Master 512 has a 16-bit processor and 512K **ram** and uses icon interaction with the computer. The Master Turbo uses a combination of co-processor language and system architecture which allows for extremely fast execution times. The language is hi-**BASIC**. The Master Et is the Master Econet terminal which allows the setting up of a network system. The Master Compact has similar features to the Master 128 except all the ports have been removed except for the monitor port. There are interface points for the disc drive, a mouse and a parallel interface for printers. It uses 3½″ discs and the Advanced Disc Filing System. The welcome suite of programs is called up using the icon system. It has been designed principally for use in schools and in the home. *See manuals for particular type of BBC computer.*

Address. The specific area in the computer where information may be kept, for example, each part of the computer's memory has an address, so the information which goes into the memory has a specific location.

Algorithm. Some computer programs use algorithms for problem-solving in a particular way.

Amstrad. Amstrad produces self-contained word processors such as the PCW 8256. This model has 256K **ram** computer memory and integral 3″ discs.

Apple. Apple have produced many microcomputers such as the Apple II, IIc, IIe, Apple Mac and Apple IIIc.

Array. A list of items in a **program** from which one item has to be chosen. The computer can do this by comparing the wanted item in the array with the other items in the same array.

ASCII. American Standard Code for Information Interchange. The computer uses codes to represent characters which are stored in memory or put on the screen. The **ASCII** characters are those found on the tops of the keys on the keyboard.

Assembly. The organization of a program which is converted from a symbolic language into a whole program written in **machine language**. This conversion is carried out by an assembly language which is used in an assembly program.

B

Backup. A **disc** onto which another disc is copied. For example, a 'welcome disc' often comes with a newly bought computer with examples of various types of **computer programs**. If the information on the disc is corrupted or the disc destroyed, some of the important information would be lost for all time, so it is advised to copy the welcome disc and create a backup disc.

BASIC. An acronym for Beginner's All-Purpose Symbolic Instruction Code.

BASIC is one of several **languages** used for programming. It is very versatile and easy to use. Most manufacturers of microcomputers produce the computer able to accept BASIC. It works on a line-by-line basis, with each line numbered, so as the computer can follow the program logically. The lines can be changed as the program is being written. There are certain command words which are important in any form of BASIC which must be typed in upper case:

PRINT—written into a program, the computer will produce on the screen anything following this command placed inside inverted commas, e.g., PRINT 'My name is John!';

INPUT—a command put into a program which stops the execution of the program until the operator types something;

LIST—the program will be listed, so that the programmer can check for errors in the program and edit it accordingly;

SAVE—a command which sends a program to a **disc**;

LOAD—a command which recalls a program from the **file** on disc and places it in the computer's memory;

RUN—a command which makes the program work;

DELETE—in some forms of BASIC, this command should be preceded by an asterisk, it removes a file from disc;

NEW—this command wipes out any program in the computer's **memory** to prepare it for a new program. If the program is to be kept it should be placed on disc.

REM—some programs can become very long and involved, so this command allows the programmer to make the program clearer not only for him but also for others who may want to change certain aspects of the program. When running the program, the computer ignores these lines. Rem is an abbreviation for remark, e.g., 10 rem Find the missing word.

Each make of computer has its own version of **BASIC**, e.g., **BBC BASIC** is used for all **Acorn computers**; Applesoft **BASIC** for **Apple computers**. However, they all use the command words already given. *See appropriate computer manuals.*

Baud. The rate at which **data** moves from one processor to another, e.g., from computer to **printer**.

BBC microcomputers. See **Acorn computers**.

Bit. An acronym which stands for binary digit. This refers to one of the two numbers used in binary notation (i.e., 0,1). A bit could just be a small part of the computer's **memory**.

Block. Any grouping together of **characters** into one unit of **data**. This data can be moved from the computer's **memory** to a **printer** or **disc drive**.

Branch. The part of a **computer program** which is not part of the main program. It is often called a **subroutine**. The branching part of the program appears between branch instructions which direct the program to carry out a particular branch of the program.

Branch instruction. See **branch**.

Buffer. Part of a **peripheral unit** where **data** is stored temporarily when transferred from the computer. The buffer will hold information sent to it and act on it depending on the speed at which the information reaches the unit.

Bug. Any error or part of a **computer program** which does not work as it should.

Byte. A group of **bits**, usually eight, which is similar to a single unit of information.

C

Capacity. The amount of **data** which can be held on a disc or in any other unit which stores data.

Ceefax. A teletext system operated by the BBC.

Central processor. A unit which is used to operate other units. For example, a computer can be described as a central processor for the information which appears on a monitor screen, or for information which goes to a printer. It can also be used to describe a unit which is used to operate other environmental units.

Character. Letters, numerals and other symbols used in **word processing** or in writing a **program** (see **BASIC** and **computer program**) for a computer.

Every character has its own code made up of **bits**. The codes are those of the **ASCII**.

Command. See **BASIC**.

Compatibility. A phenomenon which, if it exists, would mean **computer programs** could be used on two different computers without the programs having to be altered. Normally, it is impossible to write a program on a BBC microcomputer using **BBC BASIC** and run it on the **Apple** microcomputer.

Computer. A machine which takes in information, processes it and sends it out in a specific way. There are three types of computer—digital computer, analog computer and hybrid computer. The first type of computer includes **main frame computers**, **minicomputers** and **personal/microcomputers**.

Computer aided learning. A system which uses **computer programs** designed especially for remediation and/or teaching purposes.

Computer program. A set of instructions given in a logical order to help solve almost any problem. When writing a program, it is important to remember the computer does not have a mind of its own and will operate only on the instructions it is given. It accepts instructions written in a specific language. Possible languages to be used are **BASIC** (the commonest, simplest and most versatile computer language), **Pascal** (a language using **algorithms** for fast processing of the program), COBOL (stands for Common Business Oriented Language used in commerce), FORTRAN (stands for FORmula TRANslation and used for mathematical and scientific purposes). Most programs for therapeutic use in speech therapy will be written in **BASIC**. Many program listings may

have **loops**, **subroutines** and certain **commands**.

Programmers begin by drawing a **flowchart** which they map into the instructions allowed by the language they decide to use. However careful programmers are in writing a particular program, there are usually errors in it which cause it not to operate correctly. These errors are **bugs** and the process to get rid of them is **debugging**. *See White (1985)*.

Concept keyboard. An **input device** for operating **software** without having to use the **computer's** keyboard. It is a touch-sensitive pad and comes in A4, A3 and A2 sizes.

Configuration. The way in which the computer is set up to accept information and run **computer programs** or operate printers, disc drives and other **peripheral units**. For example, the BBC Master 128 has to be reconfigured to accept discs designed for use with the BBC B +, or it may be the computer has to be configured especially for use with a **parallel** or serial printer.

Continuous paper. Paper designed for use with a printer. It is made up of several hundred sheets of paper folded along perforations. Down each side of the paper are strips of paper with holes for the tractor feed. These can be torn off when printing is completed.

Crash. Occurs when the system breaks down because of the failure of the **computer program** and so the programmer has to alter it before the program can be continued.

Cursor. The little, flashing line which moves across the screen and produces characters, graphics or text at certain points on the screen.

D

Daisywheel printer. A type of printer which produces printouts by means of a wheel placed on the print unit with spokes emanating from its centre which are hit by a hammer against a ribbon cartridge. It is the print wheel which, to some people, looks like a daisy.

Data. A grouping of characters, symbols and words into a text or **computer program**.

Data transmission. The process of sending data from computer to computer by the use of telegraphic or telephonic means. This usually involves the use of **modems**.

Debugging. The process of finding and correcting errors found in a **computer program** which may prevent it from being **run** (see **BASIC**). Errors can be of two types—those which are produced because of a lack of logic in the writing of the program, and those which are produced by a mistake in the codes used during the programs. The latter are known as **syntax errors**. These can be caused by failing to use the correct **command** (see **BASIC**) word or the failure to put in a comma or other punctuation mark in the correct place of the program.

Disc. Discs are used for saving **computer programs** (see also **BASIC**) for future use and text for **word processors**. When discs are bought, they are completely blank and are known as unformatted discs. In this state, they will not save any information and will have to be formatted. There will be information in the manual that comes with the computer so that the discs can be formatted. There are different types of disc which can be single/double sided and can have 40 or 80 tracks. Thus, they are similar to music discs and like these discs, information is stored on the tracks, so the more tracks the disc has, the more information can be stored on it. The discs are placed in a disc drive which rotates the disc at a particular speed and can **read** from or **write** the information to the disc. The **commands** used to operate the disc drive are SAVE, LOAD, RUN and *DELETE (see **BASIC**). There is usually a single disc drive but there can be a double disc drive which makes it easier to copy from one disc to another. During the process of copying the operator will be asked about the source disc and destination disc. The former refers to the disc which has the information to be copied, while the latter refers to the disc to which the information will be copied. Discs come in various sizes. The most common are floppy discs of 5¼″. Some smaller discs measure 3½″ or 3″. The latter are in a harder covering than the floppy disc which is just covered by plastic.

Dot matrix printers. A printer which forms letters or **graphics** with a system of dots on the paper made up by a matrix of wires or styluses. **Thermal paper** can be used with these printers or an ink ribbon.

Dynamic memory. See **random access memory**.

E

Electronic book. An alternative input system to the **BBC microcomputer**. It is an A4 ring binder which can be connected to the computer with 12 touch-sensitive cells at the back. An overlay is placed on top and the **operator** touches the required picture and the computer responds accordingly.

F

File. Information found on different parts of the **disc**. Each particular grouping of information is thought of as a file. Each file is given a file name so that it can be easily identified by the disc drive. This name is given when a program or text from a **word processor** is stored on disc. The **command** (see **BASIC**) is typed in the form SAVE "MICRO" and the reciprocal command to retrieve the file from **disc** is LOAD "MICRO". With word processors, the inverted commas may not be necessary. It is possible to find out what files are on a disc by typing *CAT or CATALOG. Files can be printed out straight from the disc without loading them into the computer's **memory**.

Filing system. **BBC** microcomputers use filing systems to store files for easy **access**. The **BBC B** used the **disc filing system** while the master series (see **Acorn computers**) uses the Advanced Disc Filing System. The latter uses 'directories' which are similar to an all-embracing title. Within a directory, there could be 'subdirectories' which are similar to subtitles, and within these, there can be more 'subdirectories'. The system is similar to a filing cabinet in any office. On the front of the drawer is the name which describes what all the files in the drawer concern, e.g., finance. In the drawer, there may be several files concerning different aspects of a person's finances, e.g., income, expenditure, etc., while within these files, there may be more detailed files of information concerning these areas of finance, e.g., mortgage, rates, bank statement, etc. The ADFS is designed to make it easy to recall programs written to it.

Floppy disc. See **disc**.

Floppy disc drive. See **disc**.

Flowchart. See **computer program**.

Font. The kind of typeface produced by different kinds of printer depending on whether it has a fixed size of typeface, e.g., **daisywheel printer**, or whether it will accept all styles of typeface, e.g., **dot matrix printers**. Fount may also be found.

Format. The way in which information or text is presented for printing on a **word processor** or in a **computer program** when it is run.

Formatting. See **disc**.

Form feed. The way in which **continuous paper** is put into a printer.

For....next. A **loop** used in a **computer program** written in **BASIC**. *See White (1985): ch. 5.*

FORTRAN. See **computer program**.

Function key. Most microcomputers have function keys and are marked (f0, f1, f2, etc.). They have a specific function and can be used in various **computer programs**. In **word processing**, they may be used for editing text; in programming, they themselves can be programmed to give a **command** (see **BASIC**) word, e.g., PRINT, INPUT, PLOT, etc., or the operator can reprogram them for a specific purpose.

G

Games. Some computer games are designed to be recreational while others are designed to be educational. The former type usually test the person's dexterity and skill to hit or avoid moving objects about a screen or test the person's logic, imagination and knowledge. There are three types of game:

1. Strategy, e.g., chess;
2. Adventure, e.g., those where directions have to be followed to find some items, etc.;

3. Arcade, e.g., those just for amusement and usually **scroll** across the screen. Home computers and personal computers have many such games designed for them and can have joysticks or paddles for playing the game.

Graphics. The production of pictures from a **computer program** which appear on a monitor screen and which can be printed out.

H

Hard copy. Information which is both printed out on paper as well as appearing on a monitor screen. It is opposed to **soft copy**.

Hardware. The actual units which make up a computer system such as the microcomputer itself, the monitor, the disc drive, printer and any other peripheral unit. It is opposed to **software**.

High-level language. A type of computer **language**, e.g., **BASIC**, which looks more like English than the kind of coded **language** which the computer prefers to process, e.g., **machine code**.

Host computer. A computer from which **data** is sent to other computers being used as terminals. These terminals may have a direct link to the host computer or be linked by telegraph or telephone systems.

I

Icon. Instead of using the keyboard to operate the computer, icon programs can now be used for this purpose. When icons are called up, they appear in windows and the operator has to use a pointer to operate the computer. In some programs, the cursor keys can be used, others may require the use of a **mouse**, **touch screen** or **light pen**. Icon programs are also known as Icon software.

Input devices. Various means for the operator to communicate commands to the **computer**. These include the use of a **mouse, light pen, concept keyboard, touch sensitive screens, micromike,** micro voice, Quinkey keyboard and **toucan communicator** (7). Such devices are used if the operator suffers from a physical handicap and finds it difficult to operate a normal QWERTY keyboard.

Interface. The attachment of a **central processor** to various **peripheral units**. For example, when a **printer** or **disc drive** (see **disc**) is linked to a **computer**, they are said to interface with the computer. This type of interface is sometimes called a master/slave interface because one machine, e.g., computer, has control over one or more machines, e.g., disc drive and printer.

J

Jack. A place for fitting in a plug usually found at the back of the **computer**. It can also be called a socket.

Joystick. An **input device** used with a **computer** especially in Arcade **games** for moving objects around the screen. It may also be used with **icon software** (see **Icon**).

Justification. The positioning of text in such a way that both right and left-hand margins are equal. This occurs in **word processing**.

Justify. See **justification**.

K

K. An abbreviation for **kilo** (thousand) and stands for the amount of **memory** which a **computer** contains. When used in this way, K is 1024. So, a computer with a 2K memory will have 2048 **bytes** of storage.

Keypad. It is similar to a keyboard but is smaller as it may only contain number keys or **function keys**.

L

Languages. See **computer program**.

LED. Light Emitting Diode.

Light emitting diode. A light which shows that a machine is functioning. It is usually placed on the control panels of machines.

Light pen. An **input device** to operate a computer instead of using the keyboard. The device looks like a pen but has a light sensitive end. An example of the light pen is the 'Robin Light Pen' which can be used with the **BBC** Micro/Master computers.

List. See **BASIC**.

Liveware. Those people who work with **computers** such as programmers, operators and so on. It is opposed to **hardware** and **software**.

Load. See **BASIC** and **computer program**.

Logotron logo. **Software** developed for use by children. It is designed to allow the child to learn how to operate a computer rather than to allow the child to be overcome by the computer. Thus, it follows **Piaget's** (4) beliefs that a child learns from experience. When the child enters into a logo program, he will find a small triangle called a **turtle**. By using a simple computer **language**, the child finds he can move the turtle forwards, backwards, left and right, draw a white line, draw a coloured line or not draw a line at all. Thus, the child learns a form of language for moving the turtle. The designs which the child can produce with the turtle are known as Turtle Graphics. It has been designed for the **Apple computers** in the US and for **BBC computers** in the UK.

Loop. A process found in a **computer program** which allows instructions given to the **computer** to be repeated until a particular condition is satisfied. The types of loops may differ from computer to computer. The loops most often found in **BASIC** are **for....next** and **repeat....until**.

Low-level language. A **computer language** which is closer to the type of language which a computer can understand without translation as it is close to **machine code**. It is opposed to a **high-level language** such as **BASIC**.

M

Machine code. The internal language used by the **computer** to translate a **computer program** written in a **high-level language** such as **BASIC** into a form which it can understand and so operate on the instructions given to it within the program. It is this translation which slows down the processing time of the computer. It is possible to write programs directly in machine code which allows the same program in machine code to be processed much faster than the one written in **BASIC**.

Machine language. The language for writing in **machine code**.

Magnetic disk. See **disc**.

Main frame. A **central processor** or **host computer** with various terminals linked up to it. It is often used to distinguish between large computers and **microcomputers**.

Main memory. The **memory** of the computer which can be accessed immediately.

Main program. The principal part of a **computer program** which may **branch** to **subroutines**.

Maltron keyboard. A keyboard which has been designed to be more suitable for use because of its comfort and accuracy. The keyboard has been divided into two parts with two groupings of 26 switches on each side. The thumbs are left to operate 'SPACE', 'RETURN', 'E', '&' and full stop. The way the two groupings are set up takes away the strain on wrists and keeps them straight. The Maltron can be attached to the normal BBC keyboard. There is a single-handed keyboard for those who have a physical handicap and can not use even the standard Maltron. Again it has been specially manufactured for comfort and accuracy. Maltron have produced a keyboard which can be mounted on a stand and operated by a head or mouth stick if the patient can not use any other limbs for operating the computer. All the keyboards have been designed for use with the **BBC microcomputer**. It is produced by PCD Maltron.

Memory. The part of the **computer** in which a **computer program** is stored until it is transferred to **disc** or printed out on paper. It also holds text for **word processors** until it is sent to the **disc drive** (see **disc**) or printed out on paper. It is important to remember that programs and text can be edited when in memory, but if being saved on disc, the edited text or program must be resaved or the old program/piece of text on disc will remain as it will not have been changed.

Menu. At the beginning of most **software** packages, the operator finds a list of what is on the disc. He usually needs to press only one key to obtain the **computer program** he wishes from the disc.

Microcomputer. It is opposed to **main frame**, as a microcomputer is smaller. See **computer**.

Micromike. An **input device** for the **BBC** Micro/Master series. It comprises a hand-held microphone which is attached to a control box. It fits into the analog port of the computer. The patient has to use voice to make things happen on screen, e.g., helicopter rescuing a drowning man. It encourages a young child to use vocal play and his voice.

Micronose. A device which can be attached to a **BBC computer** to show a child how much nasality there is in his speech. A flat switch is placed between the mouth and the nose and he speaks to calibrate the computer to recognize his speech. When the **computer program** is **run** (see **BASIC**), a **graphic** of a face appears. If the child is suffering from **hypernasality** (5), the nose on the face becomes bigger, while if he is **hyponasal** (5), the mouth becomes bigger. There is also a graph at the bottom which shows the amount of nasality the child produces. The teacher or therapist can give a pattern for the patient to copy and it can be superimposed on top of the patient's graph to show more easily the difference between the two graphs.

Micro voice. An **input device** for the BBC Micro/Master series. It comprises a grey control box, a ROM, a microphone and a demonstration disc. The unit plugs into the 1Mhz bus. It can only distinguish ten words at a time but blocks of ten words can be loaded as required. These words are stored on a template. The one major problem, a problem from which most voice recognition systems suffer, is that it can only recognize the voice of the speaker and the word must be spoken in the same way for it to be accepted. It is operated by four **commands**:

1. *TRAIN teaches the template to recognize new words or voices. They have to be given in blocks of ten;
2. *LISTEN puts the unit into its recognition mode. When it 'hears' a word it gives it a value and places it in a particular memory location in the computer;
3. *RSAVE and *RLOAD save and load blocks of words to tape or disc.

There is also a built-in speech synthesis system but the words to be used have to be sent away to the manufacturers so that the words can be given the necessary code. The speech synthesis is activated by the *TALK COMMAND. The quality of speech is very good. It is produced by R & D Technology.

Modem. A device for transmitting **data**. It stands for MOdulator/DEModulator. There are many on the market presently. They can be connected to the person's telephone system, so that data can be transmitted over long distances.

Mouse. An **input device** which can move the cursor about a screen. It can be used with **icon software** (see **Icon**) as the keyboard does not need to be used. It can be held under the hand and requires the touch of only two or three buttons.

N

Nesting loops. When a **loop** is written into a **computer program** and has within it one or more other loops, they are said to nest in the main loop.

Network. A series of **computers** all linked to a **host computer** so that information can be transferred to them. This could be used in business such as the Stock Exchange where all the terminals will have the relevant data supplied from the main computer.

New. See **BASIC**.

Numeric keypad. On the BBC Master series computers, there is a group of 19 keys which allow for arithmetic functions to be carried out. Although there are keys on the main keyboard, this separate block of keys makes the use of keys for such arithmetic functions easier. It can cope with adding (+), subtraction (−), multiplication (*), division (/) and use of decimal numbers. It should be noted that all calculations should be preceded by the **command** (see **BASIC**) word PRINT, e.g., PRINT 45 + 8 − 2, and RETURN should be pressed to obtain the answer rather than (=).

O

Operating systems. The way in which computers operate different functions within themselves, other pieces of **hardware, computer programs** and data. These can be controlled manually from the keyboard or by use of **software**. When BBC computers are switched on, the operator will find the message in the top left-hand corner of the screen MOS (machine operating system). MOS functions all the time time a computer is switched on as it controls the production of characters onto a monitor screen and sending data and information to **disc drives** (see **disc**) and/or **printers**. It is also responsible for the functioning of various bits of **software**. For example, if there is a **word processor** in the computer, this can be called up by the use of MOS. However, it can only call up one system at a time, so **BASIC** is its default setting usually. Error messages which the operator receives are because the **language** used by the computer, e.g., **BASIC**, could not understand the line supplied by MOS although it was MOS which put the error message in the screen. The operator can communicate directly with MOS by the use of *****commands**. These are called direct **operating system commands** and can be used at any time when the system is being used in the computer.

Operating system commands. The direct communication between **operator** and the **computer**. These command words must be preceded by an asterisk (*****). These commands can be used in the **BBC** master series:

*****HELP will list the **software** and its version contained in the **computer**;
*****ROMS will list the systems and **languages** contained in **read-only memory** (ROM) sockets and 'sideways' **random access memory** (RAM) areas.
*****BASIC will return the computer to the **BASIC** language.
*****KEY will make the MOS associate various functions with a particular **function key**;
*****FX COMMANDS (also known as osbyte calls) change the **configuration** of the computer. For example, different types of printer can be selected, the speed of repeating characters can be slowed down or the auto-repeat function can be switched off. These commands can be used in **computer programs** written in **BASIC** (written as *****FX12, 1) to produce special effects when the program is **run** (see **BASIC**).

Operator. The person who works a computer or other machine.

Oracle. A **teletext** system produced by Independent Television for users in the United Kingdom.

Osbyte calls. See **operating systems commands**.

Output. The information which comes out of the computer. The results from running a program or the production of a printout, text on screen or sending **data** to a **disc** are all types of output.

Output devices. Machines which will accept **data** or information from a computer. These include the various types of **printer, disc drive** (see **disc**), **visual display units** and **modems**.

P

Paddle. An **input device** for moving objects around a monitor screen, usually used when playing Arcade **games**.

Paper advance mechanism. The part of a **printer** which moves the paper while printing is taking place. It may be that the number of lines which the paper is advanced is determined by the **word processing** program.

Parallel. Items of information dealt with simultaneously. It is opposed to **serial**.

Parallel interface. An **interface** where there is a parallel exchange of information from the **central processor** to other **peripheral units**. It is opposed to **serial interface**.

Parameter. Information which is written into a **computer program, subroutine, loop**, etc., the value of which can be changed each time it is encountered in the program.

Pascal. See **computer program**.

PEL. See **pixel**.

Peripheral units. Any device which can

be connected to a **computer** and, hence can be controlled by the computer. These include **disc drives, printers, visual display units, modems** and all kinds of **input, output** and **storage devices**.

Personal computers. A **microcomputer** which has sufficient memory to carry out business applications, **word processing** and the use of **spreadsheets**. They are opposed to home computer.

Photonic wand. An **input device** for those people who are too physically handicapped to use a conventional keyboard. The patient places the wand on his head. He sits back in front of the screen and points the wand at it and moves a **cursor** around the screen. This is the tip of an invisible beam of light which comes from the wand and moves over the screen as the patient moves his head. It is possible to produce **graphics**, text and music. **Computer programs** have been written for these purposes. It attaches to the computer's analog port at the back of the **computer**. It can be used with the **BBC microcomputer** (see **Acorn computers**).

Picture element. See **pixel**.

Pin. The legs on a chip which fit into little pin holes in the chip's socket.

Pixel. The smallest unit used for forming a computer **graphic**. It can also be referred to as picture element or PEL.

Plot. A **command word** (see **BASIC**) used in some forms of **BASIC** to join two or more points to form a **graphic** display.

Port. Sockets which can be found on a **computer** so that **input** and **output devices** can be connected to it. See **Acorn computers**.

Prestel. Launched in 1980 by British Telecom as the first videotex system in the world.

Print. See **BASIC**.

Printer. An **output device** for producing **data** as a **printout**. The information usually comes from a **word processor** in the **computer**. The two principal and commonest printers used are **daisy-wheel printers** and **dot matrix printers**.

Printout. The result of sending **data** to a **printer**. It is the printed sheets of paper which come out of the printer after printing has been completed.

Prodos. A recent **operating system** for use with the **Apple** II series of **microcomputers**. *See Katz (1986)*.

Program. See **computer program**.

Q

Quinkey keyboard. An **input device** for the **BBC microcomputer** for those who cannot use a conventional keyboard. It is a one-handed keyboard which bypasses the **QWERTY** keyboard. The **operator** produces combinations of keys to produce different **characters**. The Quinkey keyboard plugs into the Analog port at the back of the computer. When the **software** which comes with Quinkey is loaded, the keyboard becomes totally operational. There is a Quinkey unit which can have four keyboards all interfaced into the computer for multi-users.

Quit. An option given in many **computer programs** which allows the operator to terminate the program at any time. It is often included in a **menu**.

QWERTY. The usual keyboard layout found on typewriters, computer keyboards and other **electronic devices** manufactured in the UK. The name comes from the first six letters of the top alphabetic row of the keyboard. Similarly, on the Continent some keyboards are known as AZERTY keyboards. The positioning of letters on such keyboards depends on the frequency with which letters are used. It is opposed to keyboards which are set alphabetically from A to Z.

R

RAM. See **random access memory**.

Random access memory. An area of the computer which is reserved for holding **data** in **memory**. There are two types of

RAM memory:
1. Static RAM holds information in memory when the computer is switched off;
2. Dynamic RAM will only retain information in memory while the computer is switched on.
It is opposed to ROM (**read-only memory**).

Read. When information is stored on a **disc**, the **disc drive** can be commanded by the **computer** to produce the information. This is done by a head in the drive reading the information from the disc and putting it in the computer's **memory**. It is a similar process to the one of a stylus in a record player picking up what is said or sung from a record.

Read-only memory. An area of the **computer** which is reserved for holding **data** or information in **memory**. It is not possible to **write** to this memory, the information can only be **read** from it. Thus, **software** which comes with a **ROM**, e.g., the **micro voice**, cannot accept information, it can only produce the information stored on the chip. It is opposed to RAM (**random access memory**).

Reconfiguration. See **configuration**.
REM. See **BASIC**.

Repeat...until. See **loop**.
Return key. This key should always be pressed when the operator wants to communicate to the computer that a **command** has to be carried out when writing a **program**, carrying out an arithmetic function or when sending **data** or information to **input**, **output** and **storage devices**.

RGB. These are the first three letters of the three primary colours used in a cathode ray display to make up pictures in colour—Red, Green and Blue. An **RGB monitor** is one which uses these three colours to produce a very clear display in colour by use of a cathode ray tube.

RGB monitor. See **RGB**.

Robotics. The capability of giving a machine commands via a **computer**. In education and speech therapy, the machine is often referred to as a **turtle** which the child can move by giving commands to it by the use of a computer keyboard or some other **input device**.

ROM. See **read-only memory**.

Routine. Often used to refer to a **computer program** although, more precisely, it can refer to part of such a program.

Run. See **BASIC**.

S

Save. See **BASIC**.

Screen. The part of a monitor on which information appears after being transferred from the **computer**. It is operated by a cathode ray tube.

Scroll. The continuous movement of **characters** forming lines of text which begin at the bottom of the **screen** and make the others move up the screen. This occurs when a **computer program** is **list**ed, text is being produced on a **word processor** and in some **games**. **Graphics** often scroll across the **screen** in games.

Serial. Items of information dealt with in sequence. It is opposed to **parallel**.

Serial interface. An **interface** where there is a **serial** exchange of information from the **central processor** to **peripheral units**. It is opposed to **parallel interface**.

Shift key. When this key is pressed, it changes lower case letters into upper case.

Soft copy. Information which is produced from the keyboard and appears on the monitor only. It is opposed to **hard copy**.

Software. The **computer programs** which can be stored on **disc**. It can also refer to published programs which the operator may require to **assemble** his program in **machine code**, to **debug** his programs, to copy one **file** to another using utility programs and so on. It is also possible to obtain software for particular purposes such as making up wages or annual accounts for which the **operator** can use a **spreadsheet**.

Source disc. See **disc**.

Speech synthesis. The production of speech by the use of a microprocessor to simulate the human voice. It is also called voice synthesis.

Split screen. The process by which information can be put on screen from two separate **computer programs** but which can appear together on the same **screen**.

Spreadsheet. A piece of **software** which can be used for a particular purpose, e.g., annual accounts. It can **scroll** both horizontally and vertically if there is not enough space on the screen to take the full spreadsheet.

Starset. **Software** which allows the **operator** to produce or adapt **computer programs** for use with the **concept keyboard**.

Statement line. The line of a **computer program** giving an instruction for the computer to carry out.

Statement number. The number given at the beginning of an instruction in **computer programs** to provide the logical processing of such a program. See also **BASIC**.

Static memory. See **random access memory**.

Storage devices. See **disc**.

String. A set of **characters** or digits used in a computer program. If strings are used which consist of characters only, i.e., words, and are given a code, it is always followed by the dollar sign ($). The characters in a string are always placed between inverted commas, e.g., 10 PRINT "My name is John."

Structured programming. A type of **computer program** (see also **BASIC**) which looks at the problem to be solved by the program systematically step by step until the final step is reached. This is also called top-down programming.

Subroutine. The part of a **computer program** in which specific functions take place which do not occur in the **main program**. It can be entered at any time during the main program. The usual command for such a routine is GOSUB followed by the **statement line** in which the subroutine begins. *See White (1985)*.

Suite. A group of **computer programs** which are all of a similar nature and sometimes sold together.

Syntax error. An error which will appear while a **computer program** is being tested because the programmer has misspelled a **command word** (see **BASIC**), left out a punctuation mark or the computer has failed to recognize the instruction for a similar reason. Syntax errors are always caused by a failure in the programmer not in the **computer**.

T

Tab. See **tabulation**.

Tabulation. The movement of a typewriter carriage or **cursor** on a **word processor** to predetermined positions. This is often abbreviated to **tab** and the **operator** should use the tab key.

Teletext. In the UK, there are two teletext systems in use—**Ceefax** and **Oracle**. Television produces picture images on lines but some lines are not used for producing such images; it is these spare lines which the television uses to produce the text when switched to the teletext mode. These systems can also be used with a **computer** if a suitable converter is purchased. It is possible to store teletext information on **disc** or print it out by this means.

Terminal. **Data** can be fed to or taken from these machines. Thus, a monitor is often thought of as a terminal or a computer which is connected to a **host computer**.

Thermal paper. Special paper which is used with **dot matrix printers**. The paper has a special coating which is removed by the electric current from the styluses to produce the required **character**.

Toggle switch. A switch which when pressed can perform two functions. For example, in some **word processors**, the escape key can be used to switch from the **screen** where commands are given to **save** or **print** text to the screen on which the text is written.

Touch sensitive screen. An **input device** which allows a **computer program** to be operated without the use of the keyboard. Some touch sensitive screens consist of a frame which can be fitted to the front of the monitor producing infra-red beams which are broken by the person putting their finger on a particular part of the screen.

Trackball. An **input device** which can be used instead of the **QWERTY keyboard** to operate a **computer program**. It consists of a ball which can be rolled by the palm of the hand to move the **cursor**

or draw lines to make **graphics**.

Turtle. Either a robotic machine which can be moved by a child giving it **commands** from the **computer** or a small triangle which can be moved about the **screen**. The latter is described under **logotron**.

Twinkle eye-controlled switch. An **input device** which can be used for both the **BBC** and **Apple microcomputers**. Two sensors are put on the person's temples close to the eyes which produce electrical signals when the eyes move. When the eyes move to the right, the left sensor is closed and vice versa. There is a connection to the analog port of the BBC C and BBC Master and to the games port in the Apple II.

V

VDU. Visual display unit.

Visispeech. A real-time analysis and display system. It can be used with the BBC B, BBC Master and **Apple microcomputer**. Visispeech shows many aspects of speech visually. It can help in assessment of the voice quality of people suffering from **hearing loss** (6) or **dysphonia** (1) and those **dysarthric** patients who have **pitch** problems (1 and 3). There are three displays:

1. **pitch** (3) display;
2. **energy** (3) display;
3. **voicing** (3) display.

Visispeech II has an easy-key access as it operates with one press of each of the **function keys** on a **BBC microcomputer**. There is also a histogram **computer program** which provides a graphical representation of the frequency distribution. Histograms and the three energy displays can be saved on **disc** as well as being transferred to a **printer**, so that the therapist can keep a **hard copy** of the assessment and progress during therapy. It is produced by SCI Instruments Ltd.

Visual display unit. A unit which operates with a cathode ray tube to show text or graphics produced from the **memory** of the **computer**. It is also called a **terminal**.

Voice synthesis. See **speech synthesis**.

Volatile memory. See **dynamic memory**.

W

Window. Used in **icon software** (see **Icon**) to show the choices on a **menu**. It can also be used with **graphics** where text can be written in a window to explain features of the graphics or as a bit of text referring to the graphic.

Word processor. A machine for typing any kind of document by the use of computer technology. Some of the advantages in using a word processor instead of a manual or electronic typewriter include:

1. The text appears on the **screen** and can be edited before it is printed or **save**d on **disc**.

2. Corrections, which are quickly made, can be carried out on text which is on disc and then resaved to disc.

3. A letter format can be put on disc and used time after time.

Write. The opposite process from **read**. **Data** are transferred to a **storage device** such as a **disc**. Data can only be read from a disc, if they have already been written to the **disc**.

REFERENCES

Fitch, J. L. (1986). *Clinical Applications of Microcomputers in Communication Disorders*. Academic Press.

Katz, R. C. (1986). *Aphasia Treatment and Microcomputers*. Taylor and Francis.

White, M. (1985). *Good BASIC Programming with the BBC Microcomputer*. Macmillan.

More advanced terminology can be found in:

Chandor, A., Graham, J. and Williamson, R. (1985). *The Penguin Dictionary of Computers*. Penguin.

Appendices

A: Assessments of Speech and Language

The following assessments are all explained in section 1:

Action Picture Test
Apraxia Battery for Adults
Articulation Attainment Test
Assessment of Phonological Processes
Aston Index
Auditory Discrimination Tests

Biber's Test
Boston Diagnostic Aphasia Examination (BDAE)
British Picture Vocabulary Scale (BPVS)
Bus Story

Communicative Abilities in Daily Living (CADL)

Derbyshire Language Scheme (DLS)
Detailed Test of Comprehension (DTC)

Edinburgh Articulation Test (EAT)
Edinburgh Functional Communication Profile (EFCP)
English Picture Vocabulary Test (EPVT)

Frenchay Aphasia Screening Test (FAST)
Frenchay Dysarthria Assessment
Functional Communication Profile (FCP)

Goldman-Fristoe Articulation Test

Illinois Test of Psycholinguistic Abilities (ITPA)

Language, Assessment, Remediation and Screening Procedure (LARSP)
Language Imitation Test
Lexical Understanding with Visual and Semantic Distractors (LUVS)

Minnesota Test for the Differential Diagnosis of Aphasia (MTDDA)
Monterey Fluency Programme

Natural Process Analysis
Northwestern Syntax Screening Test

Phonological Assessment of Child Speech (PACS)
Peabody Picture Vocabulary Test (PPVT)
Perceptions of Stuttering Inventory (PSI)
Personal Construct Theory (PCT)
Phonological Assessment of Child Speech (PACS)
Phonological Process Analysis
Porch Index of Communicative Abilities (PICA)
Porch Index of Communicative Abilities in Children (PICAC)
Portage Checklist in Early Education
Profile of Phonology (PROPH)
Profile of Prosody (PROP)
Profile in Semantics (PRISM)

Rapid Screening Test (RST)
Raven's Progressive Matrices
Repertory Grids
Reporter's Test
Renfrew Test Battery
Revised Token Test
Reynell Developmental Language Scales (RDLS)
Robertson Dysarthria Profile

S-24
Self-Characterization
Sentence Comprehension Test (SCT)
Short Token Test
Symbolic Play Test

Test for Auditory Comprehension of Language
Test for Reception of Grammar (TROG)
Token Test

Wessex Revised Language Checklist
Whurr Screening Test
Word-finding Vocabulary Scale

B: Speech and Language Development

AGE   DESCRIPTION
0;0–0;3   Cries and reflexive sounds.
0;3–1;00   Babbling begins; babbling and intonation sounds like human language (i.e., babbling drift).
1;03–2;06   Lexical overgeneralisation (i.e., protowords or vocables).
1;00–1;09   First word stage; later in this stage, intonation is used meaningfully.
1;09–2;03   Second word stage the child begins to use semantic categories; his language begins to become more complex.

Acquisition of specific parts of grammar:
VERB PHRASE — tense, aspect, mood
   a. simple present
   b. progressive
   c. past tense (use of 'did')
   d. future (use of 'going to')
   e. passive (develops between 6;00–9;00)
AUXILIARY
   a. can't ⎫ used as
   b. don't ⎭ negatives
   c. no/not — alternatives
   d. did
   e. will
   f. can
NEGATION
   a. no/not (used at start of sentence)
   b. can't ⎫ used as
   c. don't ⎭ negatives
   d. no/not — alternatives
     (e.g., I no eat meat)
     (e.g., I not eat meat)
NOUN PHRASE — demonstratives/ articles, pronouns, adjectives.
Order of appearance in:
   1. Demonstratives/articles —
     a. this/that
     b. indefinite article
     c. definite article
   2. Pronouns —
     a. (i) 1st person subject — I (me/mine)
     (ii) 3rd person inanimate — it object
     b. (i) 1st person object — me, mine
     (ii) 3rd person inanimate — it subject
     c. he, she, him, her
     d. remainder includes second person and plurals
   3. Adjectives —
     a. adjectives of size
     b. adjectives of affection
     c. adjectives of colour
Some adjectives appear at two-word stage
ADVERBIALS
   a. Location — two word stage

   b. Time — 6 months after start of two-word stage
   c. Manner — end of first year of developing syntax
   d. Sentence adverbials — 4;00
PREPOSITIONS
   a. in, on, order
   b. back, front, between (+ featured object)
   c. back, front (+ unfeatured object)
   d. left, right
INTERROGATIVE
   a. yes/no questions
   — marked by intonation and gesture
   — auxiliaries added not necessarily correctly formed (e.g., does lions walk?)
   — auxiliary-subject inversion correctly used.
   b. wh- questions
   — wh- word without auxiliary or inversion (e.g., where me sleep?)
   — wh- word with auxiliary but without inversion (e.g., where me sleep?)
   — wh- words used correctly with both auxiliary and inversion.
ACQUISITION OF Wh- WORDS:
   a. what
   b. where — used for locatives in two word stages
   c. ⎫
   why ⎪ large gap between development of these three and
   what ⎬ first two seem to reflect
   where ⎪ cognitive/social
     ⎭ development
CONJUNCTIONS
   a. and, but (early)
   b. so, if, because, when ⎫ developed by
   c. before, after   ⎭ almost 4;00
Acquisition of morphology:
INFLECTIONAL MORPHOLOGY
   1. The form of morpheme occurs as a free variant with the root form:
   a. Third person simple present

$$\{z\} \Bigg\langle \begin{array}{ll} /s/ & \text{after voiceless C} \\ /z/ & \text{after voiced C} \\ /\text{ɪz}/ & \text{after sibilants} \end{array}$$

   b. past tense

$$\{D\} \Bigg\langle \begin{array}{ll} /t/ & \text{after voiceless C} \\ /d/ & \text{after voiced C} \\ /\text{ɪd}/ & \text{after } /t, d/ \end{array}$$

   2. The morpheme occurs correctly and consistently but not always used where it would be obligatory in adult language.
   3. The morpheme occurs correctly and consistently although the actual phonological form may vary.
Note: The transition from (2)—(3) may take several months so it is difficult to say when the morpheme is used correctly; it

is best to say it is present when it occurs on 90 percent of occasions it would occur in adult language. Using such a criterion, the order of inflectional morphemes:

a. Present progressive {be...ing}
b. Plural
c. Past
d. 3rd personal singular present.

Note: these forms are only acquired in this order, not necessarily with meaning. (See also **Main Length of Utterance (MLU),** (2).

ACQUISITION OF LEXIS:

The comprehension of the words is very likely to be ahead of their production.

1. Production averages (words)
By 1;06 — 100–200
By 2;06 — 500
By 5;00 — 2,000
By 6;00–7;00 — 4,000.

Words learnt first in order:
a. Names for classes of food
b. for parts of the body
c. for articles of clothing
d. for small household/garden objects
e. for animals
f. for vehicles
g. for toys
h. for things in picture books.

Word meaning:
a. Reference — most words learnt this way. The object is present when named but could lead to mislearning.
b. Linguistic induction — at 3;00–4;00. The children begin to guess the meaning of the new word by knowing the meaning of the words in the immediate vicinity of the new one.
c. Learning by deduction comes later, perhaps not until the child's early years at school.

Note: These have been found in research and are based on Cruttenden (1979). As there is variation in children's acquisition of speech and language, all ages given and the order of various items should be treated with caution.

DATE DE RETOUR
Veuillez rapporter ce volume avant ou
à la dernière date ci-dessous indiquée.

R			

No 16 – "Bibliofiches"